SECRETS
OF FEEDING
A HEALTHY FAMILY

How to Eat, How to Raise Good Eaters, How to Cook

Second Edition

ELLYN SATTER
MS RD LCSW BCD

KELCY PRESS
MADISON, WISCONSIN

Secrets of Feeding a Healthy Family
How to Eat, How to Raise Good Eaters, How to Cook
Second Edition

Kelcy Press
4226 Mandan Crescent
Madison, WI 53711-3062

800-808-7976

ISBN 978-0-9671189-2-5

Library of Congress Cataloging-in-Publication Data

Satter, Ellyn
Secrets of feeding a healthy family/Ellyn Satter.
p. cm.
Includes index
ISBN 978-0-9671189-2-5
1. Children-Nutrition Popular works. 2. Nutrition Popular works.
3. Diet Popular works. 4. Food habits Popular works. I. Title.
RJ206.S247   2008
613.2-dc21   99-33165

Printed in the U.S.

Distributed to the book trade by:
Publishers Group West
(800)788-3123
www.PGW.com

Also distributed by:
Ellyn Satter Associates
800-808-7976
www.EllynSatter.com

Developmental editor: Clio Bushland
Cover, typography and illustrations: Karen Foget
Author photo: Marcia Hansen
Typesetting: Maureen Forys, Happenstance Type-O-Rama
10 9 8 7 6 5 4 3 2 1

To the nifty people who, against all odds, still love to eat.

ALSO BY ELLYN SATTER

Your Child's Weight:
Helping Without Harming

Child of Mine:
Feeding with Love and Good Sense

How to Get Your Kid to Eat...
But Not Too Much

ELLYN SATTER'S FEEDING IN PRIMARY CARE
PREGNANCY THROUGH PRESCHOOL:
Easy-to-Read Reproducible Masters

ELLYN SATTER'S NUTRITION AND
FEEDING FOR INFANTS AND CHILDREN:
Handout Masters

ELLYN SATTER'S FEEDING WITH LOVE
AND GOOD SENSE:
Video and Teacher's Guide

ELLYN SATTER'S FEEDING WITH LOVE
AND GOOD SENSE:
Vignettes and PowerPoints

Ellyn Satter's
Montana FEEDING RELATIONSHIP
Training Package

For more materials based on the
Satter Eating Competence Model and Satter Feeding Dynamics Model,
see www.EllynSatter.com

Contents

Figures

Recipe Listing

To help you with your planning and cooking, here is a list of all the recipes in the book. Recipes that are indented are variations.

es to be satisfied, and let your body
hat it will in accordance with your life-
l genetic endowment.

grand tradition of sawing legs off a
uplifying the adult section of *Secrets*
d me to amplify the child section. "The
Relationship" chapter, in part II, "How
Good Eaters," boils feeding dynamics
the essentials of what parents need to
he second chapter in part II, "Stuff to
Have Family Meals," addresses the ins
of parenting with food.

ot of reasons, part III, "How to Cook,"
as before. The main reason is that I do
to tamper with success. My readers tell
nformation on cooking, planning, and
g has helped them greatly. *Secrets* is a
mer, not a cookbook. I carefully chose
es and crafted the background infor-
o teach cooking lore as well as eating
ing lore. There actually are a lot of new
but they are in the form of variations on
ing recipes—simple modifications to
your cooking repertory without compli-
The names of the variations are now
ldface, and they are catalogued in the
sting to make them easy to find. You
more tips and supplementary infor-
han before, and there are now figure
s on the informational boxes to make
sier to catalog so you can retrieve the
tion. Tables of contents for the figures
s for the recipes appear in the front of

se *Secrets* has so much to do, I elimi-
e previous edition's chapter 10, "Raising
y Eater in Your Community." I distilled
oter into appendix H, "Nutrition Educa-
he Schools." I have also posted the for-
oter 10 at www.EllynSatter.com. Click
rces, then scroll down to *Educational*

optimistic view, there is a profound
mation coming with respect to the way
bout our eating and the way we man-
all goes well, we will go back to the
days when people matter-of-factly
eding themselves a priority and looked
to mealtime with a comfortable sense
oation. To achieve that, we will have to
day's negative and scary nutritional
e can break those rules thoughtfully and
bly—by working toward eating com-
—rather than resorting to nutritional
The research on eating competence is

highly encouraging. Competent eaters do well
nutritionally and even emotionally. There is
strong evidence that eating competence supports health and vitality. Organizing our relationship with food around providing and
pleasure certainly supports eating competence.
At the same time, the evidence is weakening
that restricting fat, salt, and calories—the
cornerstone of conventional nutritional
guidance—prevents heart disease, cancer,
and other degenerative diseases. To see the
evidence, look for my interpretive reviews of
the literature (as well as other technical information) in the appendixes. As before, my
approach to food management contradicts
conventional advice about nutrition and food
selection. As before, I break today's nutritional
rules, but I do it carefully and sensibly. As in the
subtitle to my first book, *Child of Mine*, I do it
with love and good sense.

Secrets 2008 is even firmer than before about
the importance of meals. New research makes it
even more clear that structure is the backbone
of doing well with eating and feeding. Structure is fundamental to any educational or clinical intervention that addresses food
management. For adults, meals support stable
body weight, positive nutritional status, and
positive health indicators. Children who have
family meals do better in all ways—socially,
emotionally, nutritionally, and with respect to
avoidance of overweight, eating disorders, and
early sexual behavior. The list goes on. Young
adults who have family meals as adolescents
take good care of themselves with food when
they get out on their own.

Secrets has taken me places I hadn't expected
to go. This time, it was into elaborating in concrete and practical terms the eating competence
model. *Secrets* introduces eating competence to
the general public. *Secrets*, like all of my books,
is a crossover book—it is read by professionals
as well as non-professionals. Professionals who
read this book will gain a greater understanding of what competent eating is all about and
will be in a better position to help you with
your eating and feeding dilemmas.

As before, *Secrets* took me back to my young-
mother roots and my early dietitian days. Now
that I have become eligible for Social Security,
those personal and professional memories are
well peopled with the next generation—and the
next. It is so rewarding to see all my children—
both biological and honorary—taking so
seriously feeding *their* children and doing such

Preface

quanti
weigh
style a
In tl
table, a
promp
Feedi
to Rai
down
know.
Know
and ou
For
is muc
not wi
me the
shopp
food p
the rec
matior
and fe
recipe
the ex
expan
cating
set in l
recipe
will fi
matio
numb
them (
inforr
as wel
the bc
Bec
nated
a Hea.
that c
tion ir
mer c
on Res
Mater.
In :
transf
we fec
age it.
good
made
forwa
of ant
break
rules.
respo
peten
anarc

Eating is supposed to be enjoyable. For too many of us, it represents trouble: trouble with eating, trouble with feeding, trouble with cooking. We continue to enjoy eating but we worry about getting carried away and eating too much, especially of the "wrong" kinds of food. We value cooking but have lost the skills to allow us to be matter-of-fact about managing food and feeling successful at it. We have high standards for feeding our children but find those standards slipping in the face of time pressures and our children's reluctance to eat what is "good" for them.

Secrets of Feeding a Healthy Family takes the trouble out and puts the joy back in. "It's like you are standing at my shoulder, telling me what to do," e-mailed a reader. "I was so proud of the meal I made that I prepared it the next day for a shut-in neighbor," wrote another. "Your message, 'Everyone gets offered the same meal' has made all the difference to our family mealtimes," a relieved mother told me over the phone. "I loved the part about 'You are a family when you take care of yourself,' " said a young husband who was still waiting and hoping to become a father.

To take the trouble out and put the joy back in, make feeding yourself a priority. To that end, *Secrets of Feeding a Healthy Family* addresses all sorts of families: adults living alone, couples without children, singles, couples and even-unrelated groups of people with or without children. In both the "How to Eat" and "How to Cook" parts, *Secrets* gives lots of practical advice and encouragement about feeding yourself

singly. The "Fast
"How to Keep Co
especially fine. I s
wished I had had
when they left ho
Secrets is organ
Eat," "How to Rai
Cook." Each part
The prologues pro
and give you the o
The epilogues add
and how to apply
In the previous
ing attitudes and
"You and Your Ea
eating in four cha
"Honor Your App
Want," and "Feed
based on the Satt
The professional
were published ir
2007 issue of the *J*
and Behavior. Rese
demonstrates tha
achievable and re
eating that is con
cal, and emotiona
The eating com
even stronger fou
the previous editi
tionship with foo
deprive; seek foo
competence mode
tive about your ea
yourself, eat the f

a fine job of it. It is so rewarding to give my blessing to my professional protégés as they take over the feeding dynamics and eating competence work that has been so important to me. Among those protégés I am proud to note the members of the Ellyn Satter Foundation (ESF), a group of creative and responsible professionals who are taking leadership with feeding dynamics and eating competence research, training, writing, and mentoring. You can find ESF members, photos, and vitas at www.EllynSatter.com.

Clio Bushland, my very important right-hand woman, is a member of ESF and an integral part of my business. We laugh that Clio is the Chief Operations Officer and I am the Chief Executive Officer. We find that funny because there are just the two of us! Clio is currently working early and late right along with me to get *Secrets* ready to go to press. Clio has also contributed our COB—that would be Chief Office Baby—Sebastian. You will hear more about both later.

Secrets is woven with the threads of my entire life. I start with the attitudes and skills I learned from the dear and sturdy women I grew up with: my mother, my grandmothers, a coven of aunts, the church ladies. They cooked and kept on cooking, many times beginning by catching the chickens or climbing a ladder to pick the cherries. My country grade school teacher Betty Wynia straightened me out and made me behave after a string of way-too-strict and way-too-permissive teachers taught me that I might as well do exactly as I pleased. My vivid memories of Mrs. Wynia's hairy eyeball remain my gold standard for authoritative parenting. My high school home economics teacher, Mrs. Beatrice Clark, told me I would go far, and many days she must have felt it couldn't possibly be far enough. Miss Zora Colburn, my South Dakota State University nutrition professor, shared her passion for nutrition. Now gone to her reward, Miss Colburn's high standards live on. Mrs. Betty Jordan, my University of Wisconsin Hospitals internship director, resisted my diet therapy zeal and indoctrinated me, instead, in not turning my patients into dietary cripples. Dr. Dorothy Pringle, major professor for my master's in nutrition, demonstrated through her discriminating practicality how useful and empowering it can be to cut through complexity to the essential and applicable heart of the matter.

The fabric of the eating competence model was woven from threads I accumulated during the 15 years I spent working as an outpatient

dietitian at Jackson Clinic, a private group medical practice that has long since been swallowed up by managed care. I was there in the glory days, when patients could continue to see me for as long as they liked to address their nutritional concerns. I feel so privileged to have had that marvelous opportunity to work with those wonderful people—my patients—who taught me that I did not know all the answers and that asking good questions can be the greatest help of all.

My three lively and healthy children, Kjerstin, Lucas, and Curtis, taught me a great deal about how to feed and how to eat—understanding one helps understand the other. Now all three are parents. They and their spouses do such a fine job with feeding and parenting, and their children continue to surprise me with their quirky ways with eating. During my mothering years, I had good friends who loved eating, loved cooking and swapping recipes, and loved feeding their families. I am happy to say my children are still capable and enthusiastic eaters, but since most of my friends are dodging some medical calamity, present or threatened, cooking for them isn't as much fun as it used to be. That said, I thank you, dear reader, for providing me an outlet for my frustrated nurturing needs.

My two earlier books, *Child of Mine: Feeding with Love and Good Sense* and *How to Get Your Kid to Eat … But Not Too Much*, helped to bring me here. I wrote *Child of Mine* intending it to be a goodbye gift to a part of my life that I cherished—raising young children. My children were in the upper grades, and I was no longer working as a pediatric dietitian. Imagine my surprise when *Child of Mine* gained me a reputation as an authority in child nutrition and kept me in the field. Writing a book is truly the magic carpet ride to wonderful people and opportunities. It was only after I wrote *Child of Mine* that I discovered the area of feeding dynamics, which led me to write *How to Get Your Kid to Eat* and to make feeding dynamics my niche. My curiosity about parent–child interactions around feeding led me to graduate school in social work, and graduate school led me to Donald Williams, LCSW, long-time therapist, then consultant and collaborator, who demonstrated how empowering it can be to tell people what is bugging them and let them decide what to do about it.

Since the last edition of *Secrets of Feeding a Healthy Family* was published, I wrote *Your Child's Weight: Helping without Harming*. I mentioned earlier my conviction about the importance of family meals. A big part of that conviction comes from working with concerned parents of large children who are *so* relieved to learn that they can help without harming by emphasizing family meals.

There were many reviewers who helped with *Secrets* and I thank them all. I am happy to say they have let me use their names. I introduce them throughout *Secrets* along with a bit of their advice. I introduce them more fully in the Acknowledgments, just below.

And finally, I thank you, dear reader, for giving me the opportunity to write. The story of food is the story of life. Like writing a good story, writing *Secrets* has helped me to integrate, understand, and pull together the threads of my life in a most gratifying way.

Acknowledgments

There were many reviewers who helped with *Secrets* and I thank them all. They carefully read the many pages of the penultimate version and made thoughtful comments and suggestions that much improved this final copy.

Many are nutrition professionals, others are professionals in other areas, most are both professionals and parents. All are committed making a contribution to helping you find your way to wise and rewarding feeding and eating.

Elizabeth Jackson, MS RD
Laurel Reiman Henneman, JD
Nancy Pekar
Joy Lenz, RD
Michael Lenz, MD
Pam Estes, MS RD CD
Patty Nell Morse, RD CDE
Clio Bushland, MS
Paul Bushland
Lora Beth Brown, EdD RD
Yvonne Bushland, MS
Barbara Lohse, PhD RD
Edie Applegate, MS RD CDE LD

Chapter
1
The Secret in a Nutshell

The secret to feeding a healthy family is to love good food, trust yourself, and share that love and trust with your child. Eating is a complex brew of preference, habit, attitude, intuition, knowledge, and physical necessity. All must be considered in addressing eating, and critical to them all is *enjoyment*. Enjoyment of food and reward from eating are essential to having eating and feeding turn out well. When the joy goes out of eating, nutrition suffers.

Eating is more than throwing wood on a fire or pumping gas into a car. Feeding is more than picking out food and getting it into a child. Eating and feeding reflect our attitudes and relationships with ourselves and others, as well as our histories. Eating is about our regard for ourselves, our connection with our bodies, and our commitment to life itself. Feeding is about the love and connection between you and your child, about trusting or controlling, providing or neglecting, accepting or rejecting.

Cooking and eating can be about the happiness, comfort, and passion of celebrating wonderful food, enjoying it with others, and leaving the table filled with peace and well-being. Instead, cooking and eating today are too often about applying the rules; about consternation and avoidance; about struggling with conflict, shame, and deprivation; and about trying to forgo pleasure in the name of health.

Secrets of Feeding a Healthy Family is about good food, joyful eating, successful feeding, rewarding food preparation, and emotionally gratifying family meals. *Secrets* is written for everyone who eats. In my view as both a nutrition and mental health professional, you are a family when you take care of yourself. From that perspective, you can be a family whether you live by yourself, with a partner, or with roommates; whether you have lots of children or no children; and whether you are young, middle-aged, or elderly. *Secrets* is about emotional health and a positive relationship, whether that relationship is with yourself or with other people. The structure of rewarding family meals gives you a framework on which to hang the foods and connections that you absolutely have to have. Grazing won't give it; grabbing on the run won't give it; trying to forgo enjoyment in the name of health won't give it.

The bottom line is family meals. Whether your family numbers one or ten, meals are as essential for nurturing as they are for nutrition. Research with adults shows that meals support us in eating what is good for us, maintaining desirable body weight, and supporting positive health indicators.[1] Children and adolescents who have regular family meals do better in all ways—nutritionally, academically, socially, emotionally, and with respect to the avoidance of overweight, eating disorders, drug abuse, and early sexual behavior. Family meals have more to do with positive outcomes for children and adolescents than any other factor—extracurricular activities, church, tutoring, music lessons—you name it. For more information, see appendix B, "What the Research Says about Meals."

The Trouble with Our Eating

It isn't easy, nowadays, to *be* a good eater or to *raise* a good eater. People are upset and anxious about their own eating and confused by lots of advice—much of it counterproductive—about how to feed their children. Family meals are eroding, with too many demands on everyone's time and too little value being placed on ensuring that families get this reliable time together. Events get scheduled at dinnertime, and so many rules have piled up about "healthy" eating that meals aren't fun anymore.

At one time—probably in our grandparents' day and before—people thought about eating with a comfortable sense of anticipation and pleasure. They made feeding themselves a priority and saw to it that what they had to eat was prepared in ways that were familiar, rewarding, and satisfying. Based on their cultural heritage, they had appealing—and nutritionally sound—ways of preparing and combining the available foods. They knew how to eat: They could go to the table hungry and eat until they got full. Then they would stop, knowing they could soon do it all again. Family meals were a given. Children took pride in joining in with family meals, and they gradually learned to like the food their parents ate.

Now, we have trouble with our eating and trouble with feeding our children. As a society, we are abominable about feeding ourselves and only marginally better about feeding our children. We no longer make feeding ourselves a priority. We are offhand about eating. We eat and feed our children on the run, steal time from mealtime to do any number of other activities, and act as if time spent preparing food and eating is somehow wasted time. The norms have become haphazard, with grab-and-go eating and feeding on the one hand and food restriction and avoidance in the name of health and weight control on the other.

Lacking the routine of family meals, we orchestrate food for the primary purpose of feeding our children and end up catering to them so much that we bore ourselves with our repetitive menus and raise children who only eat what precisely suits them. In fact, since many of us were raised that way, we ourselves have short lists of foods we enjoy and have difficulty raising children to be capable with eating.

Attitudes about Food Are Negative

Whether we know it or not, in being so offhand about eating on the one hand and uptight about it on the other, we are messing up our eating attitudes and behaviors, and in the process we are doing the same to our children. We continually try to eat less and less-rewarding food than we really want. We worry that our food is poisoning us—or at least relegating us to a premature old age. We scrutinize and criticize our food and ourselves for eating it. We carry on an unrelenting love-hate relationship with our eating.

With tiresome regularity, the media incites us to hysteria about still another component of our food supply. Weight and health prescriptions make food seem like medicine or, worse, the enemy, and make us feel ashamed of eating the foods we enjoy and know how to prepare. The aggravation is everywhere. The specifics of the advice may vary, but from the latest government directives about the "healthy diet" to media alarms warning that our food will kill us, it seems the prevailing attitude about eating is "don't." Don't eat too much fat, too much sugar, too much salt—too much food, period. We spend more time thinking about *avoiding* than we do about *eating*.

Don't get me wrong. I think nutrition is important, and I think the way you feed your child is important. When I figure out what to eat or what to serve for a meal, I automatically consider the basic food groups at the same time I consider putting together an attractive meal that will taste good. But I have found that thinking about what is good for them sends most people off on an ambivalent journey of *shoulds* and *oughts*. As Patty Nell Morse, *Secrets* reviewer and registered dietitian, observes, "talking to most people about nutrition makes them feel like I do when somebody talks to me about income tax." Clinically, I spend more time calming people about nutrition than I do teaching it. Such negative responses to nutritional guidance are so ingrained in today's consumers that even the most benign messages take on a negative and moralistic spin. For many, the perfectly acceptable world *healthy*, for example, has been spoiled by its current implication of "don't eat so much, and don't eat the foods you like."

Having good nutrition doesn't mean taking the fun out of eating. In today's world, however, you are likely to feel otherwise. Today's consumers experience a fundamental contradiction between *wants* and *shoulds* with respect to food selection. If you are typical, you feel deprived if you eat the foods you *should* and guilty if you eat the foods you *want*.

Parents feel they must orchestrate "healthy" food on behalf of their child. It doesn't work. The child won't eat, especially if the food is promoted as "healthy." Parents either make do with what they provide for their child or sneak off to eat other food that is more satisfying.

In some families, the sneaking-off part has become a ritual. I remember fondly the parents who brought their chubby 10-year-old into treatment, complaining they were finding food wrappers under her mattress. Soon, she spilled the beans: Family meals were righteously boring and "acky," and everyone in the family had a food stash. The father's was the best—he kept Godiva chocolate locked in his desk drawer. To their credit, once the secret was out in the open, they all had a good laugh and got down to the business of making the food they ate in front of each other as rewarding as the food they had been eating secretly. The father became my patient. His family had shamed him about his eating and weight from the time he was a very young boy, and he had learned to be ashamed of himself. He had deputized his wife to preserve his food virtue. Once the father learned to eat in a more self-trusting and satisfying fashion, his wife happily stopped being his food cop and his daughter happily stopped sneak-eating.

Finding a Better Way

In short, today's eating dilemmas break down into the three areas addressed in the *Secrets* subtitle: How to eat, how to raise good eaters, and how to cook. *Secrets of Feeding a Healthy Family* is intended to help you feel better about food and eating and to master enough of the art and craft of food management so you can be orderly and positive about feeding yourself and your child. Part I is *how to eat*, part II is *how to feed*, and part III is *how to cook*. Address them in any order that you wish. Start where your energy and interest lie. The three areas are all interconnected, and gaining mastery in any one of them will stimulate your courage and curiosity and introduce you to the possibilities of the other two.

Part I, "How to Eat," is startling. It is well founded clinically and in the research, and it simply teaches competent eating. However, in the context of today's restrictive eating attitudes and behaviors, it will seem radical to you. If you are tired of struggling with your eating and want to find a better way, you may be ready and even eager to work your way through part I. But if it is more than you can deal with right now, skip past it and concentrate on one of the other two parts.

Several of my reviewers told me that they consider part II, "How to Raise Good Eaters," to be the place to start. Learning about positive feeding dynamics was so important to them and made such a difference in their lives that they want others to know about it *right away*. If feeding your child is your primary concern, concentrate on part II. Your doing a good job with feeding will allow your child to demonstrate what competent eating is all about. Your child's capabilities will surprise and inspire you as well as encourage you to work toward your own eating competence. Even if you don't have children, part II can be helpful for you. Most of us have children in our lives, even if we aren't responsible for raising them. Part II will help you to understand those children. It will also help you to understand yourself. Comparing and contrasting your own upbringing with the principles of optimum feeding will give you insight into your own eating attitudes and behaviors.

Your energy and interest may first take you to part III, "How to Cook." That section supports you in preparing food you enjoy and gaining expertise with cooking, planning, and shopping. Chapter 13, "Choosing Food," is way at the end, but it is not an afterthought. You will become curious about nutrition and food composition, and that will lead you to study that chapter when you are ready. Working your way through part III will encourage you to address the other two sections, as well. Providing for yourself reliably and well will support you in feeling good about your eating. That, in turn, will stimulate your curiosity about your eating and about feeding children.

How to Eat

To feed yourself and your family well, you have to make eating a priority. To be willing to make eating a priority, you have to take the guilt out and put the joy back in. In my clinical work as a registered dietitian and then later as a mental health professional specializing in eating disorders, I worked with hundreds of patients whose eating ranged from positive and functional to severely distorted and even disordered. In the process, I discovered that there are certain eating attitudes and behaviors that *work*. Those attitudes and behaviors allow people to eat in a rewarding, matter-of-fact, and responsible way—to enjoy their eating and make it a priority, but still let it keep its place as only one of life's great pleasures.

As I worked with my clinical population and observed the eaters around me, a picture emerged. To do well with eating, you need to (1) have positive attitudes about eating, (2) be able to learn to like and enjoy the food that is available to you, (3) be able to intuitively eat as much food as you need to give you energy and to allow your weight to be reasonably stable, and (4) make meals a priority and be able to provide them for yourself. Being a good eater is not about being a good *dieter*. It is far more than restricting yourself in order to lose or maintain weight and far more than striving for health by trying to get yourself to eat only "healthy" food.

People who do well with eating are positive, comfortable, and flexible with eating and make sure they get enough enjoyable, nourishing food to eat. Growing out of positive attitudes about their eating and about their weight, people who do well with eating are generally *confident* eaters. They trust their bodies to know how much to eat by tuning in to what goes on inside: how hungry and how full they are. People who do well with eating like their bodies—at least well enough—and are loyal enough to their own genetic endowment to resist buying into the cultural craziness about weight.

After 30 years' experimenting in my clinical practice, I organized my observations into a formal model and gave it a name: the Satter Eating Competence Model (ecSatter).[2] I put my name on the model to protect it—to keep others from giving it meanings different from what I intended. I designed a paper-and-pencil test, the ecSatter Inventory (ecSI), to assess the degree to which people have those positive eating attitudes and behaviors. For the last 5 years, I have collaborated with Dr. Barbara Lohse, associate professor at the Pennsylvania State University, to examine whether the test works to measure eating competence—it does—and what characteristics competent eaters show. To read more about the test, see appendix A, "Interpreting and Using the ecSatter Inventory (ecSI)."

Adults who score high on ecSI have indicators of better diets, have weights that tend toward the average—neither unusually high nor unusually low—and are more satisfied with their weights.[1] Adults who score high on ecSI also show better health indicators: They have higher HDL (high-density lipoprotein, or "good cholesterol"); lower blood pressure (even when stress-tested), lower total cholesterol and LDL (low-density lipoprotein, or "bad cholesterol"), and lower triglycerides; and show fewer of the components of "sticky plaque," today's high-tech approach to predicting the tendency toward cardiovascular disease.[3] Finally, adults who score high on ecSI appear to do better socially and emotionally, as well. They feel more effective, are more self-aware, and are more trusting and comfortable, both with themselves and with other people.[1]

Competent eating is made up of a positive tension between structure and reliability on the one hand and self-awareness and self-trust on the other.

Competent eating is made up of both *permission* and *discipline*:
- The permission to choose food you enjoy and eat it in amounts you find satisfying.
- The discipline to provide yourself with regular and reliable meals and snacks and to pay attention when you eat them.

Our remarkably positive results with defining and testing the eating competence model let us come full circle with our eating. Like previous generations, we can let eating take its place as one of life's great pleasures, and we can be matter-of-fact and reliable about feeding our children. We can consider our eating with a comfortable sense of anticipation and pleasure.

Chapters 2 through 5 in part I, "How to Eat," address each of the components of eating competence. They tell you how to develop positive attitudes and approaches that *support* rather than *undermine* eating.

How to Raise Good Eaters

A good eater is a *competent* eater. To raise your child to be a competent eater, do your jobs with feeding, and then let go of it. Today's parents have trouble with both the doing and the letting go. I have worked with children and families, in one capacity or another, for more than 40 years. I practiced as an outpatient pediatric dietitian starting in the early part of my career. My own children are in their 30s and 40s, and my grandchildren range in age from under a year to the preteens. I have been a speaker and consultant since the 1983 publication of my first book about feeding, *Child of Mine: Feeding with Love and Good Sense.* Parents in my own practice tell me of their trials and triumphs, and I get telephone calls from all over the country. I hear about parents and children when I give presentations, and I hear and read[4] about parents' dilemmas from other professionals.

My strong impression is that the incidence of feeding problems is increasing. Parents struggle with their children about eating, and those struggles both reflect and exacerbate children's negative eating attitudes and behaviors, poor nutritional status, and poor growth. Many of today's children are finicky and will accept only a short list of favorite foods—often by brand name. At times, a child's food selectivity becomes so extreme that she grows poorly. Parents panic about getting their child to eat vegetables or fruit—even if they don't know why and don't eat vegetables or fruit themselves. Parents and children struggle over "forbidden" foods. Parents feel they should purge their households of chips, sweets, and soda—and children beg, wheedle, and sneak around to get them. Parents are drifting away from seeing to it that their family has meals together and maintaining that reliable family time, particularly when the children enter their teen years. Schedules are complicated and many parents have trouble knowing how important they themselves are and how important it is to give their child regular access to family time. Hysteria about child overweight absolutely spoils feeding and even parenting. The hysteria is so bad, in fact, that parents worry about letting their *babies* eat as much as they need for fear they will be fat later in life.

In short, for many parents as well as for many children, feeding has become miserable—a confusing struggle invested with frustration and anxiety. It need not be so. If you know how to do it, feeding a child can be one of the most rewarding endeavors you will undertake. The key is knowing when to take leadership and when to let go. I have a golden rule of feeding,

and it is this: You do the *feeding* and your child does the *eating*—and growing.

> Feeding children appropriately requires a division of responsibility.
> - Parents are responsible for the *what, when,* and *where* of *feeding.*
> - Children are responsible for the *how much* and *whether* of *eating.*

If you observe the division of responsibility, you will enjoy mealtimes with your child and you will avoid 99 percent of the problems parents commonly experience in feeding their children. If you don't follow the golden rule of feeding, you will get into trouble.

The division of responsibility in feeding boils down to both *taking leadership* and *giving autonomy.* You take leadership when you maintain the structure of meals and snacks, choose the family food, and teach your child how to behave at the table. You give autonomy when you let her decide what and how much to eat of the food you have put before her. Leadership and autonomy with feeding are in direct parallel with the basic principles of eating competence: discipline and permission. The discipline is taking leadership; the permission is giving autonomy. The difference, of course, is that for your child, you provide the discipline. For yourself, you play both roles.

Chapter 6, "The Feeding Relationship," discusses how you can feed your child to ensure harmonious family meals and to allow her to grow up to be a competent eater. By the way, I say *her* because this is a *she* chapter. With each chapter I alternate between *he* and *she.* The next chapter is a *he* chapter. Chapter 7, "Stuff to Know to Have Family Meals," offers considerations and strategies for supporting meals.

How to Cook

I never thought I would write a book about cooking, but I love what the cooking chapters do for *Secrets.* The principles of feeding yourself and feeding your children come alive when they are applied to actual food and actual menus. *Secrets of Feeding a Healthy Family* aims to help you and your family rediscover the joy and security of sharing rewarding food. To help you toward that goal, I have made the "How to Cook" section a food-management primer—an instructional manual about planning and preparing family meals and including children in the kitchen and at the table. A review of my first edition said, "There are better cookbooks out there, but there isn't a better book on feeding yourself and your family." That's exactly what I set out to achieve! The recipe chapters do serve as a kind of cookbook, but I am not entering any cookbook competitions. *Secrets* isn't written for foodies or for gourmet cooks. It is a set of basic lessons on food management based on simple recipes that demonstrate the joy of eating. *Secrets* is written to convey the message, "You can do this."

The recipes are intended to help you to take your first baby steps in the kitchen, to encourage you to enjoy eating rewarding meals, and to inspire you to begin thinking of yourself as a cook. There are no goods or bads, no rights or wrongs—only what works for you and your family. If you are going to go to all the trouble of keeping up the day-in-day-out routine of family meals, those meals have to be richly rewarding to plan, prepare, and eat. The juice absolutely and positively has *got* to be worth the squeeze. Otherwise, your energy will run out, you will drift away from your best intentions, and you will go back to grabbing, eating on the run, and feeling dissatisfied and guilty. Once again, if the joy goes out of eating, nutrition suffers.

Chapter 8, "How to Get Cooking," chapter 9, "How to Keep Cooking," and chapter 10, "Enjoy Vegetables and Fruits," give fast, simple, and good-tasting recipes that include lots of nifty food management tips. To let you have some fun with food before learning the principles of food management, I put the cart before the horse by addressing cooking before considering planning. Chapter 11, "Planning to Get You Cooking," circles back around by showing you how to use your head to streamline the food management process as much as possible, thereby conserving your time and energy. Chapter 12, "Shopping to Get You Cooking," gives lists and strategies to shortcut grocery shopping as much as possible. Chapter 13, "Choosing Food," circles back around still again and considers basic nutrition principles. Because becoming neurotic about food is always impending, "Choosing Food" discusses basic food and nutrition principles from the perspective of blessing the food, thereby freeing you up to eat the foods you like, not nagging you to give them up.

Don't be in a rush to make your way around the different parts of the book. Go at your own pace. Enjoy the journey, and trust yourself to learn and grow as the possibilities unfold. The goal of all the sections and all the chapters is the same: to help you feel empowered and encouraged with food. There is no need to go on a campaign to make yourself over. You don't have to be a zealot about family meals in order to feed a healthy family, and you don't have to be a gourmet cook to have tasty meals that are worth savoring. Make feeding yourself a priority, make yourself more important than the rules, and your eating, feeding and cooking will come out just fine.

References

1. Lohse B, Satter E, Horacek T, Gebreselassie T, Oakland MJ. Measuring eating competence: psychometric properties and validity of the ecSatter Inventory. *J Nutr Educ Behav.* 2007;39(suppl):S154–S166.
2. Satter EM. Eating competence: definition and evidence for the Satter Eating Competence Model. *J Nutr Educ Behav.* 2007;39(suppl):S142–S153.
3. Psota T, Lohse B, West S. Associations between eating competence and cardiovascular disease biomarkers. *J Nutr Educ Behav.* 2007;39(suppl):S171–S178.
4. Linscheid TR, Budd KS, Rasnake LK. Pediatric feeding problems. In: Roberts MC, ed. *Handbook of Pediatric Psychology.* 3rd ed. New York, NY: Guilford; 2003: 481-498.

Part

I

How to Eat

Prologue

In part I of *Secrets of Feeding a Healthy Family*, I teach you how to become competent with your eating. Throughout *Secrets*, when I use the term *eating competence*, talk about becoming a competent eater, or construct a sentence that includes any form of the words *competent* and *eating*, I mean the whole package that makes up the Satter Eating Competence Model (ecSatter). As outlined in figure PI.1, ecSatter is a specific cluster of eating attitudes and behaviors. It is that cluster of attitudes and behaviors that is tested by the ecSatter Inventory (ecSI) and that we addressed in our research. For details about the ecSatter Inventory, see appendix A, "Interpreting and Using the ecSatter Inventory (ecSI)."

FIGURE PI.1 SATTER EATING COMPETENCE MODEL (ecSATTER)

Eating attitudes: You are positive about eating and about food. You like to eat and, not only that, you feel *comfortable* with your enjoyment of eating.

Food acceptance attitudes and skills: You are comfortable with the foods you like, you are flexible about the foods you choose, you are interested in new foods, and you have ways of learning to like them. You can be courteous but firm about turning down food you don't want to eat (to say yes, you have to be able to say no). But keep in mind that sometimes you just have to get *fed* regardless of your preferences. When that happens, you can politely tolerate and even eat food that you don't particularly enjoy.

Internal regulation attitudes and skills: You tune in on and trust your internal regulators of hunger and appetite as well as your satiety—your feelings of fullness, satisfaction, and genuine readiness to stop eating—to know how much to eat. Moreover, you are *comfortable* with eating enough. You trust your body to know how much it needs to weigh and are able to reject outside pressure—whether it is medical or aesthetic—to strive for a body weight other than the one that is right for you.

Contextual attitudes and skills: You take feeding yourself seriously, plan ahead for it, know how to prepare food, and generally see to it that you have regular meals and snacks. You make it a point to put together meals with foods that you enjoy. At the same time, you can pay attention to basic nutritional principles to guide your planning without taking the pleasure and reward out of eating.

Eating Competence Works

Despite the fact that the principles of eating competence say nothing about *what* or *how much* to eat,[1] people who have high eating competence are healthier medically, physically, and even emotionally and are more consistent about taking care of themselves with food.[2] How can that possibly be? In the context of what we are currently told about eating right for health, it doesn't make sense. How can such seemingly giddy self-indulgence with food be good for us? Instead of emphasizing *avoiding* food and forcing ourselves to eat foods we don't like in order to be healthy, eating competence does the opposite. It says to *feed* ourselves, eat what we enjoy, and trust our good sense and internal processes to guide us.

Eating competence is based on the utility and effectiveness of biological, psychological, and social processes: hunger and the drive to survive, appetite and the need for pleasure, the social reward of sharing food, and the biological propensity to maintain preferred and stable body weight. The internal contradiction that is the essence of ecSatter—discipline and permission—works by giving stability. Discipline and permission draw on both the external and the internal: maintaining structured and reliable access to a variety of food *and* trusting the body's powerful and resilient drive to maintain itself and to keep its systems in balance.

Providing structure for your eating plus trusting your body to do the fine-tuning with *what* and *how much* puts your body and mind in harmony. Making eating rewarding supports your taking time, calming down, and paying attention when you eat. Making eating a priority by having regular and reliable meals and snacks supports your eating a variety and being able to trust your internal regulators of hunger, appetite, and satiety. Together, the permission and discipline even out the peaks and valleys in eating that are produced by grabbing, grazing, going on and off calorie restriction, and alternating between being good and being bad with food selection. Your body does best with digestion and absorption when you eat what you enjoy[3] as well as tune in when you eat. Would it be so far-fetched to assume that being lovingly supportive with eating rather than guardedly antagonistic would allow your body to be healthier as well?

As one of my patients says, "If I have to count it, measure it, or weigh it, it makes me crazy." To my patients who struggle so much with their eating that their quality of life is impaired, the experience of eating competence seems like a miracle. They can eat as much as they want without going out of control. They can eat *what* they want without feeling guilty. Instead of having eating be an ordeal where they restrict and deprive and scrutinize and doubt practically everything they eat, they learn to provide. Instead of having to throw away all controls and tolerate guilt and shame in order to eat as much enjoyable food as they want, they can do it all the time in a self-respecting fashion.

Feel Good About Eating

In the next four chapters, each of the components of eating competence is addressed in turn. Take your time with each chapter, examine yourself, and apply what I advise. Keep in mind the basic principles of *permission* and *discipline*. The permission has to do with pleasure: eating joyfully, seeking out good-tasting food, and trusting yourself to eat as much as you need. The discipline is *positive* discipline, again built on pleasure and on satisfying your needs: being trustworthy about feeding yourself and paying attention while you eat. The bottom line is that eating competence encourages you to feel good about your eating.

When you read chapter 2, "Adjust Your Attitude," give yourself time to examine your own eating attitudes. Consider whether those attitudes are helping or hindering you. As you read chapter 3, "Honor Your Appetite," ask yourself, "What do I really want to eat?" Let yourself discover that, even though appetite is compelling, it *can* be satisfied. You will likely find chapter 4, "Eat as Much as You Want," to be the most challenging. It is an alarming notion to go to the table hungry and eat until you are satisfied. Only your own experience will reassure you that it is safe to do so. Chapter 5, "Feed Yourself Faithfully," is not as alarming as the other chapters, but it does demand discipline. As the chapter stresses, the trick is being disciplined without becoming negative.

The Food Hierarchy

You do not have to be motivated, nagged, or reminded in order to do well nutritionally. In my experience, people who develop eating competence gradually push themselves along to eat a greater variety of food without my saying a word about it. I trust that it will be the same for you. You will grow with food management as you gain capability with and self-confidence about satisfying your food needs. That's because it is natural for you to learn and grow.

Have you heard of Maslow's Hierarchy of Needs? Abraham Maslow taught that we all learn and grow in sequence, and that once our needs at each level are satisfied, we become aware of and address needs at the next level. From the foundation through the apex on Maslow's pyramid-shaped hierarchy, those needs are: (1) physiological needs: air, water, food, shelter, sleep, sex; (2) safety, security, order; (3) social affection: love, belonging; (4) esteem, status; self-esteem and esteem by others; and (5) self-actualization: being all the individual can be.[4]

Arranging food needs in a similar hierarchy, from the foundation through the apex, would give the sequence pictured in figure PI.2.[5]

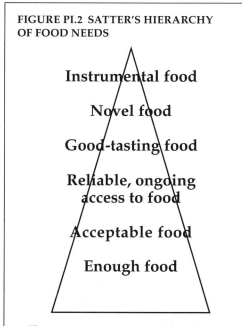

FIGURE PI.2 SATTER'S HIERARCHY OF FOOD NEEDS

Instrumental food

Novel food

Good-tasting food

Reliable, ongoing access to food

Acceptable food

Enough food

The way you position yourself on the hierarchy and move up it depends on your feelings and inclinations rather than on your thinking. Your hunger, appetite, and satiety guide you.

Enough food If you are on a tight food budget, are on a weight-reduction diet, or are caught on an airplane with no food stash, your major concern will be getting enough to eat. Your hunger will drive you to be most interested in food that is relatively high in calories—whether or not you want to allow yourself to eat that high-calorie food. Like the rest of us, you have learned from past experience that high-calorie food is filling and sustaining. While many of the foods you choose in response to pressing hunger provide nutrients, your main concern is not nutrition, but getting enough to eat.

Acceptable food After you fully reassure yourself that you won't have to go hungry—which can take a long time—your appetite will become more discriminating. Rather than being willing to eat and be satisfied with almost anything, you will reject some foods because they don't taste good or they aren't socially acceptable.

Reliable, ongoing access to food After you function comfortably at that level for a while, you will find yourself considering the next meal or the next day. You will plan for subsequent meals, accumulate a food stash, and budget for food purchases.

Good-tasting food Given the security of knowing you will be fed not just today but tomorrow and into the indefinite future, your appetite will become more prominent. Most people prioritize taste in food selection, but that is only when they know they will get enough to eat. Under starvation conditions, food preference isn't as pressing.

Novel food After you have had plenty of time to eat adequate amounts of rewarding food, you will find yourself tiring of even your favorite food and taking more of an interest in new foods or perhaps in familiar foods prepared in unfamiliar ways.

Instrumental food Having satisfied your needs at all the other levels, you will become aware of and interested in considering instrumental food—food that will do something for you in addition to satisfying your hunger and appetite. Choosing food to achieve a desired physical, intellectual, or spiritual outcome happens at this level. People have always chosen food for instrumental reasons—eating or avoiding certain foods during pregnancy to influence the baby's appearance or temperament, for example. A contemporary example of food selection for instrumental reasons is eating— or avoiding—certain foods to resist disease, prolong life, or enhance mental and emotional functioning.

I bring the hierarchy of food needs into the discussion to demonstrate that it is natural for you to learn and grow. Conversely, it is unnatural for you to try to function at a higher level than you are ready for. Moving up the food hierarchy takes time. Achieving eating competence takes time. Your growth and change will be comfortable and sustainable when you build on a solid foundation of achievement.

References

1. Satter EM. Eating Competence: definition and evidence for the Satter Eating Competence Model. *J Nutr Educ Behav.* 2007;39 (suppl):S142-S153.
2. Lohse B, Satter E, Horacek T, Gebreselassie T, Oakland MJ. Measuring Eating Competence: psychometric properties and validity of the ecSatter Inventory. *J Nutr Educ Behav.* 2007;39 (suppl):S154-S166.
3. Hallberg L, Bjorn-Rasmussen E, Rossander L, Suwanik R. Iron absorption from Southeast Asian diets. *Am J Clin Nutr.* 1977;30:539-548.
4. Maslow A. *A Theory of Human Motivations.* 1943.
5. Satter EM. Hierarchy of food needs . *J Nutr Educ Behav.* 2007;39 (suppl) :S187-188.

Chapter
2
Adjust Your Attitude

Celebrate eating. Eating is okay. Eating *enough* is okay. *Enjoying* eating is okay. Eating what you *like* is okay. Taking *time* to eat is okay. Making eating a *priority* is okay. To be consistent and effective in feeding yourself and your family, build on *enjoyment*. Optimism, pleasure, and self-trust are good motivators. Pessimism, avoidance, and self-doubt are poor motivators. Today, far too much is made of the difficulties of eating: avoiding disease, not getting fat, not *eating* fat. Today's attitudes and behaviors around eating are punishing and negative. Because they are negative, they can't be sustained. Nobody can go through life expecting not to be fed and expecting not to take pleasure from food. As I said in chapter 1, "The Secret in a Nutshell," if the joy goes out of eating, nutrition suffers. While feeding yourself requires effort and discipline, the discipline can—and must—be positive.

Consider Your Eating Attitudes

Your attitudes about eating can make or break you. Unlike what we *think*—our conscious judgment—attitudes are based on feelings and beliefs, both often unexamined. Attitudes are generally subtle and implied rather than spoken right out loud, and are, in fact, often hard to pin down. But they affect you nonetheless. They control your behavior, influence the way you feel, and dictate your priorities.

Competent eaters are relaxed about eating: They enjoy food and eating and they are *comfortable* with their enjoyment. They feel it is okay to eat food they like in amounts they find satisfying. In contrast to these perfectly normal and highly desirable attitudes about eating, most people today feel more or less ambivalent and anxious about eating and doubt their ability to do a good job with food management. They carry around some standard of what and how much they *should* eat—often ill-defined—and feel ashamed of themselves when they eat food they like, particularly when they fall short of their standards.[1]

Today's eating attitudes are negative: *Eating isn't important. Time spent eating is wasted time. You should eat and do something else at the same time. Skipping meals is good. Not eating is a sign of superiority. Being offhand about eating is trendy. Being finicky is sophisticated.* Then there are the negative attitudes about nutrition: *I shouldn't eat that. I shouldn't eat so* much *of that. If it tastes good, it can't be good for me. Eating right takes all the fun out of food.*

Social patterns reflect a lofty disregard for eating. Events for children get scheduled at dinnertime. Schools and child care centers feed in a hurry and children eat in a hurry to get out on the playground. Schools schedule children's meals at odd times. Families wolf down dinner (or eat in the car) to make time for other, "more-important" events. Ah, the irony! For children, the family meal is the most important event of all.

Eating and Emotional Competence

As I already told you, our research findings show that competent eaters do better with feeding themselves and their children and show evidence of doing well with respect to their physical health and well-being. None of that surprised me. What did surprise me, although it shouldn't have, is that competent eaters are emotionally and socially healthier than people with low levels of eating competence. They feel more effective, they are more self-aware, and they are more trusting and comfortable with themselves and with other people.[2]

Allow the psychotherapist in me to explain these findings. Consider that being emotionally and socially healthy—emotionally competent, if you will—depends on being sensitive to and comfortable with what goes on inside you— knowing what you feel, what you want, who you *are*—and being honest with yourself and with others about it. Your comfort and honesty with yourself allow you to act on your feelings in a rational and productive way. You can appreciate not only your own feelings and wishes but those of other people and, as a consequence, be reasonably adept at working things out.

Being competent with eating depends on exactly the same processes: being sensitive to and comfortable with what goes on inside you and being honest with yourself and others about it. In this case, of course, we are talking about your enjoyment of good food, your drive to get enough to eat, your excitement about eating—all of the natural feelings and urges that surround your eating. We are also talking about the sensations that regulate your eating—your hunger, appetite, and satiety. Your comfort and honesty with yourself about your inner experience related to your eating allow you to manage your eating in a rational and productive way.

We become neurotic when we don't trust our feelings and inclinations, and as a result don't feel comfortable acting on them. As a matter of fact, we suffer from a *national* neurosis about eating. Surveys find that we try not to eat the foods we enjoy in amounts that we find satisfying and instead feel obligated to eat "nutritious food" in amounts that leave us hungry—or at least unsatisfied. Eating "enjoyably" comes loaded with guilt and fear; eating "properly" comes loaded with control and dreariness. Many times we careen from one to the other, like the respondents to a 2005 *Parade* magazine survey who say they eat a healthy mix of foods, then reward themselves with "pleasure foods." (For a detailed discussion as well as references, see appendix C: "What Surveys Say about Our Eating.")

Weight and Eating Attitudes

Our national neurosis and even hysteria about weight destroys our trust in ourselves to eat the amount of food we need. Trying to force weight below its natural level undermines everything about eating competence—attitudes, patterns of food acceptance, and consistency with meals as well as the ability to internally regulate food intake. With weight, as with eating, we have trouble accepting who we *are*. While vanity enters into it, a big contributor to the problem is health and nutrition policy that arbitrarily defines anyone whose weight is above average as overweight. The cutoff point for overweight— BMI 25—is the average weight for adult men and women in this country. BMI stands for *body mass index*, if you are so lucky as to have been uninformed. It is a mathematical formula that calculates—and expresses—body density in kilograms per height in meters squared (kg/m^2).

Since the cutoff point for normal weight is set at the average weight, it is little wonder that more than 50 percent of us are defined as overweight! While policy makers and other weight-loss enthusiasts insist that maintaining a weight that is artificially low for most of us is necessary for health, a review of mortality studies indicates that the death rate is actually *lower* in the BMI 25 to 30 category than in the "normal" BMI category of 18.5 to 24.9. Deaths associated with high BMI do not increase until at least BMI 35 or even 40. Diseases that presumably are caused by overweight can be effectively addressed by improving health behaviors independent of weight loss: eating competence, activity, and routine health care. For the facts and figures on this topic, see appendix D, "BMI, Mortality, Morbidity, and Health: Resolving the Weight Dilemma."

People with high eating competence seem to have resolved the dissonance between what they *should* weigh and what they *do* weigh in favor of the latter. In our studies, it is notable that people with high eating competence are not thin. Their average BMIs range from a low of 19 to a high of 31—highs that qualify many for the health-policy-based diagnosis of over-weight and a few for a diagnosis of obesity. But here's the important part: People who are eating-competent are reasonably satisfied with their weight. When asked to rate their weight satisfaction from a high of 5 to a low of 0, they gave themselves a 3. *Three* is about as good as it gets in our weight-obsessed culture.[2]

Development of Eating Attitudes

Our attitudes come from our upbringing, which in turn reflects our traditions and our culture. Tradition and culture certainly have a powerful influence on parenting. However, to have their maximum impact, tradition and culture have to be passed along by parents.

CONSIDER YOUR UPBRINGING

Our most deeply embedded attitudes come from childhood. We learn them by osmosis—by picking up on the attitudes and behaviors of our parents and other people who are important to us. Unless we get a major attitude adjustment from life circumstances or psychotherapy, we are either self-accepting or neurotic because of the way we were raised. If our parents took an interest in us and were accepting of us, we do the same with ourselves. If our parents were primarily interested in their agendas for us, we learned that we, ourselves, were neither acceptable nor particularly interesting. As a result, we turned to developing agendas for ourselves, and we make those agendas more important than who we really *are*.

Allow me to illustrate. Thanks to my patients who showed me the error of my ways, by the time I had my own children, I had recovered from being a food cop. (I will confess in more detail later.) Thank goodness for that, because my third child, Curtis, was downright chubby. And he *loved* to eat. By the time he was 8 months old, he was using his hands to feed himself modified grownup food—soft cooked vegetables and canned fruit, strips of bread and toast, chopped-up meats mixed with potatoes and gravy, cut-up casseroles, soft fresh fruit. Curtis's eyes lit up when he got into his high chair, and he ate by the handfuls. He *adored* eating, I adored feeding him, and friends and family got a big kick out of watching him eat. "I am so glad," I thought more than once, "that I am not worried about his weight. That would spoil

all this." Today Curtis is in his 30s and still enjoys eating. He slimmed down slowly over his first 7 or 8 years, and today he is an average-sized adult. Curtis is more typical than atypical. Contrary to popular belief, most chubby children slim down as they get older. The fat infant or toddler has no greater likelihood of growing up fat than the slim one.[3]

Contrast Curtis's story with Holly's. Seven-month-old Holly also *loved* to eat. When she was put in her high chair, her eyes lit up, her arms and legs fanned, and she made little squeaking noises. While she ate, she moaned—sensuous, heartfelt moans. Enjoyment *oozed* from her very pores. Delighted friends and family gathered around to enjoy the spectacle.

Holly's mother was *mortified*. She felt that her daughter's passionate response to food was almost, if not downright, obscene. It meant Holly was self-indulgent, a glutton, and, well, not *lady-like*—and that she would get too fat. The mother's anxiety kept her from seeing that Holly was not the bottomless pit that she feared. Holly *did* get filled up, and then she lost interest in eating until she got hungry again.

From her mother's disgust, Holly learned to feel ashamed of her own exuberant response to food—and ashamed of herself. Eventually, she *did* eat too much. She tried to please her mother by eating less—and less appealing—food than she really wanted, then gave in to her love of food and ate way too much. The mother's worst fears were realized for Holly, but the problem was the mother's *attitude*, not Holly's eating.

You can only take someone else as far as you have gone yourself. Holly's mother couldn't support her daughter's enthusiasm about food because she was afraid of her own. Because the mother was so concerned about her own weight, she considered food enjoyment to be threatening: It undermined her willpower and made her eat more than she thought she should. The whole situation was part of a repeating history—the mother's parents had done to her what she was doing to Holly.

CONSIDER TRADITION

What are your most positive memories of food and eating? What are your most negative memories? What is your personal family tradition of eating and feeding? If each of us goes back far enough into our own family history, we will find positive traditions of eating and feeding that we can build on. For all of our ancestors, acquiring and enjoying food and feeding the family were centrally important. As demonstrated by the variety of ethnic and regional cuisines, few cultures have settled for basic survival and have instead found ways of making the available food taste even better. In every case, some respected person was in charge of the family cooking pot, and the mechanics of getting food were such that everyone ate together—children needed their grownups to cook for them, serve them, and eat with them.

Because of their commitment to revering and learning from elders, Native Americans show us how we can learn from and build on our traditions. When I am asked to present for groups of Native Americans, I arrange to first spend time with the elders. I say, "tell us about the old ways with food and with feeding children." I also ask them what advice they have for young people today about feeding themselves and their children. Food and feeding are so full of memory for them that even normally reticent elders love to talk about it. Most of their stories speak of joy. People loved to eat good food and they had an attitude of generosity and sharing. Food was closely linked to traditions—feasts, friends, and extended family. Meals cemented their community—they knew they could travel, arrive hungry at someone else's home, and be invited in for a meal. They were reverent about their food. They were careful to give thanks to the land, the creatures, and the spirits for providing. Because they had known hunger, they learned to be grateful, and they learned not to waste. Some stories speak of sorrow as well—of being sent off to boarding school and having to eat unfamiliar food, or of being punished by being made to go hungry. Memories of food and eating are full of feeling.

What did they recommend? To remember that feeding ourselves and our children is centrally important. To remember that feeding is about more than food—it is about love, support, and connection. Finally, to recover our respect and reverence for food.

We don't have to go back to hunting, fishing, and gathering to regain that reverence. Certainly growing a garden or understanding where food comes from helps with connection and appreciation. But most fundamental of all is examining our attitudes—the attitudes we pass along to our children. We can be mindful, joyful, and thankful as we choose, shop for, and prepare food—or even eat out at a fast-food restaurant—if we remember the central importance of it all. We can be respectful of our food and pay attention when we eat it. It doesn't take any more time to value our food than it does to take it for granted (or even slander it). But it makes all the difference—to us and to our children.

CONSIDER CULTURAL BELIEFS

In his research, Paul Rozin, a University of Pennsylvania psychologist, addresses cultural worry about food, the importance of food as a positive force in life, and the tendency to associate foods with nutritional versus culinary contexts or health versus pleasure.[4] Items in his questionnaire include:

- "Which is more important to you in choosing food?" Nutrition or taste?
- "Which word do you most associate with the term *fried egg*?" Cholesterol or pleasure?
- "Which word do you most associate with the word *food*?" Health or pleasure?
- "Which word do you most associate with the word *ice cream*?" Fattening or delicious?
- "Enjoying food is one of the most important pleasures in my life." Agree or disagree?
- "Which word do you most associate with the word *broccoli*?" Butter or vitamins?
- "Which word do you most associate with the word *milk*?" Cookies or calcium?
- "Which word do you most associate with the term *holiday dinner*?" Overeating or happiness?

Rozin's studies comparing the attitudes of adults and college students in Flemish Belgium, France, the United States, and Japan found that Americans associate food most with health and nutrition, and least with pleasure. The French and Flemish Belgians are most food-pleasure-oriented and least food-health-oriented, and the Japanese are somewhere in the middle. Now, here is the truly annoying part: We guilt-ridden and hypervigilant Americans are *least* likely to assess our diets as healthy.[5] Not only that, but although the French break what we in the United States consider the rules of healthy eating by consuming a relatively high-fat diet, they have a relatively low incidence of heart disease.

There are many theories about this so-called French paradox, including the highly appealing red-wine theory that sent wine sales through the roof when it was discussed on *60 Minutes*. An equally appealing theory is *attitude*. The French take their eating seriously, they celebrate good food, and they use fat to make it appealing. They set aside time for meals and assume that their food will be rewarding enough to make their time worthwhile. The priority they assign to pleasure in their eating leads them to seek out and enjoy a wide variety of food—the keystone of a healthy diet. When checked for *variety* the French scored far higher than we do. But when it came to adherence to the U.S. Dietary Guidelines, the French got failing grades. In fact, those who adhered to the U.S. Dietary Guidelines scored poorly on variety.[6]

Consider Your Eating Attitudes

Review the positive and negative attitudes I address in this chapter. How do you feel about eating? About eating certain foods? About eating as much as you like? How do you feel about your feelings? Are you comfortable with your love of good food? Or do you feel ashamed? When do you find yourself feeling shy or self-conscious about your eating? Is your shame and self-consciousness rational, or is it just a remnant of an earlier negative experience or a product of a no-longer-useful and trivial social constraint? For instance, some of my patients feel self-conscious if they prefer to take large bites, while others feel self-conscious about small bites. Women feel they are somehow unfeminine if they eat a lot; men feel it is somehow not masculine to have a small appetite.

What about your shoulds and oughts? How did you find yourself answering on Rozin's test—nutritional or culinary, health or pleasure? Do you believe that some of the foods you enjoy are just plain bad for you, especially if you eat a lot of them? That such foods will eventually make you sick? That you will go out of control if you eat those foods?

CHANGE YOUR ATTITUDES
Changing attitudes is difficult, but it can be done. How do you change your feelings and attitudes about eating? Acknowledging those attitudes is most of the battle. As I tell my patients, acknowledged feelings and attitudes have a half-life. They decay over time. But unacknowledged feelings and attitudes remain intense. They stick around forever, ambush you, and dominate you. As with any other neurosis, the cure is *paying attention* to feelings and desires and *respecting* them, not trying to get *rid* of them. If you don't pay attention to feelings, they rule you. You act on them impulsively, when you can't stand the pressure anymore, and in the process you are likely to behave in a way you don't feel good

about. On the other hand, if you are honest about what you feel and what you want, you can gratify yourself in self-respecting ways.

In short, it isn't our *feelings* that screw us up, but our feelings *about* our feelings. The problem wasn't Holly's sensual, celebratory delight in eating, but the shame she came to feel about that perfectly natural and even enviable delight, and the impulsive and guilty way she eventually learned to gratify it.

Build on what is positive. We still enjoy eating, although, like children, we have been scolded about it so often that we feel guilty and ashamed of our pleasure. That's a good sign, because it means we are healthy enough to still have those feelings and to be aware of them. But as I said earlier, we are neurotic: We don't trust our feelings, and we certainly don't feel comfortable acting on them.

To give you an idea of what more positive eating attitudes might be like for you, consider my definition of normal eating in figure 2.1 on the following page. This captures the essence of positive attitudes about eating. People love this definition for its unflinching *permission* to enjoy eating. It gets passed around, included in lots of books and teaching outlines, and posted on refrigerator doors. Why not copy it and post it on *your* refrigerator door?

PROTECT YOURSELF FROM NEGATIVE MESSAGES
You get lots of advice about food and eating, and you have to protect yourself against it. Sorting out the advice is a matter of *trust* versus *control*. It is good advice if it encourages you to trust yourself. It is bad advice if it encourages you to ignore yourself and overrule what lies inside.

The eating competence model is based on trust: Trust in our love of food and good eating; trust in following our inclinations to eat the food we like in amounts that are satisfying; trust that taking time to enjoy eating is time well-spent; trust that taking pleasure in eating supports being healthy; trust that behaving in such a self-respecting way is legitimate.

Today's conventional food-management advice is based on control. Control is eating by the numbers—eating certain foods whether we find them appealing or not, eating certain amounts whether we are still hungry or not, avoiding certain foods whether we want them or not. Control is following outside instructions for *what* and *how much* to eat.

FIGURE 2.1 WHAT IS NORMAL EATING?

- Normal eating is going to the table hungry and eating until you are satisfied.
- Normal eating is being able to choose food you like and to eat it and truly get enough of it—not just stopping because you think you should.
- Normal eating is being able to give some thought to your food selection so you get nutritious food, but not being so wary and restrictive that you miss out on enjoyable food.
- Normal eating is sometimes giving yourself permission to eat because you are happy, sad, or bored, or just because it feels good.
- Normal eating is mostly three meals a day—or four or five—or it can sometimes be choosing to munch along the way.
- Normal eating is leaving some cookies on the plate because you know you can have some again tomorrow, or eating more now because they taste so wonderful.
- Normal eating is overeating at times—feeling stuffed and uncomfortable. And it can be undereating at times and wishing you had more.
- Normal eating is trusting your body to make up for your mistakes in eating.
- Normal eating takes up some of your time and attention but keeps its place as only one important area of your life.

In short, normal eating is flexible. It varies in response to your hunger, your schedule, your proximity to food, and your feelings.

Trust supports consistency with eating, following a relaxed and rewarding day-in-day-out routine. Control precipitates inconsistency—trying to adhere, having hunger and cravings build up, and then giving in and eating more and different food than we think we should. Control just doesn't work. No matter how hard we try, we rebel against agendas or fail at adhering to them, whether they are our own or those imposed on us by others.

To protect yourself from negative messages as you apply the eating competence model, be wary of the *buts*. Nutrition and health professionals are likely to say, "I support the eating competence model." They might even say they think it is wonderful. Then some will throw in a qualifier: "But … I don't think you should eat so much/use so much salt/use so much butter/eat so many sweets/drink 2 percent or whole milk/eat all that meat/(insert your food button here)." Take their advice for what it is worth, but know in

your heart of hearts that you dealing with a fence-sitter. As one of my workshop participants recently observed, "…*but* negates everything that goes before." That person can't trust and support you in finding your own way with eating. As a consequence, they feel compelled to put on the brakes when it seems, for whatever reason, that you are becoming free-wheeling in letting yourself eat what and how much you want.

In the next three chapters, I will address eating and food-management behaviors and tell you how you can be more successful with your eating. The key is being realistic about your standards so you can live up to them. Realistic standards will allow you to feel successful with your eating. As you eat in ways that you can feel comfortable with, your attitudes will become more positive. In other words, you will feel better about your eating when you bring your shoulds and wants together.

References

1. Satter EM. Eating Competence: definition and evidence for the Satter Eating Competence Model. *J Nutr Educ Behav.* 2007;39 (suppl):S142-S153.
2. Lohse B, Satter E, Horacek T, Gebreselassie T, Oakland MJ. Measuring Eating Competence: psychometric properties and validity of the ecSatter Inventory. *J Nutr Educ Behav.* 2007;39 (suppl):S154-S166.
3. Whitlock EP, Williams SB, Gold R, Smith PR, Shipman SA. Screening and interventions for childhood overweight: a summary of evidence for the US preventive services task force. *Pediatrics.* 2005;116:e125-e144.
4. Rozin P, Bauer R, Catanese D. Food and life, pleasure and worry, among American college students: gender differences and regional similarities. *J Pers Soc Psychol.* 2003;85:132-141.
5. Rozin P, Fischler C, Imada S, Sarubin A, Wrzesniewski A. Attitudes to food and the role of food in life in the U.S.A., Japan, Flemish Belgium and France: possible implications for the diet-health debate. *Appetite.* 1999;33:163-180.
6. Drewnowski A, Ahlstrom Henderson S, Shore AB, Fischler C, Preziosi P, Hercberg S. Diet quality and dietary diversity in France: implications for the French paradox. *J Am Diet Assoc.* 1996;96:663-669.

Chapter

3

Honor Your Appetite

Enjoy your food. What an alarming notion! Surely, wonder the food cops as well as the eaters, if we are given license to enjoy food, we will simply career out of control, willy-nilly gobbling every morsel that comes across our voracious paths. If appetite is addresssed at all, it is from the perspective of ignoring and overruling it. In fact, the concept of food enjoyment has been considered—and rejected—at the highest levels of nutrition policy making. According to nutrition writer Larry Lindner, during deliberations for one of the renditions of the Dietary Guidelines for Americans, a committee member suggested that the first guideline be worded, "Enjoy a variety of foods." But Lindner's source noted that including the word *enjoy* was voted down on the grounds that it was "too hedonistic." In the end, the committee opted for the "apparently less giddy 'Eat a variety of foods.' The decision wasn't just to keep the populace from the debauchery of liking what it ate. The fear was that '*enjoy*' would be translated by people as '*unlimited license*' to eat 'whatever' and even 'overeat.' "[1]

Many of us feel the same way. To calm ourselves down about the appealing but alarming possibility of enjoying our food, let us begin by identifying the beliefs that frighten us. Consider the meaning of the word *hedonistic*. My online dictionary gives the narrowest meaning as "selfish preoccupation with happiness and pleasure." A word treasure hunt yields verbiage further clarifying today's consternation about eating. *Hedonistic* is closely related to *epicure*: "One devoted to sensual pleasure." *Epicure*

takes a definite turn for the worse due to its close relationship to *sybarite*, one who lives "for his wine or women or feasts continually," as well as to its relationship to *glutton*: "A voracious eater having a very heavy and quite indiscriminate appetite."[2] The thesaurus even throws in *voluptuous*, an alarming possibility that requires no definition.[3] I think that about sums it up, don't you? We are afraid we are bottomless pits—that if we get encouragement to eat foods we enjoy, we will eat without stopping. And if we do that, we are bad-bad-bad! While we are at it, *consternation* means "fear resulting from the awareness of danger," or, better still, "amazement or dismay that hinders or throws into confusion."[2]

But that is the dark side. What about the aspect of appetite that works *for* us, rather than against us? Appetite is a natural and life-giving inclination. The interest in eating based on its aesthetic and gustatory rewards is a powerful motivator for food-seeking. Even though appetite is compelling, it *can* be satisfied. Being an epicure—valuing and experiencing sensual pleasure—is a critical factor in becoming satisfied. It is normal to get enough and to stop eating, even of highly enjoyable food. If you pay attention when you eat, you will notice that at some point you lose interest. Food stops tasting as good. That might be a sudden or a gradual cutoff for you—it is very individual. As one of my patients put it, "I am ready to stop when my mouth is finished as well as my stomach." Another called this subjective endpoint "a feeling of nuffness." I can't improve on those descriptions. They were both saying that *appetite* was satisfied. But to satisfy appetite, you have to find the food appealing and it has to taste good. Eating a whole package of rice cakes won't satisfy you if what you really want is chocolate chip cookies—or vice versa.

Certainly, there *are* people who can't get enough, but they are the ones who have been denied. Let me tell you about Wesley, one of my adult patients.

Wesley's Epiphany

There is a glowing moment in eating treatment when the person *gets* it. After weeks of going through the motions of being deliberate, relaxed, and tuned in with eating, the kaleidoscope shifts. The individual's whole experience of eating and of himself in relation to food realigns. For Wesley, that moment came when he discovered he could trust his appetite.

Wesley remembered his mother as a horrible cook who would load up his plate with food he loathed and insist he eat it all—or else. He did. In the process, Wesley learned to put himself on automatic pilot when he ate. He tuned out his sensations of hunger, fullness, and pleasure—and, as much as he could, his discomfort with feeling stuffed—and simply got the food down.

Through no fault of his own, Wesley's chronic overeating made him fat as a child and fat as an adult. When he grew up, he tried to stop overeating and turned instead to dieting. Over and over, he restricted his food intake and forced his weight down, only to give up the diet and gain the weight back—almost without exception to a higher level. By the time he came into my office, his eating was totally out of control. He could no longer stand to diet, and his internal regulators had been so obliterated that he was only vaguely aware of being famished on the one hand and stuffed on the other.

Systematically, I coached Wesley in giving himself permission to eat; tuning in on his internal regulators of hunger, appetite, and satiety; and addressing the feelings he encountered when he did that. Gradually, he sorted out his hunger from his appetite, his sensation of satiety from his experience of being stuffed. As he did, he discovered that his drab food was interfering with his food regulation. Fearing that good-tasting food would send him out of

control, Wesley had asked his wife to cook only the most uninteresting food with few seasonings and little or no fat. But rather than keeping him from overeating, the drab food made him overeat. Because the food didn't satisfy his appetite, he ate and ate and still didn't feel like stopping. To his delight, Wesley discovered that good-tasting food let him feel like stopping. He could get satisfied and stop eating, not because he thought he should, but because he genuinely felt he had had enough. Wesley and his wife became good and adventurous cooks as well as epicures—in the very best sense—with their food. Together they applied what he had learned about tuning in to the process of eating and savoring food.

Let Your Appetite Work for You

Wesley took a leap of faith: He allowed himself to have good-tasting food and he took the considerable risk that he could get enough. But Wesley's leap wasn't just a flying header. Week after week, he worked hard to calm himself down in the presence of food, and he worked just as hard to increase his ability to pay attention when he ate.

Figure 3.1 describes how you can give yourself good-tasting food and get enough when you eat it.

Base Meals on Pleasure

We are getting along so well, I hesitate to arouse your suspicion by approaching you about having meals. "Oh, yeah," you may think, "I *knew* there was a catch! You are just like all the others!"

Settle down. We can handle this.

It is hard for people to hang on to the concept of permission when they consider meals. Meal preparation and conscience seem to come in the same package, and people find themselves planning dreary meals based on good-for-you food that is low-fat, low-salt, low-calorie, low-who-knows-what-else. Then sooner or later, virtue goes out the window and they give in to good-tasting "forbidden" food. In fact, there is a regrettable and totally unnecessary pattern: Meals are for duty; snacks are for fun.

TO STRUCTURE OR NOT TO STRUCTURE
To stay out of this conscience-driven trap, some eating "gurus" recommend eating on demand—cruising for food, being vigilant for internal signs of readiness to eat, and then finding the food that "hums." For the uninformed, the questions that drive a quest for humming food are, "Am I hungry? What am I hungry *for*?" A food that "hums" is one that really hits the spot—a food that exquisitely satisfies that moment's precise craving.

If you want to manage your own eating that way, it is up to you. If you are feeding a family, it is not a good idea. Eating on demand mimics the demand feeding of early infancy, and it is impractical for anyone over a year old. Eating on demand makes food an issue all the time, as one continually asks, "Am I hungry? What am I hungry *for*?" Eating on demand isolates you, because you must eat at the critical moment, whether others join in or not.

In my experience, structure is key to being able to eat in a positive and orderly fashion and to allowing eating to take its place as only one of life's great pleasures. Structure is also critical to feeding children and, indeed, providing them with a secure overall environment. Eating is a social activity. After the first year or two, rather than expecting others to drop everything and feed them when they get hungry, children learn to tolerate modest levels of hunger and so they can join in when others eat. As they do with everything else as they grow from being an infant to being a child, they lose some and gain some. They give up being the center of the universe, but they gain becoming part of the family. If all goes well, the gain is worth the loss.

With my patients, I have found it unnecessary and even counterproductive to settle for demand eating. When I helped Wesley learn to feed himself in a more positive and nurturing way, I encouraged him to have regular meals. This brought us right up against his well-developed pattern of freaking himself out with the food rules, and together we apprehended him again and again when he went chasing off after the food rules and neglected to provide himself with foods he enjoyed. When his eating became chaotic, we traced it to his out-of-control virtue. You understand the dilemma of the overdeveloped conscience if you order broiled fish when you really want it fried, and then give in to cheesecake when the dessert tray comes around. If you *truly* enjoy broiled fish, you will have to come up with some other example of out-of-control virtue, but the point stands: If you can't give yourself permission to eat the foods you enjoy, you will have to rely on impulse to get them. Can you trust yourself to gratify your desire for good-tasting food, rather than battling against it? Those restrictive patterns are deeply embedded, and they will trap you when you least expect.

Eventually, Wesley learned to deliberately choose food he liked, and you can, too. Put together meals including foods you enjoy and pay attention when you eat. Don't feel you have to eat everything. Pick and choose from what you have made available and eat what tastes good. Even if you planned it and prepared it, you can't necessarily predict what will taste good at any one meal on any one day.

Shun Virtue

Most of us crave pleasure from eating and will go to some length to achieve it, even if we have to cheat and play little mind games with ourselves. The problem is out-of-control virtue. Guard against it! Nutrition suffers when the rules get the upper hand over enjoyment. If you have to break your rules to eat what you like,

you are being too strict and withholding. In the long run, you will come out behind, not ahead. Eating is not a moral issue.

Do you remember those Rozin questions about nutrition and health versus pleasure that I shared with you in chapter 2, "Adjust Your Attitude"? Those questions address our unconscious virtue—our restrictive knee-jerks. When you think of broccoli, do you think "vitamins" or "butter"? If you think butter, or cheese sauce, or ranch dip, you have your priorities in order, and those priorities will encourage you to eat broccoli. What about milk? Do you think "calcium" or "cookies"? Thinking about cookies brings along the pleasure. Thinking about calcium introduces the obligation. The point? You will do better nutritionally if you eat broccoli or drink milk because you *enjoy* them, not because you *ought* to. Eating for enjoyment is more durable.

Truth be told, we eat what we like anyway, and we get plenty of help feeling guilty about it. A University of Hawaii nutrition professor got a lot of attention for her survey finding that taste is our most important influence on food choices, followed by cost, nutrition, and then convenience. Unfortunately, she went on to say, "… nutrition education programs should attempt to design and promote nutritious diets as being tasty and inexpensive."[4] There is that fear again: that eating for enjoyment is contradictory to good nutrition. Instead, we must be persuaded to eat what is good for us—and persuaded that we enjoy it. Our role as the target of these persuasions is to force a grin and lie that *naked* broccoli—no salt, no fat—tastes really *quite* good.

The idea of taking pleasure from eating is so difficult for so many of us that I will belabor the point. There is nothing wrong with eating broiled fish for dinner, then savoring cheesecake for dessert. In fact, the combination is good menu planning because the high-fat, high-calorie cheesecake balances off the low-fat, low-calorie fish. I will say more about this in chapter 7, "Stuff to Know to Have Family Meals." The problem lies in trying and failing to resist what you really want, which is likely to send your eating out of control and make you feel bad about it. Pam Estes, registered dietitian and content reviewer, observes—truthfully—that she is fond of lightly steamed naked broccoli. However, she always plans it with a higher-fat entrée such as tamale pie with sour cream or chicken with mashed potatoes and gravy. She says if she ate the broccoli by itself, she would have to have some ranch dressing with it.

Cultivate Variety

From the perspective of ecSatter, the key to nutritional excellence is variety growing out of genuine food enjoyment. Our research shows that people who have high overall eating competence scores, and particularly those who have high scores on the food acceptance subscale, enjoy a greater variety of food and are more likely to plan and cook meals that include all the food groups.[5] We have known for a long time that variety supports nutritional adequacy. Eating a variety of food increases your chances of getting what you need and decreases the chances of getting what you *don't* need or what might not be good for you. Consuming too much of anything can make you sick. Sugar won't hurt you, but a steady diet of sugar—because it crowds out the essentials—will. If you eat too much cauliflower, it interferes with thyroid functioning. Eating too many raw soybeans interferes with protein metabolism. For all foods, it's a dosage-and-frequency issue. You protect yourself by eating a variety; you increase your risk by eating the same foods all the time.

Emphasizing variety is the best way to hedge your bets against disease. Our understanding of the connections between nutrition and disease is far from complete and is always changing. Emerging research questions what we did in response to earlier research. For example, all-vegetable shortenings were emphasized; now we are told the trans fats they contain are bad for us. Polyunsaturated fat was emphasized; now we are told that monounsaturates are better. We were told to avoid eggs (actually, we are still told that); now we find that the cholesterol in egg yolks has little to do with blood cholesterol. Emphasizing variety rather than jumping on the latest bandwagon increases the chances that you are doing something right and decreases the chances that you are doing something wrong—and it dilutes the negative effects of whatever that wrong thing may be. For more on this topic, see appendix L, "Diet and Degenerative Disease: It's Not as Bad as You Think."

ENJOYMENT COMES FIRST

However, the way you *arrive* at variety makes all the difference. Do you eat a variety of foods because they are "good for you," or do you eat a variety of foods because you *like* them? From the perspective of the eating competence model, *liking* food is critical. Food preferences predict the nutritional quality of the diet. In our eating competence research, we found that people with positive food-acceptance capabilities have a longer list of foods they like, and like them more, and a shorter list of foods they don't like, and dislike them less, than people who are not so eating-competent.[5] Food preferences are a predictor of dietary intakes.[6]

Lest you should fear that license to eat the food you like will make you eat the same things all the time, keep in mind that seeking variety is natural. The process of sensory-specific satiety and our own experience tell us that we tire of even favorite foods and eat alternatives. That process works well in "overweight" people as well as in "lean" people.[7]

Ironically, enjoying food makes it more nutritious. In a classical study, Thai and Swedish women were fed a Thai meal of rice and vegetables flavored with spicy chili paste, fish sauce, and coconut cream. The Thai women absorbed almost 50 percent more iron in the meal than the Swedes, who had mixed feelings about the meal—they liked it but considered it very spicy. Pureeing the preferred meal to a pasty consistency decreased iron absorption by 70 percent compared with the same meal served in the traditional manner. This held true for Thai women eating a traditional Thai meal and for Swedish women eating a familiar meal of hamburger, string beans, and mashed potatoes.[8]

This absorptive discrepancy is likely explained by variation in the "cephalic phase of digestion." This is the physiological process whereby your body reacts to the sight and smell of appealing food and prepares to receive it with increased activity in your digestive tract. You will likely notice this process when you salivate more and your stomach growls in the anticipation of enjoyable food. The cephalic phase of digestion responds to appetite: Appealing food triggers it, but unappealing food does not. As a side note, it says a lot about prevailing eating attitudes that the current interest in the cephalic phase of digestion is driven by the goal of finding a drug that blunts the body's response to appealing food.

The research tells us that we seek novelty *and* do best with familiar food. Is there a contradiction? I don't think so. We are merely dealing with the human condition: We seek novelty and challenge on the one hand; we seek predictability and peace on the other. The solution, of course, is finding a balance between the two. We need predictability in order to free ourselves to seek novelty.

Food Acceptance Is Innate

It is natural to take an interest in new food and learn to like it. You did, too, at one time. As I will explain in chapter 6, "The Feeding Relationship," learning to enjoy and eat the foods his parents eat is a child's basic survival skill—until his parents train it out of him, that is. To learn to eat what parents eat, children need opportunities to learn and independence. They get opportunities to learn from family meals that offer a variety of food. They get support for their independence when parents let them decide what and how much to eat of what is on the table. Children lose food acceptance skills when they don't get support and when they do get interference. Exposing children to the same foods all the time limits their opportunities to learn. Getting pushy about what and how much they eat undermines their independence. For details and research, see appendix J, "Children and Food Acceptance: The Research."

FIGURE 3.2 FOOD ACCEPTANCE ATTITUDES AND SKILLS
These attitudes and skills are more important than what you eat on any given day. They allow you to be comfortable in the presence of unfamiliar food and gradually learn to like it.

- Being calm in the presence of food, including unfamiliar and disliked foods.

- Being comfortable with eating the foods you like, including foods that are high in fat, salt, and sugar.

- Being able to pick and choose from available foods, politely and matter-of-factly accepting or turning down what is offered to you.

- Being able to settle for food you don't much like when need be, just to get something to eat.

- Being curious about novel food.

- Being inclined to experiment with novel food by examining it, watching others eat it, and repeatedly tasting it (perhaps not swallowing early tastes).

- Eventually becoming familiar enough with the taste and texture of novel food to enjoy it and include it as part of a personal food repertoire.

Consider yourself. What kind of upbringing did you get with respect to your food acceptance attitudes and skills, and how does that upbringing affect you today? The food acceptance attitudes and skills listed in figure 3.2 are more important for you than what you eat on any given day. They support you over the long haul in consistently eating a variety of food as well as encouraging you to seek out novel food and gradually increase your food repertoire. Best of all, those skills will allow you to be comfortable at even unfamiliar tables. Think of it! You will be able to travel the world and eat the food there! If all went well for you, you developed those attitudes and skills as a child. If it didn't go so well, you can develop those attitudes and skills now.

THE CASE OF THE FINICKY FATHER
The story of one of my patients illustrates the lifelong impact of food acceptance attitudes and skills. A couple asked me to consult with them about feeding their four finicky preadolescents. Both parents were committed to good nutrition and were concerned about their children's short lists of acceptable foods. Unfortunately, their commitment to getting food into their children had led them to become food-caterers. They restricted family menus to food the children would readily accept, and frequently short-order cooked a different meal for each child. In the process, they raised a whole houseful of food prima donnas.

As we talked, the parents came to realize they were angry and out of patience with their demanding brood. Isn't that the way of us parents? We raise kids to be a certain way, then get angry and impatient with them for being just that way! Oh well, we live and learn, and they were prepared to learn. So we talked about how to take back control of family menus without doing sadistic menu-planning—how to be considerate without catering. For more on the topic, see figure 5.1, "Being Considerate without Catering," on page 48. In brief, the idea is to avoid limiting the menu to foods that children and other eaters readily accept by putting a variety of food on the table so even the pickiest eater can find something to eat—even if it is only one food item. Having provided that variety, the parents were to let their children pick and choose from what was on the table—again, even if it was only one food item, even if they didn't eat at all. As long as the parents provided something each child could ordinarily eat, they had done their job of providing the meal. More detail about feeding children is outlined in chapter 6, "The Feeding Relationship," and chapter 7, "Stuff to Know to Have Family Meals."

Then we turned to the heart of the matter: the parents' own eating attitudes and behaviors. Both parents said they ate a variety of food and felt they had nutritionally superior diets. When I asked whether they *enjoyed* their food, however, a different picture emerged. The mother said she liked the food well enough, which was a lukewarm response if I ever heard one. But the shame-faced father's response was downright negative. He had been a finicky child and still ate from a sense of obligation rather than because he enjoyed food. But his finickiness had a history. His parents were absolutely rigid about their family menus and insisted he eat all of what was put before him. The forcing ended when his parents made him eat peas and he threw up on his plate. After that, they didn't force him to eat anymore, but then they shamed him for being *a finicky child,* a label that was painful to him but that he, of course, had no reason to doubt.

In the process, the father had lost his food-acceptance skills. Not only that, but he was so careful to avoid doing to his children what had been done to him that he didn't give them opportunities to learn. It didn't occur to him that he could make a variety of food available to his children without forcing them to eat it.

We made a plan: He and his wife would include a variety of food on the table, including at least one food that each child ordinarily ate—such as bread—and reassure the children that they didn't have to eat anything they didn't want to. They would teach the children to be polite. They were to learn to say "yes, please" and "no, thank you" and to pick and choose from what was available. If the children had negative feelings about something that was on the table, they were to keep those feelings to themselves. No disrespecting the food or the cook. And no raiding the kitchen right after the meal.

The parents could only enforce the rules. They had no control over whether or not their children ate a greater variety of food. Given the plan, the likelihood was that sooner or later the children *would* learn to eat most foods that their parents ate. However, given the children's ages, it would take quite a while—younger children learn faster. Be that as it may, the parents' job was to enforce the mealtime rules. It was up to the children to decide whether or not to eat.

But, back to the father's learning about food acceptance. As so many children do, when the father was around 11 or 12 years old, he woke up to the fact that he was missing out on a lot of food and handicapping himself at school and at friends' homes with his inability to eat what was offered. He made up his mind to eat a wider variety of food, and he did. But he didn't enjoy it. He forced it down.

I gave him my blessing and let him off the hook. Stop forcing yourself to eat, I told him. Instead, do what children do to sneak up on new food and learn to like it. Look at the food, watch others eat it, put it on your plate and ignore it, put it in your mouth and take it out again. Before he could get grossed out by the idea, I taught him the napkin trick: Use a paper napkin or tissue to get the food out without making a fuss.

He was encouraged by the concept of food acceptance as a set of attitudes and behaviors he could learn, and he was especially encouraged by the napkin trick. He had tried the maneuver a few times as a boy and had been roundly scolded for it. He was relieved that he still had a chance to genuinely enjoy the foods that he had been forcing himself to eat. Best of all, he found out he really hadn't been a bad boy for refusing to eat. The situation had simply been set up so he *couldn't* eat. Now, he could set it up for himself so he *could.*

Address Your Food Acceptance Skills

What if your food acceptance skills are really bad? What if you are alarmed by unfamiliar food, are disinclined to try new foods, and have such a short list of foods you like that you have trouble eating in polite company? You have lots of company. My Google search on the term *picky eaters* yielded more than a million hits, among them a Web-based support group for adult picky eaters. I applaud their efforts to help themselves, although from their descriptions I think they are more *finicky* than *picky.* In my view, *picky* is children's normally erratic eating behavior. *Finicky* is picky gone awry. Finicky is being overly difficult to please. Finicky is extremely limited food acceptance driven by negative eating attitudes and behaviors. In short, it is eating *in*competence.

Finicky eaters have difficulty remaining calm in the presence of unfamiliar food and therefore can't provide themselves with the repeated neutral exposure they need to learn to like new food. In my experience, most adult finicky eaters haven't had opportunities to learn or have been forced to eat new food rather than trusted to sneak up on it and learn to like it. As a result, their food acceptance skills have been obliterated. I am also finding that an increasing number of people become finicky because of the rigid and prescriptive rules about food selection they accumulate as adults. That kind of finickiness has less to do with poor food acceptance skills than with the rules themselves.

RITA'S VICTORY

Although Rita was far more handicapped with food acceptance than I hope you are, her dilemma is instructive. Rita was way beyond finicky: She was phobic about eating. She could only eat when she was really hungry and even then she distracted herself by reading a book or watching television. Then she got eating over with as fast as she could. She ate rapidly and took in as little food as possible to sustain life.

When she was little, Rita's parents were downright sadistic in their insistence that she eat the food they deemed wholesome. They often forced her to sit for hours in front of a plate of congealing food—liver was the worst—until she finally choked it down. The legacy for her was so much internal conflict when she approached eating that she could get food down only by going on automatic pilot. I have seen that unconscious, mindless eating in many people, but she helped me most to understand it. She could only deal with her inner conflict about eating by doing what I have come to call *eating-without-eating*: eating without connecting with the experience of eating.

To help Rita build a more positive relationship with food, I used desensitization training. I coached her in relaxing, then gradually introduced her to food and helped her to focus her attention on it. Focusing her attention on the food would upset her, and I encouraged her to put down the food, relax again, then talk about her feelings. She was flooded with her feelings from childhood: Feeling abandoned, feeling ashamed, feeling angry and overwhelmed by being expected to eat food that she found repulsive. Talking about her feelings helped to take

away their sting, and eventually her upset around eating went away. Rita started with a strawberry, the least threatening food she could think of. It took 3 weeks for her to get to the point where she could put the strawberry in her mouth, and then she couldn't swallow it or even chew it. She had to take it back out again. But after a couple of more weeks she was able to chew and swallow the strawberry. Then she learned to enjoy it. From there, she moved on to other foods. By the end of the 5 months we worked together, she was eating and enjoying a variety of food.

You are unlikely to have such impaired food acceptance skills that you need an eating specialist to help you. But if you do, go for it. It can change your life.

HELP YOURSELF WITH FOOD ACCEPTANCE

While Rita's story is extreme, it is encouraging as well as instructive. If Rita can do it, so can you. Rita gained capability by giving herself lots of time and exposing herself to new food in such small doses that she wasn't overwhelmed by it. You can do the same for yourself by not overwhelming yourself. Base your meals on foods you enjoy. To experiment with the unfamiliar, you need the reassurance of the familiar. Plan meals to give yourself an out. Always have bread on the table. Bread is easy to like and you can eat it when all else fails. Pair familiar food with unfamiliar, favorite with not-so-favorite. You'll be braver about trying new foods if you have something familiar to fall back on.

When you are ready to experiment with a new food, give yourself time and an escape hatch. You may back out at any point. Keep in mind that your poor food acceptance skills likely grew out of one or both of two things: too few opportunities to learn or too much pressure. In order to improve your food acceptance, do the opposite: Give yourself lots of opportunities to learn and stow the pressure. Examine foods at the market without buying them. Read recipes without trying them. Buy a small amount, and prepare it without eating it. Put it in your mouth without swallowing it, and keep the tissues handy. Putting something in your mouth is one thing; swallowing is quite another. Do it over and over again until you are truly ready to swallow. Take another bite if you want to—and another—or not. Keep trying. Studies show that adults give up on a new food after only three tries. That's not enough. You need 10 or 15 or 20 tries, or even more.

Like a new song, new food will grow on you until you get to the point where you truly enjoy it. Ever so gradually, you will expand your food repertory.

References

1. Lindner L. A measure of pleasure. *Health at Every Size.* 2005;19(3):155-160.
2. Webster's Third New International Dictionary, Unabridged, 2002 [Web page]. Miriam-Webster Web site. http://unabridged.merriam-webster.com. Accessed December 15, 2007.
3. Thinkmap Visual Thesaurus [Web page]. Thinkmap Web site. http://www.visualthesaurus.com. Accessed December 15, 2007.
4. Glanz K, Basil M, Maibach E, Goldberg J, Snyder D. Why Americans eat what they do: taste, nutrition, cost, convenience, and weight control concerns as influences on food consumption. *J Am Diet Assoc.* 1998;98:1118-1126.
5. Lohse B, Satter E, Horacek T, Gebreselassie T, Oakland MJ. Measuring Eating Competence: psychometric properties and validity of the ecSatter Inventory. *J Nutr Educ Behav .* 2007;39 (suppl):S154-S166.
6. Drewnowski A, Hann C. Food preferences and reported frequencies of food consumption as predictors of current diet in young women. *Am J Clin Nutr.* 1999;70:28-36.
7. Brondel L, Romer M, Van Wymelbeke V, et al. Sensory-specific satiety with simple foods in humans: no influence of BMI? *Int J Obes (Lond).* 2007;31:987-995.
8. Hallberg L, Bjorn-Rasmussen E, Rossander L, Suwanik R. Iron absorption from Southeast Asian diets. *Am J Clin Nutr.* 1977;30:539-548.

Chapter
4
Eat as Much as You Want

Eat as much as you want? It just gets curiouser and curiouser! Are we to throw caution to the wind and let every meal be Thanksgiving dinner? Won't we just eat ourselves sick? Or at least gain a lot of weight?

Certainly, the nutrition policy makers feel that way. Why do you think MyPyramid, the current version of the Food Guide Pyramid and the official nutrition education document of nutrition policy, makes such an issue about "proper" portion sizes? Why do you think the official statement of national nutrition policy, the Dietary Guidelines, tells us to eat *nine* fruits and vegetables a day? That is 4 1/2 cups of virtually *naked* fruits and vegetables—with only the smallest amounts of salt, fat, or sugar. The intent, of course, isn't to satisfy nutritional requirements—we could do that with four or five well-chosen vegetables and fruits a day. It is to get us to fill up on relatively low-calorie food *so we don't eat so much.*

The people who actually *proudly* call themselves the food cops are on a vendetta against food-related big business, convinced that we use the availability and advertising of "bad" food as a license to eat too much. A lot of those food cops appear in *Super Size Me*, the popular 2004 documentary by Morgan Spurlock. Spurlock capitalizes on our fear of being sent out of control by food. His hypothesis is that if he eats every meal at McDonalds for 30 days, he will eat himself sick and gain a lot of weight. He does. He gains weight, his blood lipids go up, and his liver function tests deteriorate.

In reality, Spurlock doesn't just *eat* at McDonald's—he *overeats* there. In fact, he *forces* himself to overeat. Whether or not he wants the food, he eats every morsel and drinks every drop served to him. He consumes it all even if they super-size his portions, which he obligates himself to accept if it is offered. In an early and memorable scene, Spurlock eats to the point of obvious misery, then throws up. By the end of the 30 days, he appears to be accustomed to overeating, so he doesn't seem as miserable, and he doesn't throw up. But he is still going by what he is served, not the way he feels inside, to determine how much to eat. Little wonder he makes himself sick!

The idea that eating as much as we want creates nutritional mayhem leaves out an essential part of the equation: the body's wisdom.

Why Do We Overeat?

Essential to eating's rich reward is having *enough* to eat. Being hungry and eager to eat can feel positive and exciting on the one hand or negative and distressing on the other. The difference lies in whether or not you are confident that your hunger will be satisfied—that you can look forward to getting enough to eat of food that you find rewarding. The irony, in this land of plenty, is that most of us fear hunger, not because we lack the financial resources to provide for ourselves, but because we obligate ourselves to undereat. At any one time roughly three-quarters of both men and women are dieting to lose weight or maintain weight loss.[1]

As a result, most of us, like Morgan Spurlock, *are* potential overeaters. However, unlike Morgan Spurlock, we don't set out to gorge ourselves. Contrary to the fears of the food cops—both internal and external—we don't have a slothful inclination toward overindulgence. Rather, we overeat because we are *restrained* eaters—we chronically restrict ourselves. We restrict ourselves until we can't stand it anymore, then we overeat.

We eat less and less-appealing food than we really want. Why? Because we think we *should*. Why should we? Health or weight concerns? Some general idea about proper nutrition? In response to what we learned at our parents' table? In my clinical work, I find that my patients' long and often-contradictory lists of food rules—their shoulds and should-nots about food management—come from earliest memory and from bits and pieces of old diets, reports from the media, and advice from friends. Their food rules keep them continually in a tizzy about eating and continually feeling deprived.

Try yourself out on the list of restrained feeding tactics in figure 4.1. How many of them do you use?

FIGURE 4.1 RESTRAINED EATING
As originally defined, restrained eating is trying to get yourself to eat less food or less-desirable food than you really want in pursuit of thinness. In my experience, the goal can also be health.

- Imposing absolute limits: so many calories, so many helpings. Going by portion sizes or a food pattern.
- Making yourself hurdle: "I have to eat this before I can eat that."
- Avoiding certain foods, such as sweets, chips, or snacks.
- Limiting your menus to drab, uninspiring food.
- Trying to fill up on low-fat, low-calorie, "healthy" food.
- Trying to eat only low-carbohydrate or low-glycemic-index food.
- Substituting low-calorie butter, margarine, or salad dressing for the real thing in order to save calories.
- Asking yourself, "Do I really need that?" "Do I *want* that?" is a self-trusting question; "Do I *need* that?" is a restrained eating question.
- Your method?

So we restrict. Or feel we *should* restrict. Then, when we can't stand the restriction any more, we overeat. We identify overeating as the problem, but the fundamental cause is undereating—or the *threat* of undereating. In fact, a lot of people have gotten so sick and tired of restricting themselves with all the negativity that it entails that they only have to *think* of going without in order to make themselves overeat.

It is wonderful to take an interest in food and nutrition and to try to make sense of it. However, when that interest leads you to restrict and avoid and makes you distrust yourself and your food, it becomes more negative than positive. It puts you in the quandary of having a too-long list of foods-to-avoid. To eat the foods-to-avoid, you must throw away your rules, and in throwing away your rules, you are likely to not just eat *enough*, but to eat *way too much*. It's the "I blew it today but I will be good tomorrow" syndrome. Food avoidance leads to a cyclical pattern of eating that is not rewarding and not good for you.

RESTRAINT AND DISINHIBITION

It's striking that the pattern of cycling between "being good" and "being bad" is common enough to have a term: *restraint and disinhibition*. It means eating less and less-appealing food than you really want, on the one hand, then throwing away those controls on the other. Disinhibiting isn't just stopping restriction; it is catapulting way over it, often with a sense of careening out of control. We might disinhibit at a given meal, when we try to be virtuous with food selection and then discover that dessert is just too good to pass up. We might disinhibit once a week, as we take weekend vacations from the food rules. Or we might disinhibit over a longer cycle as we regain lost weight. We disinhibit because our fundamental need is to be fully nourished and fully satisfied, and the rules we go by—whether we realize it or not—say we shouldn't. To get around the rules, we periodically throw them away.

I have said it before, and I will say it again, because it is so important: The *rules* are the problem, not us. Rules are unrealistic when they say we have to go without—either in amount or type of food—and we have to do it forever. Restraint is profoundly unrealistic. Going without is painful. Going without *forever* in the name of weight management or disease avoidance is unthinkable. But that is what we expect of ourselves, so we find ways to cheat.

Address *How,* Not *What*

Having outlined our dilemma, we arrive at the heart of the matter.

> The problem is the *how* of eating, not the *what* or the *how much.* There is absolutely nothing wrong with deliberately eating what you want in quantities that satisfy. However, eating in response to impulse—disconnecting with the self that restricts—means you have to disconnect with the self that tunes in and enjoys, as well. You have to go on automatic pilot.
> The solution is to stop restricting.

Your eating will fall into place when you learn to trust yourself, accept that taking pleasure in eating is natural, and acknowledge that eating *enough* is essential.

"You can't say that, can you?" worries a dietitian correspondent. "Won't they just eat way too much of the wrong food?" "You can't let people just give in to their desires," warns an obesity researcher. "They will just get fatter and fatter." "They don't have any idea of proper eating," insist the food cops. "The high-calorie foods and big portion sizes make people overeat."

In my experience, none of it is true. I wish I had a nickel for every patient who said to me, "I know *what* to do, I just can't do it." What they *can't* do is fight against their perfectly legitimate interest in good-tasting food and their natural drive to eat until they feel satisfied. What they *can* do is learn to honor and trust their own needs. It doesn't happen overnight, but when people eat in a tuned-in, self-trusting fashion, they get to the point where they truly get enough to eat without overeating. Because it is so *hugely* important, let's emphasize that last point.

> Self-trusting eaters truly get enough to eat without overeating.
> While many fear that giving permission to eat preferred foods in satisfying amounts will promote gluttony, in practice quite the opposite occurs.
> • Foods that are no longer forbidden become ordinary foods that can be consumed in ordinary ways.
> • Large portion sizes become less appealing in the context of regular and reliable meals and snacks featuring adequate amounts of rewarding food.

Setting aside food restriction is like nutritional judo—going with the energy (the natural drive to eat as much as you want) rather than fighting against it. When my patients trust and honor their true and legitimate needs, they find that rather than periodically cutting loose and eating a great deal of high-calorie food, they eat moderately and consistently of all food, all the time, and find it genuinely satisfying. Check yourself. You are being restrained if you feel deprived. You are disinhibiting when you sneak off to eat. The solution? Trust your body to help you find the middle ground between the two extremes. Feed yourself reliably and well, and eat as much as you are hungry for.

Trust Your Body

I have said this before and I will say it again—and again—and again. Your body knows how much you need to eat. To recover your internal regulators of hunger, appetite, and satiety, learn to work *with* your body rather than against it. As I emphasized in chapter 1, "The Secret in a Nutshell," eating competence is made up of both permission and discipline. To trust your body to eat as much as you need, you require both:

- The *permission* is letting yourself choose foods you enjoy and eat them in amounts you find satisfying by depending on your internal regulators of hunger, appetite, and satiety.
- The *discipline* is providing yourself with the structure of regular and reliable meals and sit-down snacks and paying attention to your food and to yourself while you eat.

Structure is discipline, but it is positive discipline that is built on permission. Structure provides support and reassurance for your eating. To be able to have meals, you need to be able to tolerate your hunger long enough to get to the table. To be able to tolerate your hunger, you have to know that there is a good-tasting meal coming soon, when you can eat as much as you want.

STAY IN TOUCH

Once you get settled down and start to eat, stay in touch with your feelings of hunger and eagerness to eat. That takes effort, but it is rewarding effort. Tolerating your feelings and sensations lets you tune in on the taste-enhancing effect of hunger. As you eat, pay attention to how the food tastes and feels in your mouth, and how your stomach and your whole body feel as you begin to nourish yourself. Keep trying, even if at first it all feels the same.

Your eventual goal is to be able to pay attention to your eating through most meals, most of the time, whether you are alone or with other people, whether you are at home or eating in a restaurant. My smug little secret is that, when need be and given the right food, I can eat in a tuned-in fashion in the *car*. When I am on a long trip and am loathe to stop for food that will be ordinary anyway (on a not-so-crowded road such as we still have here in the Midwest), I can tune in on a quarter-pounder with cheese, fries, and a diet soda. Sometimes I eat it all, other times I don't. With time and practice, you too can reach such an elevated level of focused eating!

Eating behavior is deeply ingrained and habitual. It takes time and effort to change it. Take your time, or it can become so overwhelming that you will give it up and go back to eating on automatic pilot. In figure 4.3, "Steps to Internal Regulation," on page 33, I have outlined an approach for breaking the process into simple steps and building up focused eating a little at a time.

DISCOVER SATIETY

You will find your stopping place—your point of satiety—when you are ready. Reassure yourself that you aren't using your slowed-down, tuned-in eating as a way of tricking yourself into eating less. Keep eating until you genuinely feel like stopping. Notice when your hunger goes away and when your appetite goes away—when food stops tasting as good.

Don't worry if you eat more or less than someone else does. You could naturally require twice as many—or half as many—calories as someone else of the same sex, age, height, weight, and apparent physical activity. The difference is body metabolism. Whether your metabolism is set up to require a lot of calories or a few, being tuned in to your internal cues of hunger, appetite, and satiety means you will be satisfied on the amount *your* body needs. For more on this fascinating topic, see appendix E, "Energy Balance and Weight."

Meal after meal, day after day, as you stay in touch with your eating, your internal regulators will become more prominent. Depending on how consistent you are in giving yourself

permission to eat and tuning in on your eating and on yourself, within two to four months you will discover a trustworthy sensation of *truly* feeling like stopping. That natural stopping place is quite different from forcing yourself to stop and different from quitting because you are so full you can't take another bite. As one of my delighted patients exclaimed, "I can get enough to eat without overeating! It's like there is sanity in the midst of insanity!"

NOTICE THE PARTS OF SATIETY

Notice that there are stages in getting enough to eat. First, your hunger—your physical sense of food deficit—goes away. When I train my patients to eat in a tuned-in, self-aware fashion, they say they feel they *should* stop eating when their hunger goes away. But they are only *truly* willing to stop when the food stops *tasting* good. Eating to the point of satisfying your appetite as well as your hunger is a durable endpoint. But I have no rules for when to stop eating. You can eat past the point of satisfying your appetite. Next comes the point of feeling quite full. Most people find the too-full sensation generally pleasant and seek it out once in a while or eat to that point when the food is particularly good. Stopping at this point is okay, too.

If you continue to eat beyond the *full* feeling, you will arrive at *stuffed*. For most people, this is an unpleasant feeling. It is the feast-day syndrome, the point at which you would like to make it all go away. There is nothing wrong with eating to the point of feeling stuffed. You need only make a *choice* about whether it is positive or negative for you and whether you want to seek or avoid it. The issue is *choice. Awareness brings choice.*

Part of learning to internally regulate food intake is gaining experience with tolerating and accepting the feelings of satiety—including feeling too full or even stuffed—as normal and natural. Restrained eaters expect themselves to stop eating when they are still more-or-less hungry and still have food cravings. They interpret feelings of being satisfied and uninterested in food as overeating and therefore bad and even shameful. Amy, one of my University-student patients who was suffering from bulimia, had an almost irrepressible impulse to throw up when she felt at all full and satisfied. Because she expected herself to stop eating when she was still hungry, her internal conflict about eating was enormous.

Her chronic food restriction had left her terribly hungry, but her guilt and anxiety about eating were just as terrible. Sometimes she starved, sometimes she binged. Whether she starved or binged appeared to be determined by her level of stress. If her stress level was too high, she couldn't tolerate the starvation. To allow herself to binge, she put herself on automatic pilot and ate as much as she could hold. Then she felt stuffed. Her stomach bulged, her pants were too tight, and she felt revolted by the food that she had just gorged on. Again, when her stress level was too high to avoid the impulse, she threw up.

In treatment, Amy worked hard to be deliberate and tuned in when she ate. Gradually, she learned to intentionally let herself eat as much as she was hungry for, and that cut the pressure for gorging and vomiting way down. Before, she could only get enough to eat when she went out of control. But she still had to work hard to calm herself down when she felt at all satisfied. "It is normal for my belt to be a little tighter after I eat," she would reassure herself. "So my stomach isn't as flat as before. That's just natural."

Amy learned to expect that her body would tell her how much she needed to eat. She even got to the point where she could trust her body to make up for her errors in food regulation. So she ate too much. Her body would deal with it. The body has no need to resort to such drastic measures as purging to compensate for variations or even outright errors in food intake. Amy discovered she had hungry days or strings-of-days, followed by not-so-hungry days or strings-of-days. If she ate an unusually large amount, she wasn't as hungry for a while. She learned by experience that food regulation functions not just within a given day or even within two or three days. It functions week-to-week, month-to-month, or even seasonally.[2]

Your body remembers, just like Amy's. It makes up for eating more or less one time by cuing you to eat less or more another time. But if you try to compensate with your *head* by saying, "Today I have to cut down," or "Today I get to eat more," you will perpetuate the restraint-disinhibition cycle and interfere with the natural processes of food regulation. Figure 4.2 on the next page summarizes what I just told you about food regulation cues.

Boiling down our discussion about trusting your body, here is the basic kernel of take-it-with-you information.

> Trusting your body requires both permission and discipline. To translate those principles into eating the amount of food that is right for you:
> • Have meals that include foods you enjoy.
> • Calm yourself down.
> • Give yourself permission to eat.
> • Tune in while you eat.

That may be all the information you need in order to go back to regulating your food intake based on your hunger, appetite, and satiety. If that is the case, the next three sections, "How to Eat," "Recovering Internal Regulation," and "How Judy Found Her Freedom," will be useful to you primarily for reinforcing your capability—and your conviction that preserving that capability is essential. On the other hand, your sensitivity to internal regulators may be so deeply buried that you have to work hard to recover them. If that is the case, the next three sections are important. They will help you go through the motions and recover your ability to internally regulate food intake.

How to Eat

In telling you how to recover internally regulated food intake, I am depending on my clinical experience. My methods come from my 40 years of clinical practice as a registered dietitian and mental health professional. Much of that time, I have worked with people I have come to call dieting casualties: people who had been hurt by repeated failed attempts at weight reduction dieting—often for many years, not infrequently from childhood onward. I must confess that during the early part of my career, I helped to *create* those dieting casualties, a shameful bit of my past that I share in hopes that it will encourage other professionals and dieters to forgive themselves, as well. I learned the error of my ways, and so can you.

My patients demonstrated eating attitudes and behaviors that simply didn't work. Working with them, I experimented and pruned and surprised myself until I developed a remarkably effective method of helping people to develop eating attitudes and behaviors that *do* work. The method, *How to Eat*, applies the antithesis of food restriction and food avoidance and systematically builds competence with internally regulated food intake and food acceptance, improves attitudes about eating, and improves physical self-esteem. How to Eat is clinical—it is a treatment

FIGURE 4.2 FOOD REGULATION CUES

What are your food regulation cues, and what do they tell you? There are no rights or wrongs, shoulds or oughts. The goal is to tune in and experiment to find out what works for you. Your experiments will work best if you have meals and snacks at predictable times, and if you provide yourself with ample amounts of food at those times. Your food regulation cues will adjust to those set eating times so you will be comfortably hungry but not famished when it is time to eat.

Depending on your prior eating experiences, your internal cues will be either coarsely or finely tuned. Even if you haven't paid much attention to your eating cues, you will probably still be aware of the coarsely tuned extremes of feeling famished and feeling stuffed. However, you may have to do some work to gain access to the stages between the extremes: the subtle fine-tuning.

Famished	Extreme hunger, pronounced uneasiness: shakiness, fatigue, headache. You are likely to feel urgency and desperation to eat, especially if you can't be sure of getting enough to eat. People often become famished as a result of food insecurity, extreme self-restraint, or poor planning.
Hunger and appetite	The physical experience of moderate emptiness, perhaps *mild* uneasiness. Provided you know that you will soon have access to adequate amounts of rewarding food, your hunger and appetite can be tolerable and comfortable and, in fact, contribute to the enjoyment of eating. As the old saying goes, "Hunger is the best spice."
Hunger goes away	The physical experience of emptiness subsides along with uneasiness from energy deficit; sense of relief accumulates. However, eating is still rewarding and most people are reluctant to stop eating at this point.
Appetite goes away	Satiety, or stopping place: positive experience of readiness to stop eating. This is a comfortable and trustworthy endpoint to eating for most people. Food stops tasting as good (but is by no means repulsive) and your interest in eating decreases.
Full	For most, this is a pleasant, if occasional, endpoint to eating. It is a positive state of feeling filled up. Eating past satiety can be pleasant for you if you make a deliberate decision to eat more than usual, perhaps on a holiday, because the food tastes exceptionally good, or because your energy needs have suddenly increased. However, eating past satiety will feel negative if you do it because you have impulsively thrown away your constraints.
Stuffed	Almost everyone experiences feeling stuffed as being negative. This is extreme fullness, lethargy, physical discomfort, and perhaps nausea. Food may seem revolting and you may feel ashamed of overindulging. You may arrive at this point accidentally, out of habit, or because on some level you decided to throw away all controls.

Keep in mind that while the descriptions of internal regulators are useful, you learn internally regulated eating with your *body*, not with your *head*. You have to go through the motions.

protocol that I have tested many times with my own patients, have taught to others, and have had tested by others.[3,4] The tools for change in the How to Eat approach include focused eating exercises in sessions, in-session discussions, and progressive take-home assignments.

The basic principles of How to Eat, *permission* and *discipline*, are identical to those of the eating competence model. The goal of treatment is to develop eating competence. The difference is that my patients have been so traumatized for so long by their struggles with eating that they need systematic professional help to find their way out. And they *do* find their way out. I have successfully used How to Eat with men and women, from teenagers through people in their 60s. How to Eat is positive and achievable, but it is not easy. When my patients do their work, they are successful. When they don't do the work or are afraid to let go, they are not.

Often, my patients' eating has been interfered with since they were young and when they got older they have interfered with it themselves. They have been left with only coarsely tuned internal regulators and a lot of conflict and anxiety about eating. When they try to tune in on their food regulation cues, they find that those cues come packaged with upsetting memories and negative feelings. They need help processing those memories and feelings in order to become competent with eating. You may or may not need systematic, expert help to recover your internal regulators. Whether you can learn internally regulated eating on your own from the instructions in these pages depends on how much conflict and anxiety surround your eating. If you get stuck in spite of your best efforts, you need outside help.

Recovering Internal Regulation

In How to Eat, I use a stepwise approach to help a patient learn to internally regulate food intake and disconnect from restrained eating. That stepwise approach is outlined in figure 4.3.

FIGURE 4.3 STEPS TO INTERNAL REGULATION

1. **Center and give permission before eating. Try for meals with foods you like.** Get everything on the table, declare the kitchen closed, and get comfortable in your chair. Use a centering breath to bring your attention to yourself. A yoga centering breath works well, as does paying attention to 5 or 10 slow breath cycles. The idea is to give yourself a minute or so to interrupt your hurry-up and your distraction, relax a little, and bring your attention to yourself and to your meal.

    To give permission, say to yourself, "I can eat as much as I want; I just have to center myself first."

    That's it. Once you center and give permission, go back to eating the way you usually do. Try to center and give permission whenever, however, and wherever you eat—at your desk, leaning against the kitchen counter, at the mall.

2. **Increase the frequency of step 1.** Wait to move on to step 3 until you are doing step 1 half of the time or more. The payoff is that you will be more aware of your eating and of yourself. With subsequent steps, do the same: Wait until you can do the behavior half of the time or more before you move on. Be patient but firm with yourself. Keep working at it. Mastering each step can take several weeks.

3. **Do step 1, plus pay careful attention to each mouthful for *1 minute*.** Focus your whole attention on what is going on in your mouth while you eat. Ignore what is on your plate. Notice how you chew, how the food tastes, what helps you to savor. Wait to take another bite until your mouth is empty. What makes you swallow? Is it letting the food get on the back of your tongue so it slips down automatically? To savor more, keep the food farther forward in your mouth.

    Be sure to limit your focused attention to 1 minute. At first, trying to focus for too long may overwhelm you and make focused eating seem impossible. Keep yourself at this step until you are doing it half of the time or more.

4. **Do steps 1 and 3, plus have a focused snack daily.** For the focused snack, go through the whole routine—center, give permission, then be exquisitely aware of each bite of food. Focus your whole attention on what is going on in your mouth while you eat. For the focused snack, disregard my advice about eating as much as you want. Instead, make the snack small enough so you can eat it in 2 to 3 minutes. The goal is to sustain your undivided attention, and 2 to 3 minutes is long enough at this stage to do that.

5. **Continue with steps 1 and 4 and increase step 3 to 2 minutes.** Maintain 2 minutes of focused attention half of the time or more before you move on.

    Continue with steps 1 and 4 and increase step 3 to 3 minutes, then 4 minutes, then 5 minutes.

    Keep yourself at each step until you are doing it half of the time or more.

6. **Identify your stopping place.** If you are systematic about pacing yourself through the steps, somewhere between weeks 6 and 10 you will discover your stopping place—the place where you truly feel satisfied and ready to stop eating. This will feel entirely different from stopping because you think you should or stopping because you are too full to take another bite. Depending on how much you have struggled with your eating, you may experience finding your stopping place as an epiphany—an intuitive grasp of your innate capability with eating. On the other hand, you may find it helpful but not particularly thrilling. For me, being with my patients when they discover their stopping place is like seeing them be reborn. Appendix F, "The Story of Sharon," tells the story of how one woman found her stopping place.

If all goes well, you will be able to work through the sequence in a way that is helpful to you. If you get stuck, find someone who can help. Reading the steps and enacting them on your own isn't the same as working with a knowledgeable and supportive eating therapist who can coach you, discuss your experiences, and help you process your feelings.

By the time you have worked your way up to focusing 4 or 5 minutes at the beginning of each meal, you will likely find yourself paying attention on some level most of the time throughout the meal. Your attention may not have the same sustained, exquisitely tuned-in quality as when you were first learning focused eating, but you will have your moments. For the most part, you will be tuned in enough to be aware of your internal regulators.

You will be able to maintain this tuned-in eating when you are with other people and eating in other places, but it doesn't happen automatically. You will have to work yourself through the steps, the same as you did when you were first learning. However, you will learn faster each time you apply it to a new situation.

Over the long term, give your eating enough attention to maintain your focus. Your old attitudes and behaviors have been with you for a long time, and they will come sneaking back if you let them. Continue to begin your meals with a centering breath, permission to eat, and a reminder to tune in and enjoy your food.

How Judy Found Her Freedom

While I hope your negative experiences with eating have been less traumatic than my patient Judy's, I think her process of mastering internally regulated eating will be instructive for you. Because Judy had been the object of family scorn and ridicule throughout her life because of her eating and weight, a big part of her treatment was dismantling her self-criticism about weight as well as food-restriction thoughts, attitudes, and patterns. Judy's food intake had been restricted by her parents from the time she was small, and she began restricting herself when she was a preadolescent. With each weight loss, Judy regained to a higher level until, at age 30, she appeared to be a *lot* fatter than nature had intended her to be.

I started her with step 1: centering breath, permission to eat, and eating meals with foods you like. Judy came back the next week to report that she hadn't done the centering breath (it *is* hard to remember) but that she thought it was *such* a good idea. "If I did that, I wouldn't eat so much," she observed.

"So you are going to punish yourself for centering?" I asked. She looked puzzled, and cautiously hopeful. "The punishment is eating less than you want. You have restricted yourself all this time—or tried to," I reminded her. "Now you are learning to eat until you feel satisfied. Paying attention is part of that. Paying attention is *not* a way of tricking yourself into eating less." So I gave the assignment again: "Center, and tell yourself, 'I can eat as much as I want; I just have to center myself first.' Oh, yes, and have meals with the foods you like."

This reminded Judy that she had trouble deciding what to order when she stopped for dinner after our previous appointment. "What I really wanted was the lasagna," she said, "but I just couldn't order it. I felt everyone was looking at me and saying, 'Look at that fat woman eating that lasagna. No wonder she is fat.' So I ordered the broiled chicken, salad, and vegetables. It was okay, but what I really wanted was lasagna."

"I can understand," I told her. "People do look and criticize, but perhaps less than you think. They are interested in their own meals and their own lives more than they are in you. But even if they look, are you willing to let that spoil your meal? What about tonight? Are you stopping for dinner tonight? What are you hungry for?" Judy allowed as how she wanted Rocky Rococo pizza. I gave her the firm instruction to stop to get it and told her how to find the closest Rocky's.

I was giving Judy lots of permission to eat as well as blessing her food—telling her it was all right to eat the food she enjoyed. As a result, when we did the focused eating exercise, which involved relaxing and tuning in on her feelings and sensations as she prepared to eat, she was able to admit that she was excited about eating her Triscuit. But, because she was so intensely ashamed of her excitement, Judy cried. Judy was a grown-up version of Holly, the toddler I talked about in chapter 2, "Adjust Your Attitude," who moaned when she ate. Judy, like Holly, had been taught that it was wrong to enjoy her eating. Her inclinations toward eating had been so rejected by so many (including herself) for so long, she even felt ashamed that these inclinations *existed*. Because she couldn't forgive herself for the way she was, at first she depended on me to accept and support her joyful interest in food and eating. Later on, she learned to accept herself.

This was still only session 2, and already Judy was catching on that her work with me was entirely different from anything she had done before. She was being encouraged to *eat*, not to restrict herself. Her excitement about eating was a good thing, not something to feel ashamed about. But her inclination to restrict didn't go away easily or quickly. At each step along the way, Judy's impulse was to use the tasks to get herself to eat less. "After I did that, I wasn't hungry anymore so I thought I should stop eating," she would report. "Did you feel like stopping eating?" I would ask. "No, I still felt like eating."

"First you have to give yourself permission to eat," I would tell her. "Later on, you can give yourself permission to stop eating."

"But I should stop," objected Judy, "because otherwise I will get too fat." Over and over again, as Judy became more and more deliberate about her eating, she tripped over her weight talk. "I shouldn't eat that," she would scold herself. "I am too fat and that is why. *Because* I eat that." Getting herself off automatic pilot left an opening for Judy to torment herself about her eating and weight—and explained her pattern of putting herself on automatic pilot in the first place. Digging into her food and eating without awareness spared her the torment. If you think the word *torment* is too strong, you haven't been there.

Weight talk is always there. The fix for it is to bring it out in the open so it can be addressed and set aside. "What happens when you get into weight talk?" I asked Judy on many occasions. The story was always the same: She tried not to eat it, whatever it was, or tried not to eat as much as she wanted. Then she felt deprived. Then she overate. "So does weight talk help you?" I asked her. "No, it doesn't," she acknowledged. "It just makes my eating worse." It came to seem as if the weight talk was something she felt obligated to do. It was almost like magical thinking: If she tormented herself about her weight, she was doing something about it. Eventually, we agreed on a little mantra she could use to extinguish her weight talk: "I can't control my weight, but I can control my eating." *That* was helpful. Judy was discovering that her weight talk didn't help her. A study from Yale says the same thing: Most people respond to put-downs and criticisms about weight by eating more than usual and gaining weight.[5] If shaming made people thin, we wouldn't have any fat people.

At times Judy reported binge-eating. Then, we put on our detective hats and tracked down what led up to the binge. It wasn't difficult, because it was always the same. Judy had taken away permission to eat—she had tried to get herself to eat less or less-appealing food than she really wanted. Underneath that was the knee-jerk notion that she should lose weight.

POSITION, PLACE, AND ASSOCIATED ACTIVITY

Judy was typical in that when she got to about step 4, she wondered whether she should do the "position, place, and associated activity" behaviors: Eat only sitting down, in only one designated place, and don't do anything else while eating. Being a veteran dieter, Judy had been exposed to about every weight-management technique, including these typical behavioral weight-control techniques. The behavioral weight-control idea is to complicate eating to the point where you reduce calorie intake and produce weight loss.

We were using behavioral techniques, but we were using them to make Judy's eating positive and deliberate, not to complicate and ultimately decrease her food intake. "Someday you may decide you want to get rid of other activities while you eat, but it has to be because you want to, not because you think you should," I told her. "You are new to paying attention to your eating, and you haven't yet discovered that you can trust yourself to eat as much as you want. Right now, trying to use those tactics will feel like taking away permission."

A few weeks later, Judy began complaining that she almost always ate dinner in the living room in front of the TV, and when she did, her food would be gone before she even noticed she was eating. Judy was ready to address the way she distracted herself while she ate. However, we weren't going to jump into it. "For a long time, you have been watching TV while you eat dinner," I told her. "It must have some benefit for you, or you wouldn't do it. Let's see if we can find out what that benefit is."

So we set up a little experiment. We agreed she would do step 3—center, permission, focused eating for 1 minute—before she turned on the TV. Then she would pay attention to what she was feeling. She discovered she was upset about what was going on in her life, and that she was zoning out by eating in front of the TV. Bringing this automatic behavior up to a conscious level allowed Judy to realize that, unlike when she was younger and had first developed the pattern, she now had ways of dealing with her stress. She didn't have to be afraid of her feelings, and she no longer had to zone out. Having made that discovery, however, eating to zone out was still one of her choices, as was eating in front of the TV. Judy continued to work on her focused eating, and she continued to eat in the living room. She got to the point where she could get most of the way through her meal before she turned on the TV.

THE STOPPING PLACE

Then one grand day, about 7 weeks into treatment, Judy found her stopping place. When she described it at our next session, she went right by it, not realizing the significance of what she was telling me. "Wait a minute," I told her. "Did you hear what you just said? What made you decide to stop eating?" I asked her. She looked puzzled. "I don't really know," she said. "I had a piece of pumpkin pie and then another piece and then I stopped. I really didn't want any more. I didn't feel stuffed or anything. I just felt like I had had enough."

"It seems to me you found your stopping place," I told her. Her face lit up and she was delighted. Judy was the person who said, "I can get enough to eat without overeating! It's like there is sanity in the midst of insanity!"

As a result of treatment, Judy has become competent with her eating and has gained new self-respect relative to her eating. She isn't the out-of-control glutton she had thought, but instead feels proud of her ability to manage her eating. She no longer uses her weight as evidence that she is out is out of control and lacking in self-discipline. Judy would like to be thinner, but she enjoys her eating. She is delighted with being free of the enslavement of struggling to lose weight and scrutinizing every mouthful she eats, and she knows if she gets back into weight-loss endeavors, it will spoil her eating. Being a relatively heavy person in our weight-obsessed culture is not easy for her, but she is willing and ready to act on her own behalf.

Emotional Eating

Earlier, I talked about Amy's insight that stress exacerbated her tendency to binge-eat as well as Judy's discovery that she ate in front of the TV

for emotional reasons. The first step for both of them was to get rid of the food restriction. After that, we addressed the feelings. "There is nothing wrong with using food for emotional reasons," I told them both. "It can bring up your spirits when you are low, soothe you when you are tense, and distract you when you are upset. The problem is that you are doing it poorly. You have no idea what you are feeling, other than generally upset or stressed. You reach for something to eat to feel better, you feel guilty while you are doing it, and you eat to push down or blot out your feelings. Often you eat fast and eat too much. So you end up feeling guilty and out of control."

It is unrealistic and even undesirable to get rid of eating for emotional reasons. When I am feeling down and discouraged, there is nothing like a good meal to lift my spirits. When I am weary from struggling with a difficult life issue, eating a bowl of chicken soup or Cheerios while I sit in my dining room rocking chair with my feet up is one of the ways I take care of myself. When I am in a celebratory mood, cooking and eating with others extends and heightens the celebration. I don't try to ignore my feelings—I stay with them, let them teach me what I need to learn, and take care of myself while I do that. Feeding myself well is one of the ways I take care of myself.

Many eating practitioners say that emotional eating is to blame for overeating and weight gain and that the key to weight loss is to get rid of emotional eating. That idea is oversimplified and physiologically naive. To gain weight from emotional eating, even if that emotional eating leads you to eat quite a lot, you would have to overwhelm your body's natural regulatory abilities by overeating day after day without stopping. There are few people who do that.

In my clinical experience, as well as in the research, people who overeat for emotional reasons tend to be restrained eaters. People who are not restrained eaters are far less likely to use food for emotional reasons. Conversely, eating in a restrained fashion increases the tendency to use food for emotional reasons.[6] In reality, rather than overeating in response to stress, the restrained eater disinhibits. The end result is still overeating, but the root cause is the *under-eating* rather than the emotional arousal. Hunger and emotional arousal exert pressure in tandem with one another. Stress undermines the ability to tolerate the symptoms of under-eating, and hunger undermines the ability to deal appropriately with stress. The solution has two parts: setting aside the restrained eating and becoming more comfortable with feelings. Rather than grabbing food on impulse or trying to tough it out and separate food from emotion, learn to productively use food for emotional reasons. Figure 4.4 offers an approach to help you do that.

FIGURE 4.4 CENTERED EMOTIONAL EATING

- Make sure you are regularly getting enough to eat.
- Center yourself. Relax, and pay attention to your breath and to yourself.
- Reassure yourself. "It is all right to eat. But first I will find out what I am feeling."
- Take a few moments to know what you are feeling and what you want.
- Be clear about what eating can do. Eating in a focused fashion is likely to soothe or calm you. It won't resolve the problem—unless the problem is being hungry!
- Then eat—positively, deliberately, soothingly, cheeringly.

Sylvia, another of my University-student patients who, like Amy, was a seriously out-of-control bulimic, was able to discontinue her bulimia when she learned to consciously use her eating to soothe herself. To give herself that great and wonderful gift, she first had to go through the How to Eat program to learn to feed herself reliably and well and to internally regulate her food intake. Letting herself eat enough neutralized most of the pressure that led her to gorge and then vomit. She herself discovered the key that allowed her to set aside her bulimia altogether: using her eating as a kind of meditative practice, to calm herself and to take good care of herself emotionally.

With emotional eating as with eating for every other reason, you will find that you eat in a more controlled fashion when you give yourself permission to eat rather than withhold it.

With Awareness Comes Choice

As I said earlier in this chapter, with awareness comes choice. Eating attentively again and again, and paying attention to how you feel again and again, lets you decide what works for you. While I tell you that paying attention most of the time and making eating a priority most of the time is necessary for letting your internal regulators work for you, you are entitled to find that out for yourself. Unless you find through your own experience that eating competence helps you manage your eating, it will be just another set of rules. You don't need a whole new set of rules to impose on yourself with regards to your eating.

Pay attention. How do you feel physically when you slow down and tune in with your eating? When you don't? What happens to the orderly and positive nature of your eating when you set aside time to eat? When you don't? When you let yourself become famished? Do you like that desperate feeling of having to eat *right now*, or would you rather avoid it?

What happens to your tuned-in eating when you decide you have to cut down on your eating and lose weight? Are you able to go to meals hungry but not famished? Can you sustain your orderly, attentive, and focused eating when you are overly hungry? Do you trust your satiety cues when you try to eat less? What happens to your attitudes about eating? Are you still relaxed about eating? Do you feel it is okay to eat food you like? Are you still comfortable with eating enough and with your enjoyment of food and eating?

Will you decide to be just tuned in enough to enjoy your food and to support food regulation? Or will you continue to pay the kind of exquisite attention I teach in figure 4.3, "Steps to Internal Regulation," on page 33. Eating that attentively could open up the possibility of making your eating a kind of meditative practice, where you connect with yourself and with the process of taking in food. Do it if you want to and if it is rewarding for you. Don't do it if paying such exquisite attention to eating feels enslaving and rigid.

Learn How to Feast

The eating competence model is built on pleasure. Loving to eat is a special sensitivity that offers heightened experience and particular pleasure. Loving to eat doesn't mean that you will overeat, as long as you know how to handle it. People who love to eat are often extremely tuned in to textures and tastes and smells. People who love to eat savor their food—they take conscious pleasure in it. They appreciate it by *tuning in* a great deal, not necessarily by *eating* a great deal.

Often, people feel that the only way to fully appreciate great-tasting or freely available food is to eat a lot—to eat to the point of being very full or even stuffed. As I have said before, that is one of the choices. If you like feeling stuffed, you have my blessing. Do, however, pay attention while you eat to the point of feeling stuffed so you can enjoy the process.

But think about it. Does the pursuit of eating-a-lot transform your eating pleasure into an unconnected, unaware urgency to eat more and more? Do you continue to savor your food, paying attention to what is in your mouth so you can get all the enjoyment out of it? Or do you lose track of pleasure as you focus on the next bite or the next helping rather than on what is in your mouth? Many times when people set out to eat a lot they get caught in conveyor-belt eating, like that old Lucy-and-Ethel-in-the-chocolate-factory routine. In case you missed that episode of *I Love Lucy*, Lucy and Ethel get behind on their candy-packaging and resort to eating the excess. In their desperation to clean off the conveyor belt, they stop enjoying the chocolates and just eat them to get rid of them. It's funny to watch, but it's not funny when you get caught in conveyor-belt eating. Sooner or later, it hurts. We get to the point where we can't eat another bite, we are turned off to the food that seemed so appealing to start with, and we feel ashamed.

It's a real trick—*truly* getting enough without eating so much that you feel turned off to the whole experience and mad at yourself; being conscious of your eating without feeling obligated to cut down. How can you learn that trick? *Permission* and *discipline*. Say to yourself, "I can eat as much as I want. I can eat a lot if I want. I just have to pay attention."

Beverages and Activity

Sweetened beverages and activity are two important topics related to helping yourself be successful with eating as much as you want. It is challenging to address them without getting negative and prescriptive. Let's see what we can do.

DRINK DELIBERATELY
Sweetened beverages such as soda, juice, sweet tea, fruit drinks, and sports drinks can be culprits with respect to regulating food intake. Sipping calorie-containing beverages between meals can take the edge off your hunger and appetite and make it more difficult for you to detect your internal regulatory cues. Sugar-free beverages interfere to a lesser extent, but they still interfere.

So there are good reasons for cutting down on soda. Other good reasons are to save your teeth and to leave an opening for drinking more milk. But let's not pack you up for a guilt trip. Consumption data indicate that people *love* their soda, and in the context of a lot of other vices, it is not such a big one. Think about it, and make your choices. Don't just *do* it. Many times people get into a beverage habit because they are trying to undereat, and they drink soda to stave off hunger. Others seek a caffeine fix or habitually use beverages for comfort—to smooth transitions back to the computer or to provide a reliable treat to help compensate for the rough spots of the day.

Whatever your reason for drinking soda, do it deliberately and wisely. Drink Coke with your breakfast to get your caffeine fix. I *never* thought I would say that, but hey, how different is it from drinking coffee? I have consumed tanker trucks of coffee in my day, so who am I to preach? Consider including soda at your other meals or snacks and paying attention while you drink it. If your Friday night pizza just doesn't taste right without soda, for heaven's sake, have soda! If you don't want your children to get hooked on soda, let them have it for the occasional snack and do your conveyor-belt soda-drinking when they aren't around. You watch gory movies on TV when they aren't around, don't you?

Do try to figure out other times to drink your milk or orange juice, however. You need them.

BE GOOD TO YOURSELF WITH ACTIVITY
You can help your body regulate by getting some activity—not to burn off calories, but to support your internal food regulation capabilities. Moderate levels of activity make internal regulation cues more prominent and therefore easier to read. Moderate activity also appears to make those cues more accurate. An observational study done years ago by a Harvard researcher shows that as long as they are moderately active, people balance activity with

energy intake and maintain stable body weights. However, people whose activity is below the minimum are more hungry, eat more, and gain weight.[7]

Your level of activity is up to you, but do make it enjoyable enough so it can be sustainable. Some people are naturally more or less active than others. To find the level of activity that is right for you, experiment. Start at a level you can sustain. Gradually increase until you get hooked—until you enjoy it and don't feel as good without it. Maintain a level of activity that is realistic. The American College of Sports Medicine and the American Heart Association recommend 30 minutes of moderate activity a day, 5 days a week, or vigorous-intensity aerobic physical activity for a minimum of 20 minutes, 3 days a week.[8] That might be right for you—or it might not. A recent study at the Cooper Institute in Dallas indicates that overweight and obese people show improvements in fitness levels on as little as 10 minutes of activity a day.[9]

Be careful about controlling messages associated with activity, as well. Weight-loss folks who have given up on diets have yet to give up on activity, so you will hear overly ambitious messages that encourage using activity for weight loss. MyPyramid recommends 90 minutes a day to lose weight, 60 minutes a day to maintain weight loss. That's a lot. If it is your thing, go for it. But don't try to impose it on your child.

Trying to push beyond what is realistic for you will put you behind, not ahead. You will go on binges with activity, then revert to being a couch potato until your conscience forces you to your feet to activity-binge again. It doesn't work any better with activity than it does with eating.

Beware of Counterfeits

More and more consumers as well as professionals are catching on that food restriction is counterproductive. Adults who have been trying to manage their weight through restriction, deprivation, and good-food-bad-food thinking are coming to realize that such tactics make their weight problem worse. Even weight loss businesses have picked up on consumer skepticism and reluctance to engage in weight-reduction dieting. All of that seems good, right? The problem is that there is an increasing number of phony non-dieting schemes that conceal the ulterior motive of weight loss. They are counterfeits.

Consider any food plan that outlines what to eat, how much to eat, and when to eat. This is not a diet? Consider Healthful Weight Management, which encourages you to fill up on low-calorie foods such as fruits, vegetables, and whole grains; to limit fat and sugar; and to restrict portion sizes of everything. Exactly *how* is this not a diet? Consider behavioral weight control, which teaches position, place, associated activity, putting in a delay before having a second helping, putting your fork down between bites … I could go on. The idea is to complicate eating to the point where you eat less and weigh less. Consider "mindful eating," which in some hands genuinely supports internally regulated food intake and in other hands is a thinly veiled scheme for getting you to eat less and weigh less.

In many cases, the counterfeiting is unintentional. Many practitioners I train to support eating competence come into training genuinely feeling they support internally regulated eating. But because food restriction is so deeply embedded in their thinking, they discover they unconsciously put a controlling spin on their food selection and regulation messages. Many nutrition professionals say they *love* my work, but they have no idea that telling adults what and how much to eat and teaching parents what and how much to get their children to eat absolutely contradicts my principles. In other cases, the counterfeiting is entirely intentional. Controlling portion size is near and dear to the hearts of nutrition professionals, who have bought into the limited evidence that too-big portions make people overeat. Ironically, in teaching portion size they impose food restriction and ignore the far more substantial evidence that instituting restrained eating exacerbates overeating and weight gain. Intentional or unintentional, a controlling spin encourages you to ignore and overrule your internal regulators. Figure 4.5 on the next page gives examples of negative spin-doctoring of trust messages.

Control tactics may trick your head, but they won't trick your body. In the long run, controlling tactics make you eat more and gain weight. If you try to fool yourself into eating less by

FIGURE 4.5 CONTROL OR TRUST—DETECTING THE COUNTERFEITS

Control-based practitioners can appropriate any positive and trusting eating message and turn it into a control message. The control message seems to be giving you permission to eat what you want and as much as you want, but it is really taking it away. Rather than helping you to eat in an orderly, positive, and internally regulated fashion, such negative messages are likely to precipitate out-of-control eating because they make you feel deprived.

Trust message	Control message
Go to the table hungry but not famished.	Fill up by drinking water before a meal.
Eat until you feel satisfied.	Stop eating when you are full.
You decide how much to put on your plate.	Pay attention to portion size.
To be sure everyone will have enough, make enough to have leftovers.	Eat off smaller plates.
Savor sweets; eat until you get enough.	Eat sweets in small amounts.
"C" is for cookie.	Cookies are a sometime food.
Go to some trouble to get foods you enjoy.	Don't keep sweet foods at home.
Make eating important by taking time to enjoy meals.	Every time you eat a meal, sit down and chew slowly.
Pay attention to how good the food tastes.	Remind everyone to enjoy every bite.
If you savor cheese and chocolate, you will get enough.	Cut cheese and chocolate into small pieces and only eat a few pieces.
Trust your hunger, appetite, and satiety to guide you at buffets.	Skip buffets.
Eat as much as you are hungry for.	Don't have seconds.
Eat as much as you are hungry for.	Serve food portions no larger than your fist.

Since I couldn't possibly list all the counterfeit non-dieting messages, here is a litmus test: If the message or tactic encourages you to eat less, to avoid foods you like, or to lose weight, it is negative and controlling and will undermine eating competence.

---

drinking water before a meal, filling up on low-calorie food, or eating off a smaller plate, you will eat more some other time. Often, the distinctions are subtle: "Make eating important by taking time to enjoy meals" is a trust message because it encourages you to tune in on yourself and enjoy eating. "Sit down and chew slowly" is a control message because it encourages you to eat mechanically with the aim of eating less.

You simply can't have it both ways. If you try to be a little bit controlling and a little bit trusting, you will end up controlling, utterly confuse yourself, and make your child unhappy. With professionals, I use the term *paradigm straddling* to describe approaches that give permission and take it away at the same time.

The Matter of Weight

People who show high eating competence tend to be somewhat slimmer than those who do not. Forty-two percent of people who are competent with eating have BMIs over 25, compared with 57% of people who are not eating competent. Competent eaters show a moderately lower range of BMIs than the general population. Their average BMI is 25, with a range of 20–31. Those who are not competent eaters have an average BMI of 27, with a range of 21–33.[10]

Despite the modest statistical differences, the eating competence model is not a weight-loss method. In fact, striving for weight loss impairs competence with eating in all areas. You can't trust your internal regulators of hunger, appetite, and satiety when you diet. The point of dieting is to ignore and overrule those regulators in order to eat less and lose weight. Taking too much pleasure from eating is a threat when you are trying to lose weight because stimulating the appetite can make you eat more than you think you should. Rather than having a relaxed and positive attitude about your eating, when you are on a diet you have to be vigilant and critical. The only way that dieting may seem to improve eating competence is in the matter of context. Many people get serious about feeding themselves only when they are on a weight-reduction regimen. Then, they have regular and reliable meals. But when they abandon the diet, they abandon regular meals, as well, and nothing changes.

To become competent with your eating, you have to be willing to take risks with your weight. You have to take the leap of faith that you can internally regulate your eating and that your weight will be all right. Trying for any stated weight, even if it is your current weight, will tip you into restrained eating and undermine your competence with eating. I can't promise you that if you become competent with your eating that you will lose weight. In fact, I can't promise you *anything* about your weight, because your genetics and body metabolism dictate what that weight will be. I can only make general observations. Your weight is likely to stabilize if it is at its current usual point. Your weight is unlikely to stabilize if you have just lost weight. Your biological pressure will be to regain; to maintain weight loss, you will have to continue to eat less than you are hungry for. If your weight is unusually high, you might lose a little. On the other hand, your body may have metabolically equilibrated at that higher weight level and will defend that new, higher weight level.

Even my treatment protocol, How to Eat, is not a weight-loss method. I must admit that once in a great while, a person who goes through the How to Eat treatment loses 10 percent or so of body weight and keeps it off. However, that is the exception, not the rule. In my experience, most people stabilize their weight right where it is, even if they come into treatment showing extremes of restraint/disinhibition behavior such as binging and purging.

WEIGHT AND HEALTH

Health can be improved independent of weight loss by developing positive behaviors and attitudes: competent eating, rewarding and sustainable activity, and physical self-esteem. Survey data indicate that people who are more competent with eating have better health indicators—blood lipids, blood glucose, and blood pressure.[11] They have higher levels of body satisfaction and lower levels of psychosocial dysfunction.[10] Clinical data indicate that people who replace restraint and disinhibition with internally regulated eating improve their attitudes about eating, stabilize weight, and have improved health indicators.[3,12] Appendix D, "BMI, Mortality, Morbidity, and Health: Resolving the Weight Dilemma," shows the evidence that weight stability produces superior health outcomes compared with major weight loss or yo-yo weight patterns secondary to yo-yo eating. People who are moderately and consistently active have higher disease resistance, irrespective of BMI: It is better to be fat and fit than thin and unfit.

DATA RESISTANCE

The idea that it is possible to lose weight and keep it off is astonishingly data-resistant. Despite overwhelming evidence to the contrary, people have a remarkably strong tendency to keep the dream alive that the next diet will work. Old professionals like me, and some who gain wisdom before they get old, have come to realize that dieting *doesn't* work. However, the young ones come out of school just like I did, with stars in their eyes, convinced that they alone can break the curse with their nifty new approach to weight management. But there is nothing new under the sun, and the "new" methods have been tried—and have failed—before.

Health policy makers are as data-resistant as the rest of us. The official policy makers continue to emphasize the dangers of high body weight and the importance of weight loss even though, when pressed, they acknowledge that weight loss is rare. However, they judge that it is better to lose and regain than to not lose at all.[13] Those policy makers can only draw such conclusions by ignoring the anguish of people who are caught in the cycle of dieting and weight regain. Instead, policy-makers judge that above-average body weight is, on some level, a matter of choice and that choice must be addressed in order to save the person of size from health catastrophe and social, emotional, and quality-of-life inferiority.

Fiddle-faddle. If people of size are miserable, it is because they are reminded over and over again that they are miserable. The data I report in appendix D, "BMI, Mortality, Morbidity, and Health: Resolving the Weight Dilemma," show that people of size can be as healthy—physically, emotionally, and socially—as anyone else. However, I have yet to help someone give up dieting by showing them the true facts and figures on weight and marshalling the evidence that it is not the serious health risk we have been led to believe. In my experience, coming to terms with body weight is an emotional issue, not an intellectual one.

"You are taking away hope," both professionals and individuals accuse in response to my naysaying about weight loss. "Your hope is too narrow," I respond. "Why confine your hopes to being a different size and shape? Why not hope for being all you can be and having joy in life?"

DIETING: COST OR BENEFIT?
Despite the fact that we alibi our dieting by saying it is a health concern, most of us do it because of *vanity*. If vanity is your reason for weight loss, it is a cost-benefit decision. How much are you willing to expend for vanity? How rigid do you want to be about your definitions of beauty? Rigid enough to devote a great deal of your time and energy to forcing your weight down and keeping it down? Rigid enough to be continually hungry and food-preoccupied and chronically tired, cranky, and even depressed? How attractive is it to be self-absorbed and surly, unwilling to join in with the rewarding meals that others are eating, and how does it affect your ability to be a good friend or spouse or parent?

Trying to get your body to be heavier than is natural for it doesn't work either. You can stuff yourself to force your weight up, but eventually you will tire of the bloated, turned-off-to-food feelings that go along with overeating, and you will give up the effort. Your body will fight you on gaining above your preferred level as well, and eventually it will return to what it was before you started trying to change it.

If you are lucky.

If you are *not* lucky—and many people, children and adults alike, are not—you will experience a rebound effect. Over my professional career, I have worked with hundreds of people who have become fatter because of their dieting. They look wistfully at their toddler, school-age, teenage, or young adult photos and say, "I was chubby, but I was fine. I wish I were as slim now as I was then." Despite the casual way many people jump on and off diets, weight-reduction dieting is serious business with the potential for considerable negative consequence. It can screw up your homeostasis, the mechanisms that keep your weight pretty stable without you having to think too much about it. Once homeostasis is corrupted, it is beastly difficult to restore it to order.

I say this in other chapters, and I will say it again. If you choose to diet, it is up to you. However, if you have children, you are being irresponsible in making that choice. Parents who diet don't do as well with feeding their children, and despite their best intentions, their children tend to go on and off diets right along with them. Consider the child of the parent on the Atkins Diet or the South Beach Diet. Is that child likely to be offered pasta prepared in interesting ways, luscious bread, and wonderful fruit desserts? Children and adolescents learn dieting from their parents. Even if the dieting parent has willpower of steel, the child will observe what her parent eats, and deep in her heart of hearts, she will say, "When I get big, that is how I will eat."

Nutrition professionals emphasize "healthful" low-calorie dieting as a way of losing and maintaining weight: Eat more fruits, vegetables, and skim milk; eat more high-fiber food such as whole grains; and hold way down on fat and sugar. In fact, if you work your way through MyPyramid and get your "personal eating plan," that is exactly what you get—a food prescription that satisfies those parameters. There is no evidence that such regimens produce weight loss. In fact, for teenagers, there is evidence to the contrary. Adolescents who diet are heavier 5 years later, whether they engage in "healthful" or unhealthful weight-control practices.[14]

Of the four chapters that discuss eating competence, this may be the most difficult for you. It is certainly the longest, and grappling with energy regulation and weight issues has spun off two appendixes. It also has the potential for being the most pivotal and rewarding chapter. Compared with trying to manage your food intake with control and avoidance, trusting your body to let you know how much you need to eat is like night and day. It is joyful.

References

1. Serdula MK, Mokdad AH, Williamson DF, Galuska DA, Mendlein JM, Heath GW. Prevalence of attempting weight loss and strategies for controlling weight. *JAMA.* 1999;282:1353-1358.

2. Mayer J. Some aspects of the problem of regulation of food intake and obesity. *N Engl J Med.* 1966;274:610-616, 662-673, 722-731.

3. Hammond-Meyer A. *Stabilizing Eating and Weight Using a Nondieting Treatment As a Means to Improve Biomedical Health Parameters in an Overweight Population of Women: A Health at Any Size Perspective [Dissertation] .* Seattle, WA: Seattle Pacific University; 2005.

4. Jackson E. Eating Order: A 13-week trust model class for dieting casualties. *J Nutr Educ Behav.* 2008;40:43-48.

5. Puhl RM, Brownell KD. Confronting and coping with weight stigma: an investigation of overweight and obese adults. *Obesity (Silver Spring).* 2006;14:1802-1815.

6. Van Strien T, Ouwens MA. Counter-regulation in female obese emotional eaters: Schachter, Goldman, and Gordon's (1968) test of psychosomatic theory revisited. *Eat Behav.* 2003;3:329-340.

7. Mayer J, Roy P, Mitra KP. Relation between caloric intake, body weight and physical work. *Am J Clin Nutr.* 1956;4(2):169-175.

8. Haskell WL, Lee IM, Pate RR, et al. Physical Activity and Public Health. Updated recommendation for adults from the American College of Sports Medicine and the American Heart Association. Circulation. 2007;116:1081-1093.

9. Church TS, Earnest CP, Skinner JS, Blair SN. Effects of different doses of physical activity on cardiorespiratory fitness among sedentary, overweight or obese post-menopausal women with elevated blood pressure: a randomized controlled trial. *JAMA.* 2007;297:2081-2091.

10. Lohse B, Satter E, Horacek T, Gebreselassie T, Oakland MJ. Measuring Eating Competence: psychometric properties and validity of the ecSatter Inventory. *J Nutr Educ Behav.* 2007;39 (suppl):S154-S166.

11. Psota T, Lohse B, West S. Associations between eating competence and cardio-vascular disease biomarkers . *J Nutr Educ Behav .* 2007;39 (suppl):S171-S178.

12. Bacon L, Stern JS, Van Loan MD, Keim NL. Size acceptance and intuitive eating improve health for obese, female chronic dieters. *J Am Diet Assoc.* 2005;105:929-936.

13. NIH Task Force on the Prevention and Treatment of Obesity. Weight cycling. *JAMA.* 1994;272(15):1196-1202.

14. Neumark-Sztainer D, Wall M, Guo J, Story M, Haines J, Eisenberg M. Obesity, disordered eating, and eating disorders in a longitudinal study of adolescents: how do dieters fare 5 years later? *J Am Diet Assoc.* 2006;106:559-568.

Chapter
5
Feed Yourself Faithfully

Structure is the backbone of eating competence. Throughout part I, I have stressed permission to eat: To feel good about eating; to eat the foods you like; to eat as much as you want. Now we arrive at the essential framework that will make your eating fall into place.

To reap the rewards of trustworthy, satisfying, internally regulated eating, you must provide yourself with regular, reliable, rewarding meals as well as sit-down snacks if you need them. To be able to trust your body to help you with the *what* and *how much* of eating, you must provide it with the support it needs. You will do a good job with eating as much as you need of a variety of food if you reliably feed yourself, go to some trouble to make food taste good, and take the time to tune in and enjoy your food. On the other hand, you won't do a good job with the *what* and *how much* of eating if you are casual about feeding yourself, grab food when you happen to think about it or when hunger drives you to it, absent-mindedly snack and nibble instead of taking time to feed yourself, or chronically restrict yourself.

The trick is being disciplined without becoming negative. There is positive discipline in feeding yourself well. It takes discipline to set up regular and predictable mealtimes, to plan the shopping list, to get the food in the house, to do the cooking and cleanup, to set aside the time to eat, to tune in when you are eating—the list goes on. On the other hand, the discipline becomes negative when you get caught up in the *shoulds* and *oughts*: what to eat, what to avoid, how much to eat. "If I made it, I should

eat it." "I mustn't let it go to waste." "It is good for me." "That is *way* too fattening." (Insert your guilt trip here.)

In part III, "How to Cook," you will learn ways to harness the chores to decrease time and preserve satisfaction. But even if you plan and cook in a hurry, do not *eat* in a hurry. Stow your rushing when you sit down at the table. Provide yourself with good-tasting food at predictable times with a mind-set and in an environment that takes care of your spirit as well as your body. In chapter 7, "Stuff to Know to Have Family Meals," and chapter 13, "Choosing Food," I address the details. This chapter is for encouragement. You can be deliberate and resourceful about feeding yourself—even when you consider nutrition—without getting caught by the food cops. Consider Clio's story.

Clio's Excellent Adventure

Clio had a rough upbringing with respect to food, one that left her with the attitude that wanting to be fed was an enormous imposition, the pattern of not regularly feeding herself, and the profound fear of going hungry. When Clio started working as my assistant in my home office, my regularly cooking myself lunch and spending time eating it both attracted and alarmed her. Since she generally arrived at work without food and with no plans for eating, I often invited her to join me for lunch. Clio was in a dilemma. The food was attractive.

On the other hand, she was afraid I would judge the way she ate. But hunger drove her to accept my invitations, and after many shared lunches, she began to relax and enjoy her food.

Clio was fascinated by the way I cooked and provided for myself—or *that* I did, perhaps. Some meals were delicious because I took the time and trouble to prepare them; others were just ho-hum, something I threw together to get the job done. Clio valued meals and tried to have them from time to time, but she had such high standards that getting a meal on the table was overwhelming.

She set out to change. Everything was hard. Remembering to feed herself was difficult. Feeling it was *okay* to feed herself was a long time in coming. Taking time for breakfast, bringing food to work, and saving time in her busy schedule to have dinner were all big changes for her, and it took her a long time to make those changes. Not only that, but as she made her eating important, she continually ran across upsetting feelings. She felt embarrassed about going to so much trouble for herself. She discovered painful memories of not being reliably fed as a child. She doubted her hunger and satiety. Sometimes we have to do things differently in order to know why we have kept them the same. Clio's failure to take care of herself with food had protected her from the hurt and anger she felt about being so neglected and from the lack of trust she had in herself.

It was hard for Clio to be realistic about feeding herself. Even though she had shared meals with me lots of times, she still had these elaborate ideas about what made up a meal. It had to be low-fat, it had to be something she cooked from scratch, it had to look attractive on the plate—it had to be a lot of work. Her standards directly contradicted her preferences. She had grown up eating fast food, convenience food, and snack food, and that is what she liked. She had to adjust her expectations to allow herself to put together enjoyable meals she could manage.

Depending on what else was going on in her life, for a while Clio would consistently feed herself, then for weeks she would be neglectful or do the eat-on-the-run thing. She married Paul, who considered himself an accomplished cook but who didn't value feeding himself regularly, and together they neglected themselves and each other with regard to food. But together they resolved to do better, and together they soldiered on, trying to find the happy medium between outright neglect and Ozzie-and-Harriet-style meals.

After years of effort, Clio has succeeded. She and Paul regularly have family meals, and those meals are generally good-tasting. They cook for themselves, eat out, and order in. They do gourmet cooking, homestyle cooking; made-from-scratch cooking; freezer-, can-, and package-based cooking; and reheating. Periodically, they make great vats of taco meat, vegetable-beef soup, red beans and sausage, or spaghetti sauce, freeze it, and actually remember to defrost it and eat it. Their enjoyment of food and their natural inclination to learn and grow has pulled them along to the point where they now eat a variety of nutritious foods and think in terms of including food groups when they plan meals.

Their son, Sebastian, is over a year old, and they do a great job with feeding him. He joins in with family meals, he insists on eating what they eat, and he takes great delight in finger-feeding himself. When Clio comes to work, she brings Sebastian and not just lunch for him and for herself, but also food for Sebastian's morning and afternoon snacks. Clio is giving Sebastian the security with food that she didn't get herself, and it is an unending labor of love. "Maintaining the division of responsibility in feeding is not for sissies," she regularly mutters, as she interrupts her schedule at least six times a day to see to it that Sebastian gets fed. (I talk about the division of responsibility in chapter 6, "The Feeding Relationship.")

Why Structure?

As I said in the two previous chapters, maintaining structure allows eating competence to fall into place.

> Structure + food acceptance skills =
> variety and therefore positive nutritional status
>
> Structure + food regulation capabilities =
> energy balance and therefore constitutionally
> appropriate body weight

People with high eating competence do a good job of managing structure and therefore taking good care of themselves with food. They manage their money to allow themselves to be fed, they take time to cook and to eat, and they plan for meals and for shopping. People with

high eating competence experience little of the misery that can surround eating. They are relatively satisfied with their bodies, their drive for thinness and their body dissatisfaction are low, and they experience little inclination to restrict food intake and to disinhibit.[1]

People who eat meals do better nutritionally. Respondents to the National Health and Nutrition Examination Survey (NHANES) who report having three meals per day plus one or two snacks show superior dietary quality compared with breakfast- or lunch-skippers.[2] For adults, a pattern of regular meals and snacks appears to be more metabolically desirable than today's increasingly common grazing pattern. Subjects who follow a regular meal pattern of six eating occasions per day compared with a random pattern of three to nine eating occasions show superior patterns of blood lipids and glucose metabolism.[3] Pregnant women who eat three meals and one or more snacks per day show a lower frequency of preterm births compared with women who miss meals and/or snacks.[4] For more about meals, see appendix B, "What the Research Says about Meals."

Work Up to Structure

When you think of meal planning, think *strategy*, not *rules*. Your eventual goal is to develop the meal habit: to come to depend on the structure of meals and snacks to do your eating and feeding. To develop that habit, you must get to the point where you can plan and provide meals and snacks that you and your eaters enjoy—at least well enough—and that support doing a good job with eating. As Clio did on her excellent adventure, first get the structure in place, then gradually incorporate principles of food management to improve the staying power and nutritional adequacy of your meals.

Keep in mind that structure is your servant, not your master. There is considerable peace and comfort in knowing you are going to be fed. If you have a meal coming, and you know it is going to be something you enjoy, you can postpone eating until it is time. Whether you know it or not, if you wait until hunger drives you to figure out what to eat, you'll scare yourself. You will grab something that is not too tasty and also not so satisfying. You are also likely to seek out high-calorie food. It is natural to seek out high-calorie food when you are hungry and desperate to eat. Think about it. When you miss a meal or two and are absolutely

starved, what do you crave? Some light food without many calories, or something more substantial? I rest my case.

Next to our need for air and water, getting fed is our most primitive and urgent creature need. Providing for that need in a trustworthy fashion frees you, gives you pleasure, and keeps eating in perspective. Failing to acknowledge and address your need to be fed makes it control you. When you have a meal and let yourself leave the table feeling satisfied, you know you've been fed. You can forget about eating for a while. When you eat on the run or graze or munch, eating is always an issue. There is no beginning, no ending. Without meals, you will find yourself thinking about food a lot of the time and rummaging to get your food needs met.

Don't avoid planning as a way of getting around your conscience! My chronic-dieter patients have many ways of deliberately booby-trapping their attempts at food restriction. They purchase ice cream, cookies, and potato chips with no intention of eating them, or they keep candy around—for company that never comes—or get themselves into such a starved state that they just can't resist super-sizing when the family goes out for a fast-food meal. Their behavior is perfectly understandable because they expect themselves to go hungry, and to do so indefinitely. If we are unrealistic about our eating, we find ways to cheat.

START WITH WHAT YOU *ARE* EATING
I tell my audiences, "The most reprehensible meal is better than no meal at all." I doubt if your meals can regularly be described as *reprehensible*, but the fact remains. Even if you do manage to put together a truly reprehensible meal, you will reap the benefits of structure, sociability, and security. Meals are *so* much work that for you to keep up the solid routine of planning, shopping, preparing, providing, and eating, you simply *must* find them rewarding.

Start out with what you and your family *currently* eat, and cluster those foods into meals and snacks. Do you cook up a box of macaroni and cheese or Tuna Helper to feed the children? Make enough for everyone, put out a plate of bread and butter and a carton of milk, and sit down together and all share the same food. Eaters can generally manage bread and butter if all else fails. If drinking milk turns your meal into a chore or a bore, drink what you drink. Do you order out for pizza and leave it on the kitchen

counter for everyone to help themselves? Arrange to have it delivered at mealtime, then sit down together to eat it. Do you nuke a couple of hot dogs and plate them up on buns with chips for you and your child—or have your child nuke a hot dog for himself—then retreat to your respective corners and your respective activities to eat? Instead, nuke two or three hot dogs for each of you and put the hot dogs, buns, fixings, and bag of chips on the table. If you wish to be truly elegant, put the chips in a bowl (make sure to have plenty), and enjoy the meal together.

PROTEIN, FAT, AND CARBOHYDRATE

Because they include the three major calorie-contributing nutrients—protein, fat, and carbohydrate—all the meals I just discussed will be satisfying to eat and keep you from being hungry for a while. These major nutrients are called *macronutrients* to distinguish them from the vitamin and mineral *micronutrients* that you need in much smaller quantities. Food combinations people often eat and call a meal lack one or more macronutrients. Consider muffins and coffee: Muffins have fat and carbohydrate but not much protein. A glass of milk or café au lait would make it a meal. Consider Mountain Dew and Oreo cookies: Cookies and soda have carbohydrate for sure, and five or six Oreos have the same amount of fat as 2 teaspoons of butter. But the meal is low in protein. Milk and Oreos would give you all three, but would skipping your Mountain Dew turn you into a food martyr and leave you with Mountain Dew cravings? Only you can say. If it is the sweet taste you crave, why not have some chocolate or strawberry milk? Appendix G, "Select Foods That Help Regulation," shows you which foods have protein, fat, and carbohydrate and explains how food composition affects satiety.

EXPAND SLOWLY

The idea is to develop the meal habit by getting the structure of meals made up of familiar food well in place. After you get used to the idea of structure, you can consider gradually expanding your menu. That will be later—*months* later—*many* months later. You will know you are ready to expand your menu when you are paying enough attention to eating to notice that you are getting tired of mac 'n' cheese, Tuna Helper, and hot dogs. You will begin to experiment—maybe open a can of peaches or dig out the dill pickles. Maybe slice up a cucumber or put out a few carrot sticks and get out the ranch

dressing to dip them in. If you have children, expanding your menus will require you to consider not only your own food preferences, but also those of other family members. To expand your menu, you must reassure yourself and anyone who eats with you that meals will still be enjoyable, will include preferred and familiar foods along with the not-so-liked and unfamiliar foods, and will *not* carry the expectation that anybody has to eat or even taste anything they don't want to. Even though food may seem good when you plan and cook it, sometimes it doesn't taste good when you eat it. Remember: You don't have to eat it if you don't want to!

ORGANIZE CAUTIOUSLY

Before long, you will be ready to apply the meal-planning guidelines that I outline in figure 5.1.

FIGURE 5.1 BEING CONSIDERATE WITHOUT CATERING

These simple strategies will help you be successful with family meals. Offer yourself and other family members a variety of food, then letting everyone—including yourself—eat what tastes good to them.

- Choose something from each of the basic food groups: Protein, cereals and grains, fruits and vegetables, dairy.
- Include protein, fat, and carbohydrate.
- Always include bread or whatever you use for bread—tortillas, pitas, chapattis. In some cultures, rice is used as routinely as bread. Most people can eat bread if all else fails.
- Pair familiar food with unfamiliar, favorite with not-so-favorite.
- Include fat in food preparation and at the table.
- Let everyone pick and choose from what is on the table.

Now you have a list, but do not get carried away! You are working toward including the components of the list, not trying to change overnight. Keep in mind: The bottom line is building the reliable and satisfying structure of meals. Don't try to do too much, too fast, and don't let your inner food cop get you, or you will spoil the whole enterprise. Here are some suggestions for gradually expanding your menus:
- Have foods you like.
- Add on rather than take away.
- Make only one change at a time.
- Always remember that for meals to be sustainable, they have to be satisfying.

Decide When You Will Eat—And Not Eat

Have meals at regular times, plan snacks so you can get comfortably through to mealtime without being famished, and then forget about eating between times. If you know you will be fed, and fed *well*, you won't want to spoil your appetite by grazing on little tidbits here and there. The tidbits are okay, but the lack of attention is not. When you graze, you miss out on good eating because it is hard to tune in and enjoy your food. Oh yes—and don't force yourself to graze to get the tidbits you want. Include them at meals.

Grazing is rapidly becoming our preferred way of eating. Foods are marketed as commuter foods—the kind you can eat with one hand while you drive. We keep foods on the counter, on the desk, in the break room—even in little dishes on the floor for toddlers to grab as they run by.

You may be reluctant to give up your grazing. Grazing is so deeply embedded in our current way of eating that in some circles, it is even seen as being superior. It's not. Grazing works for a few people, but not for most. Check yourself. Do you get a variety of food when you graze, or only the easy-to-grab, easy-to-like, high-fat, high-sugar foods? Does keeping food around so you can eat it at a moment's notice help it keep its place? Or does food sitting out constantly beg you to eat it—whether you want to or not?

Some people can eat every-which-way and still do a good job of regulating their food intake and getting the nutrients they need. They eat on the run, eat whatever is available, or go all day without eating and make up for it in the evening. If you are one of those people, structure may not be as important for you. If you graze and still eat well, you have my blessing. But not if you are raising children. Children who graze don't learn to enjoy a variety of food, but only eat their favorite foods over and over. Children who graze are likely to have trouble eating the right amount to grow well. Some eat too little and grow poorly; some eat too much and get too fat. A few are such good regulators that they eat the right amount and grow predictably. Of course, you won't know which pattern characterizes your child until it starts causing trouble, so it is best to avoid the pattern—and the problem—in the first place.

For all kinds of reasons, children need structured meals and sit-down snacks.

Feed Yourself Singly

More and more of us are choosing to live alone. If you live alone, you may do poorly with feeding yourself. You may feel it is somehow not worth it or not legitimate to go to any trouble to feed yourself. You may be embarrassed to eat out alone, feeling somehow stigmatized by your single state.

Well, isn't that just silly? If *you* won't go to any trouble for you, who will? Even if you have a life partner, nobody else can do it better. Growing up is where you learn to take responsibility for yourself. As I said in chapter 1, "The Secret in a Nutshell," you are a family when you take care of yourself. Treat yourself like your own family—you are. Moreover, if you feel comfortable, entitled, and tuned in with your eating, you will bring it off when you eat out alone. You won't feel—or come across—as if you have been ignored at the dance.

When you eat alone, being orderly and tuned in about feeding yourself can be challenging. Since the act of eating goes back to our earliest history, tuning in on eating comes loaded with memories from those earliest times. At first, eating mindfully can be painfully sharp with regard to the feelings it evokes. After a while, those memories and feelings mellow out, and being with yourself at mealtime becomes more tranquil. If you meditate, you know what I mean. Mealtime alone offers a regular opportunity to calm yourself and enter into a state of contemplation.

If you are a single parent, you will get into trouble if you fail to make feeding yourself a priority. You will prepare meals especially for your child. The next thing you know, you will be limiting menus to foods he readily accepts, boring yourself to tears and getting aggravated with him when he doesn't eat the meals you have so carefully, on his behalf, purged of interesting and potentially challenging food.

Don't forget that your child is growing up to join your table and to learn to like the food you eat. It is what children do. Plan meals based on food you like, incorporating the principles from figure 5.1 on the previous page. Cook your child's favorite food from time to time—sometimes he gets lucky, sometimes someone else does. And trust him to cope. He will.

Relax and Tune In

Whether you eat alone or with others, before you start to eat, settle down and reconnect with yourself. Saying grace works for some people. Tuning in on your breathing for a few seconds can be helpful. The idea is to disconnect from the rush of the day and the rush of getting the meal on the table, to reconnect with yourself, and to get into a relaxed and tuned-in state of mind.

You don't have time to relax, slow down, and tune in? Well, think about it! It will take you 10 or 15 minutes longer to relax and tune in to your meal than it will to rush through it. Isn't it a few minutes well spent? Consider your priorities. Is your priority to spend time with yourself and your family? For children, time spent at mealtime has more social, emotional, and nutritional value than any other activity. That's because your child benefits from time with you where he can have your undivided attention. Your making that regular time together a priority tells him louder than words can speak that he is important to you. For more, see appendix B, "What the Research Says about Meals."

Is it a priority for you to take care of your health and welfare and that of your child? With respect to the enjoyment you get from eating and the support you give to your internal regulation, digestive processes, and nutritional welfare, time spent at meals is time well spent. You consider eating to be important or you wouldn't be reading this book. Why not take time for it?

Developing the positive and self-accepting eating attitudes and behaviors that characterize eating competence is only the beginning.

With eating, as with the rest of life's endeavors, your inborn tendency is to master and gain comfort on the one hand and to learn and grow on the other. The eating competence model supports you both in seeking comfort and in exploring. You will eat in ways you find comfortable and rewarding at the same time as you increase the practicality and diversity of your eating. You will become more consistent about eating as much as you need and you will eat a wider variety of food as you feel more positive about your eating and are more reliable about seeing to it that you get fed. Working *with* rather than *against* yourself lets it all unfold.

References

1. Lohse B, Satter E, Horacek T, Gebreselassie T, Oakland MJ. Measuring Eating Competence: psychometric properties and validity of the ecSatter Inventory. *J Nutr Educ Behav .* 2007;39 (suppl):S154-S166.
2. Kerver JM, Yang EJ, Obayashi S, Bianchi L, Song WO. Meal and snack patterns are associated with dietary intake of energy and nutrients in US adults. *J Am Diet Assoc.* 2006;106:46-53.
3. Farshchi HR, Taylor MA, Macdonald IA. Beneficial metabolic effects of regular meal frequency on dietary thermogenesis, insulin sensitivity, and fasting lipid profiles in healthy obese women. *Am J Clin Nutr.* 2005;81:16-24.
4. Siega-Riz AM, Herrmann T, Savitz DA, Thorp J. The frequency of eating during pregnancy and its effect on preterm delivery. *Am J Epidemiol.* 2001;153:647-652.

Part

I

Epilogue

There you have it: four chapters outlining the four parts of eating competence:

- **Adjust your attitude.** Cultivate a positive and self-trusting attitude about eating.
- **Honor your appetite.** Eat the foods you like and develop your food acceptance abilities.
- **Eat as much as you want.** Trust yourself to know how much to eat and to weigh what nature intended for you to weigh.
- **Feed yourself faithfully.** Be reliable about providing yourself with regular and rewarding meals and sit-down snacks.

As I emphasized in chapter 1, "The Secret in a Nutshell," and reinforced in one way or another in chapters 2 through 5, the common themes with respect to competence in all four parts are *permission* and *discipline*: the permission to choose food you enjoy and eat it in amounts you find satisfying, and the discipline to provide yourself with regular and reliable meals and snacks and to pay attention when you eat them.

Are you waiting for the other shoe to drop? It won't. That's all there is to it. I think it's enough. In fact, it wouldn't be surprising if you were feeling a bit overwhelmed right now. Overhauling eating attitudes and behaviors is major. Eating is complex, and patterns of thinking, feeling, and behaving relative to eating are deeply embedded.

But it may not be as difficult as you fear. Eating competence works *with* your body rather than *against* it. It taps into your inborn capabilities and supports you in rediscovering

what is natural. Clinically, I am continually astonished at how working toward natural allows even the most negative, conflicted, out-of-control eater to rapidly bring order and pleasure into eating.

Your new attitudes and behaviors will grow to feel so comfortable that, until you stop to think about it, you may not realize that anything has changed. Here's a little self-test to help you be aware of what you have achieved. Check yourself:

❑ Do you have mealtime structure well in place?

❑ Do you usually enjoy mealtime?

❑ Would you say you have developed the meal habit?

❑ Do you provide yourself with food you enjoy?

❑ Do you regularly make use of the skeleton of meal-planning principles that I outline in figure 5.1, "Being Considerate without Catering," on page 48?

❑ Do you generally tune in and enjoy your food? Review figure 3.1, "Becoming a Kitchen Table Gourmet," on page 19.

❑ Have you recovered your internal regulators of food intake, including finding your stopping place with eating? Review figure 4.2, "Food Regulation Cues," on page 32 and figure 4.3, "Steps to Internal Regulation," on page 33.

❑ Do you depend on your internal regulators of food intake to guide you in how much to eat?

❑ Can you put unfamiliar, challenging, and "nutritious" food on the table without strong-arming yourself or anyone else to eat it?

❑ Are you generally relaxed about eating?

❑ Do you feel comfortable about enjoying food?

This is a progress report, not a pass-fail test. While the eventual goal is to check all the boxes, eating competence is a matter of degrees. That's why some of the statements say "regularly," "usually," or "generally." Your competence with eating will increase with time and life experience. Working your way through the other two main parts of *Secrets of Feeding a Healthy Family* will further increase your eating competence. Part II, "How to Raise Good Eaters," will help you raise your child to be a competent eater, and your child will demonstrate to you what competent eating is all about. Part III, "How to Cook," will support you in developing the meal habit and reassure you in concrete detail that it is all right to enjoy eating.

How Much to Eat

I don't tell you how much to eat. Telling you how much to eat would make you go by the numbers rather than going by what your body tells you. As I said in chapter 4, "Eat as Much as You Want," your body has a way of managing *how much* that is far more sophisticated than any food plan or calorie prescription. Instead, I encourage you to develop your eating capabilities in the two main areas related to *how much to eat*: structure and internal regulation. Establish the reliable structure of meals and snacks with foods you enjoy, give yourself permission to eat as much as you want, and work toward being tuned in when you eat those meals. That's important, so let's set it off:

Determining How Much to Eat
• Provide regular, reliable, and rewarding meals.
• Depend on your capabilities with internal regulation.

As I pointed out in chapter 4, you learn internally regulated eating with your *body*, not with your *head*, and going through the motions

lets your body learn. But you have to *do* the behaviors, not just *try* them. As Yoda says, there is doing or not-doing. There is no trying. (I didn't put that in quotes because Yoda needed a good editor. What he actually said went on for a full paragraph.) *Trying* means you don't expect it to work.

In my clinical work, I find that rediscovering internal regulation takes about 10 to 12 weeks. That's not long when you consider the kinds of messes my patients had gotten themselves into with their eating. Since you are working on your own, I assume it will take you somewhat longer.

Once you discover internal regulation, it will keep working for you if you continue to go through the motions: having structured, reliable, and rewarding meals and tuning in when you eat them. At times you might relapse and go back to your old ways. We all are likely to relapse when we are busy or under a lot of stress, but you can relapse and then recover your orderly eating, if you want to. Now you know how it feels to take good care of yourself with food. You also know how it feels to eat chaotically or absent-mindedly. You get to decide which you want. If you decide you want to be competent with eating, you also know how to restore order.

It wouldn't be surprising if you found yourself tempted to try to lose weight. That certainly is up to you, but consider this: What will you have to sacrifice in order to achieve weight loss? Is it worth undermining your trust in your body and giving up your ease and enjoyment with eating? You may even have to try out dieting a few times to see if it works and to find out how it feels. After that, it is up to you how you manage your eating. Unless, of course, you have children.

What to Eat

By now, even you, my loyal reader, may be getting desperate for me to tell you what to eat. While I will give more detail about meal-planning in part III, "How to Cook," I *won't* tell you what to eat and *you* can't make me! Telling you what to eat will put you in your head rather than in your body and undermine your eating competence. Instead, I encourage you to develop your eating capabilities in the two main areas related to *what to eat*: providing meals and accepting food. That's important, so let's set it off:

> Determining What to Eat
> - Provide regular, reliable, and rewarding meals.
> - Depend on your capabilities with food acceptance.

As I explain in chapter 3, "Honor Your Appetite," from the perspective of the eating competence model, the key to nutritional excellence is variety growing out of genuine food enjoyment. Food acceptance attitudes and skills that support food enjoyment are more important for you than what you eat on any one day. Being able to be comfortable in the presence of unfamiliar food; to pick and choose from what's available; and to say yes, please, and no, thank you will free you to ever-so-gradually sneak up on new food and learn to like it.

Your capabilities with the food context include knowing the food that is in the world and putting together meals that include a variety of food. I assume that you know the basic food groups and that if you have meals, you will more or less automatically provide yourself with choices from the food groups. I don't mention the food groups when I start you off with organizing your grab-and-go food into meals in the section, "Work Up to Structure," pages 47 to 48, in chapter 5, "Feed Yourself Faithfully," because getting a structure in place is enough to think about. However, I have a hunch that if you impose structure on grab-and-go eating, it's likely that you will be providing yourself with most of those basic foods anyway.

You know the basic food groups. Otherwise, you wouldn't get that tired joke, "My basic food groups are grease, sugar, salt and ..." I forget the other one. Maybe I shouldn't tell that joke! If you plan meals, you will be less likely to choose grease, sugar, and salt, and more likely to choose some approximation of the real food groups: protein, cereals, fruits and vegetables, and dairy. Every person who went through grade school learned the food groups. Unless you skipped a *lot* of school, you did, too. If all went well, you also learned that meals are supposed to include choices from all the food groups. If all went even better, you developed

the expectation at your parents' table that a meal includes protein, a starch, a fruit or vegetable, and milk. I also nudge that expectation along. In figure 5.1, "Being Considerate without Catering," I encourage you to start thinking about the food groups when you plan menus. In part III, "How to Cook," I introduce you to the Mother Principle, which gives more detailed tips about planning family meals, and I demonstrate lots of meals that include choices from the basic food groups.

The bottom line is, while I help you learn what to put on the table, I do not tell you what to eat, how much to eat, how many servings to have from each of the food groups, and what portion sizes to eat. I don't tell you to restrict fat, salt, and sugar. Unfortunately, your nutrition education lessons in school probably taught you all that, and I would just as soon you forgot it. All those directives get in the way of your being competent with eating.

Nutrition Policy

I suspect that my nutrition and health-professional readers are still looking for the missing pieces, so allow me to say "that's all there is to it" in a somewhat different way. The Dietary Guidelines emphasize maintaining nutritional adequacy, energy balance, moderation, and proportionality. In conventional nutrition practice, MyPyramid becomes formulaic in telling how to manage food to put those principles into effect. It specifies what and how much to eat. In contrast, the eating competence model operationalizes the Dietary Guidelines by encouraging regular meals and then depending on each person's capabilities with food regulation and food acceptance to determine what and how much to eat. Going by externally determined criteria for what and how much to eat is the antithesis of eating competence. However, the eating competence model does not ignore nutrition policy. Figure EI.1 on the next page illustrates that while MyPyramid and the eating competence model, ecSatter, both work toward carrying out the principles outlined by the Dietary Guidelines, they do it in quite different ways.

The Dietary Guidelines and MyPyramid also emphasize restricting fat, salt, and sugar and striving for a BMI of 24.9 or less. The eating competence model sets all that aside. It

---

**FIGURE EI.1 OPERATIONALIZING THE DIETARY GUIDELINES:
HOW DO MYPYRAMID AND ecSATTER COMPARE?**
Operationalizing a set of principles means outlining a set of processes or techniques that put those principles into effect. MyPyramid defines what and how much to eat. ecSatter emphasizes structure combined with internal processes.

	MyPyramid	ecSatter
Nutritional adequacy	What to eat, portion sizes, how many portions	Family meals, pleasure, variety
Energy balance	Control: Formulas, portions, daily food plan	Trust: Internal regulators, paying attention
Moderation	Restriction, avoidance	Pleasure: Regular access to all foods in satisfying amounts
Proportionality	What to eat, portion sizes, daily food plan	Regular, reliable, rewarding meals consumed based on hunger, appetite, and satiety

---

demonstrates that it isn't necessary to get caught up in micromanaging and avoiding with food. Healthful nutritional habits can be defined in a much looser, more rewarding, and more accessible fashion. Following the principles of eating competence, your weight has a very good chance of naturally stabilizing at a level that is right for you, and you will automatically have a moderate intake of fat, salt, and sugar. Emphasizing avoidance undermines eating competence. Food without fat, salt, and sugar doesn't taste as good, and avoiding them complicates food management.

To satisfy myself that I am not being irresponsible in advising people to set aside the restrictiveness of nutrition policy, I carefully investigated the issues of eating attitudes, body weight, dietary fat, and salt as they relate to health. I reached the conclusion that the restrictiveness recommended by nutrition policy exacts a high cost in the form of conflict and anxiety about eating and delivers a modest and by no means assured benefit with respect to disease prevention. The bottom line, from my perspective, is that it is more important to be well nourished and to maintain stable body weight than it is to strive for weight loss or to avoid fat and salt. I discuss my investigations in appendix C, "What Surveys Say about our Eating," appendix D, "BMI, Mortality, Morbidity, and Health: Resolving the Weight Dilemma," appendix L, "Diet and Degenerative Disease:

It's Not as Bad as You Think," and appendix O, "Sodium in Your Diet." Other appendixes that discuss related issues include appendix N, "A Primer on Dietary Fat," and appendix M, "Children, Dietary Fat and Heart Disease: You don't' have to Panic.

If you have a medical condition such as congestive heart failure, kidney disease, or an inherited tendency toward seriously distorted blood lipids, you may need to modify your diet to address it. But that is a medical consideration, not a nutritional one.

Attitude

Consider the statements about attitude that I made at the beginning of chapter 2, "Adjust Your Attitude": Eating is okay. Eating *enough* is okay. *Enjoying* eating is okay. Eating what you *like* is okay. Taking *time* to eat is okay. Making eating a *priority* is okay. By now, I expect that your attitude is different than it was when you first read those statements. Part of your attitude adjustment will have come about because you examined your attitudes. Part will have grown out of your discovering your capabilities with eating: that you can give yourself permission to enjoy your food and eat enough without going out of control. You feel better about your eating because you are bringing your shoulds and wants together.

Part

II

HOW TO RAISE GOOD EATERS

Prologue

Children who are good eaters have positive attitudes about eating, they are able to learn to like and enjoy the food that is available to them, and they are able to intuitively eat as much food as they need to give them energy and to grow appropriately. However, all of these capabilities depend on their receiving appropriate support from their grown-ups. Children who are good eaters are competent eaters, with one critical and entirely appropriate exception: They do not take responsibility for managing the food context—the *what, when,* and *where* of meals and snacks. Until they leave home, they depend on their grown-ups to do that.

Whether or not your child becomes a good eater depends on your doing a good job with feeding. In this part, I teach you how to do that good job based on the Satter Feeding Dynamics Model, fdSatter, a set of practice- and evidence-based principles and recommendations.[1] Throughout *Secrets of Feeding a Healthy Family,* when I give you advice about feeding your child, talk about feeding dynamics, discuss the division of responsibility in feeding, or encourage you to let your child grow in a way that is right for him, I am basing my advice on the feeding dynamics model. When I say the feeding relationship is appropriate, I mean that parents are observing a division of responsibility in feeding as defined by the model.

The fundamental principle of the feeding dynamics model is that, provided you do a reasonably good job with feeding, your child will eat as much or as little as he needs and grow predictably in the way nature intended for him

to grow. As I tell you in chapter 6, "The Feeding Relationship," effective feeding is based on a division of responsibility.[2] For the infant, the parent does the *what* of feeding and depends on information coming from the infant to determine everything else: how often, how much, at what tempo, and at what level of skill. Beyond infancy, the parent becomes responsible for the *what, when,* and *where* of *feeding* and the child is responsible for the *how much* and *whether* of *eating.* Adolescents gradually learn to manage the *what, when,* and *where* for themselves, but they continue to depend on parents to take leadership with feeding and maintain the structure of family meals.

The division of responsibility outlines authoritative parenting, which is the gold standard of parenting. Chapter 7, "Stuff to Know to Have Family Meals," discusses the ins and outs of authoritative feeding. Authoritative parents both provide leadership and give autonomy. They provide leadership when they set limits and enforce rules, and they give autonomy by paying attention to the child's point of view and giving leeway and respect. Other approaches to parenting include authoritarian, permissive, and neglectful. The distinctions lie in the manner in which parents combine the elements of *leadership* and *autonomy.* Authoritative parents balance the two. Authoritarian parents take leadership but don't give autonomy. Permissive and neglectful parents give autonomy without taking leadership. With respect to feeding, authoritative parents essentially say, "Here's what we have. You may decide what and how much to eat." Authoritarian parents say, "Here's your food. Eat it." Permissive parents say, "What do you want? When do you want it?" Neglectful parents say, "Don't bother me. Get it yourself." Research done at Boston University shows that authoritative parenting correlates with the lowest incidence of overweight in first-grade children: only 3.9% of authoritative parents had overweight children compared to 9.8% of permissive parents, 9.9% of neglectful parents, and 17.1% of authoritarian parents.[3]

Raising a good eater takes years. Children learn bite by bite, food by food, meal by meal. The goal of raising a good eater is to help your child grow up with positive eating attitudes and behaviors; it is not to get him to eat his peas for tonight's supper. I will repeat that statement, because it is important:

> Your child's eating attitudes and behavior are more important than what he actually eats on any given day.
> If his attitudes and behaviors are positive, he will eat well and get the nutrition he needs.

Raising a competent eater will enhance your own competence with eating. Even if you are still struggling to "get it" with respect to your own eating attitudes and behaviors, if you go through the motions of positive feeding—keeping your lips zipped, your fingers crossed, and the look of disbelief off your face—your child will show you what competent eating is all about. Conversely, being competent with your eating will help you to raise a competent eater. Trusting yourself to eat joyfully, seek out good-tasting food, and eat as much as you want will allow you to trust your child to do the same.

References

1. Satter E; The Satter Feeding Dynamics Model of child overweight definition, prevention and intervention . O'Donahue W, Moore BA, Scott B, . *Pediatric and Adolescent Obesity Treatment: A Comprehensive Handbook.* New York: Taylor and Francis; 2007:287-314 .
2. Satter EM. The feeding relationship. *J Am Diet Assoc.* 1986;86:352-356.
3. Rhee KE, Lumeng JC, Appugliese DP, Kaciroti N, Bradley RH. Parenting styles and overweight status in first grade. *Pediatrics.* 2006;117:2047-2054.

Chapter
6
The Feeding Relationship

Children want to eat. They can't help it. They are in the business of growing up, and they watch the adults and older children around them to find out what it's all about. They see others eating, and they assume, on whatever level they are able to assume it, that one fine day they will do the same. Sometimes, however, it starts to look like children *don't* want to eat. They turn away from the spoon, refuse to try a new vegetable unless they are made to, pitch a fit when they are asked to come to the table, or behave so poorly that no one wants them there. What makes the difference? The *feeding relationship*. The way feeding is conducted can support your child's being competent with eating, growing appropriately, and doing her part to contribute to mealtime harmony—or it can do the opposite.

To have a positive feeding relationship, maintain a division of responsibility. You do the *what*, *when*, and *where* of feeding, and your child does the *how much* and *whether* of eating.[1] Figure 6.1 on the following page outlines the division of responsibility in more detail. Copy the page (or get it off my Web site, www.EllynSatter.com) and post it on your refrigerator door. Make extra copies to give to your Aunt Fannie and Uncle Arthur when they insist that your child clean her plate, or want to make special food for her, or comment that she apparently does not miss any meals because, after all, look at how—well—*stocky* she is.

Leadership and autonomy are the two basic themes of positive feeding dynamics. If you recall, discipline and permission are the two basic themes of eating competence. To remind you, the two are in direct parallel. The discipline is taking leadership; the permission is giving autonomy. The difference, of course, is that for your child, you provide the discipline. For yourself, you play both roles.

At every presentation I give—and I give a *lot* of presentations—a proud parent stands in line to thank me for showing the way to help her child be an excellent eater. This book review captures the story I hear again and again:

Last week we went out for Chinese food and my kids (ages 4 and 6) were begging for more broccoli and carrots. "How did you do it?" asked the people at the next table who were begging their two older kids to eat "at least a few more bites." Then last night we went out with friends to a "family" restaurant where they put the kids' cookies on the plate with their dinner. Our friends took their kids' cookies and wouldn't let them have them until they had eaten what the parents considered an appropriate amount. There was a lot of fighting. Our 4 year old ate her cookie first, then her chicken and left most of her fries. Our 6 year old ate her chicken and fries first and then ate her cookie. There was no fighting. How did we "do it"? Easy. Ellyn Satter's division of responsibility in feeding

---

FIGURE 6.1 ELLYN SATTER'S DIVISION OF RESPONSIBILITY IN FEEDING
Your child will do best with eating when you provide both leadership and autonomy: You do your job of feeding and let your child do her job of eating. You provide *structure*, support, and *opportunities to learn*. You let her choose *how much* and *whether* to eat from the foods you put on the table.

The Division of Responsibility for Infants
- You are responsible for *what*.
- Your child is responsible for *how much (and everything else)*.

You help your infant be calm and awake and feed smoothly, paying attention to information coming from her about timing, tempo, frequency, and amounts.

The Division of Responsibility for Toddlers through Adolescents
- You are responsible for the *what, when*, and *where* of *feeding*.
- Your child is responsible for the *how much* and *whether* of *eating*.

Your Feeding Jobs
- Choose and prepare the food.
- Provide regular meals and snacks.
- Make eating times pleasant.
- Show your child what she has to learn about food and mealtime behavior.
- Do not let your child graze for food or beverages (except water) between meal and snack times.
- Let your child grow up to have the body that is right for her.

Fundamental to your jobs is trusting your child to decide *whether* and *how much* to eat of what you provide for her. If you do your jobs with *feeding*, your child will do her jobs with *eating*.

Your Child's Eating Jobs
- Your child will eat.
- She will eat the amount she needs.
- She will learn to eat the food you eat.
- She will eat a variety.
- She will grow predictably.
- She will learn to behave well at the table.

Your child will do best with eating when you provide both leadership and autonomy: You do your job of feeding and let your child do her job of eating.

The stories give me fond memories of one of my own family dinners, at Ginza of Tokyo. My three then-young children—probably ages 5 through 10—were fascinated by the fancy knife- and grill-work and couldn't wait to dive into their bean sprouts. As we were leaving, the older couple who had shared our cubicle commented, "Your children are such good eaters!" I was startled. I had done my jobs with feeding and trusted my children to do theirs. I had taken for granted their ready acceptance of new food and new eating experiences. It was as it should be.

Two Children Who Weren't Trusted

I no longer take children's good eating for granted. When parents do a good job with feeding, children's eating capability seems natural. When parents are confused about what that good job with feeding entails, feeding becomes difficult and even excruciating.

JEREMY WOULDN'T EAT
The fights about Jeremy's eating started before the meals began. "Come to the table," Jeremy's father insisted. "You have to eat. We can't play

catch unless you eat." "Aargh, I don't want to," whined 6-year-old Jeremy. "Feed me! I want you to feed me!" "I'm not going to feed you," insisted Father angrily. "You are a big boy! You have to feed yourself!" But eventually Father gave in and fed Jeremy because he was afraid that if he didn't, Jeremy wouldn't eat. Every bite of every meal, day after weary day, was a struggle. Jeremy's parents dreaded meals and hated the fight, but they were afraid to stop. If Jeremy ate this poorly when they put all this pressure on him, how would he eat if they stopped? The only time Jeremy ate on his own was when he got candy between meals.

The instant Jeremy's parents described their mealtime struggles, I was 99 percent positive that feeding was the problem. But they were so convinced that *Jeremy* was the problem—that he was missing the part that prompted him to eat—that I evaluated Jeremy. I reviewed his medical record from birth to see if he had a health condition that interfered with his eating, I checked his ability to chew and swallow, I watched videotapes of how he behaved at family meals, and I talked with both Jeremy and his parents.

According to the medical records, Jeremy's parents first complained about his poor eating when he was 3 months old and wouldn't eat solid foods. His parents acknowledged that he resisted eating from the spoon and they got pushy with feeding him. From then on, Jeremy's parents saw him as being an unwilling eater. As I suspected, it was the *feeding* that was the problem, not Jeremy's unwillingness to eat. Children only readily accept solid foods when they are developmentally ready—usually around age 4 months at the earliest, 6 months for most children, and even later for some. In fact, some children accept solid foods only when they are capable of finger-feeding themselves at around 8 to 12 months.

The feeding struggles had continued ever since. To their credit, the parents were doing a wonderful job with having family meals. But they were spoiling those meals by playing both sides of the net: They were doing not only their jobs with feeding, but also Jeremy's jobs with eating.

"Jeremy wants to eat," I told them, "but he wants more to be his own person. He will eat better if you do your jobs with feeding and let him do his with eating." My prescription was the division of responsibility in feeding. "At first he will eat less," I warned them. "But he will eat more when he comes to trust that you won't force him to eat."

Along with continuing to have regular meals and offering Jeremy sit-down snacks at predictable times between meals (sometimes the snacks included candy, sometimes not), Jeremy's parents were to make and enforce rules for Jeremy's mealtime behavior. Jeremy was to sit nicely (as nicely as any other squirmy six-year-old), to not whine or beg, and to politely say "yes, please" or "no, thank you" to food. They also made rules for themselves: They were to take *no* for an answer and they were to let him know—in words and behavior—that it was up to him to decide how much or how little to eat of what they put before him. And they weren't to let him panhandle for food or drink handouts between meal and snack times.

Over the next few weeks, Jeremy grew up before his parents' eyes. He stopped whining, took an interest in what was on the table, and ever-so-gradually began to experiment with new food. Jeremy ate enough to do well, but more importantly, he was pleasant to have at the table. He made conversation, listened to his parents when they talked, and asked nicely to be excused when he finished eating.

VICKY WANTED TO EAT TOO MUCH

Vicky's mother intruded on her 8-year-old daughter's prerogatives with eating, but in the opposite direction. Like Jeremy's parents, Vicky's mother cooked good meals, but she worked too hard. She doled food out carefully and refused to let Vicky have more when she asked for it. "Is that all there is?" Vicky whined as her mother set her plate in front of her. "Isn't there any more?" "That's all there is," answered her mother through gritted teeth. "I gave you lots. That should be enough."

"Every time she starts in on that, I just cringe," confessed Vicky's mother. "It seems like no matter how much I give her, she still wants more. Every time she runs out of something to do, she wants food. I am afraid if I let her eat as much as she wants, she will eat so much she will get even fatter than she is already."

Once again, I suspected that *feeding* was the problem. But since Vicky's mom was convinced that Vicky was missing the part that made her stop eating, I was careful to test her assumption. I did the same careful evaluation with Vicky as I had done with Jeremy. Vicky's problem, too, had a history. Vicky had been born a chubby infant, and from the first her mother restricted her food. Vicky begged constantly to eat, not because she lacked a stopping place, but because she was *hungry*.

Even though Jeremy seemingly ate too little and Vicky seemingly ate too much, my conclusions for both children were the same. The problem was a distortion in the feeding relationship, and the solution was to restore a division of responsibility in feeding. Vicky's mother was to put the food in serving dishes on the table and reassure Vicky she could have as much or as little as she wanted to eat. Between meals, instead of bracing herself, waiting for Vicky to beg for snacks, Mother was to take the initiative by keeping track of the time and putting the food on the table at snack time.

At meals, Vicky reassured herself that she would get enough to eat by reminding her mother to use the serving dishes. It wasn't long, however, before she stopped being so preoccupied with food. At first she ate a lot, but after a few weeks she stopped eating so much and began eating like any other 8-year-old: sometimes a lot, sometimes not much. She only became preoccupied with food when her mother got busy with other things and became casual about feeding her. Vicky's mother said that being so reliable about offering regular meals and snacks was a lot of work, but the rewards made it worthwhile. It was such a relief not to have struggles with Vicky about food. She found herself liking Vicky more—and enjoying mealtimes *lots* more. Her feeding struggles with Vicky had been wrecking their relationship.

Children Develop Eating Competence

In chapter 1, "The Secret in a Nutshell," I tell you that the secret of feeding a healthy family is to love good food, trust yourself, and share that love and trust with your child. In chapters 2 through 5 we focused on supporting your self-trust and self-confidence with eating in four areas:

• Positive eating attitudes
• Eating the food you like and gradually experimenting with unfamiliar food
• Eating as much as you need
• Managing the food context

When you feed in positive ways, your child will gradually develop those same eating capabilities as she grows up. Some of your child's capabilities are inborn; your job is to preserve them. Your child was born with positive feelings about eating, the drive to eat, the innate knowledge of how much she needs to eat, and the ability to grow in the way nature intended for her.

Some of your child's eating capabilities will be learned; your job is to model and teach them. Your child will take full responsibility for managing the food context only after she leaves home, but in the meantime she will develop the meal habit and positive mealtime behaviors. Given your positive example and parenting, your child will conform to the family meal and snack patterns and behave acceptably at the table, feel good about eating, and be relaxed and composed about trying new food and learning to like it. With respect to food context, the goal to work toward is having your child master, by the time she leaves home, the skills she needs to do basic planning and shopping, to keep food safe, to prepare a few simple meals, and to put together a reasonably balanced diet from home-prepared, pre-prepared, and restaurant food.

THE DIVISION OF RESPONSIBILITY FOR INFANTS

While Vicky's parents were loving, their feeding tactics were anything but loving. They ignored how Vicky felt and what she wanted. During your child's first 6 months, when she can only suckle and cuddle, the division of responsibility is simple: You get to decide whether to breastfeed or bottle-feed, and you get to pick out what goes into the bottle. Your child gets to decide everything else: how often, how much, how fast, and at what skill level she eats. Feed on demand during the first few months. Pay attention to information coming from your baby to guide her eating, sleeping, and comforting. Follow her lead and do what is necessary to make her comfortable and happy. That is easier for some infants than others. Some infants are regular and intelligible; others are irregular and unclear. Your consistently calming your baby and trying to figure out what she wants eventually helps even the irregular, unclear baby become regular and intelligible. During her first 6 months to a year, your child is the princess of the family. Your doing what she wants makes her feel loved. Don't worry about spoiling: You can't spoil a little baby.

THE TRANSITION TO THE TABLE

Consider your destination. By the time your child is 8 to 18 months old, she will be sitting at the family table, joining in with family meals, and finger-feeding herself soft, cooked table food. To get there, go by what your child can *do*, not by how old she is. Start semisolid food when she can sit up, willingly open her mouth when she sees something coming, get food from a spoon, and swallow it. Gradually increase the thickness and lumpiness of her food to teach her to chew. Start finger food when she can pick up soft pieces of food and put them in her mouth. With each transition in lumpiness, she will do a certain amount of gagging as she learns to move the food around in her mouth and position it between her jaws rather than sending it right down her throat the way she did semisolid food. Keep your nerve—if she can breathe, she is gagging, not choking. In a pinch, she may throw up to get the food out of her throat. Don't panic about that, either. It won't bother her if it doesn't bother you. Let her use utensils when she indicates an interest.

The Older Baby

To feed solid food, sit your child up straight and facing directly forward. Hold the spoon directly in front of her mouth and wait for her to open up before you feed her. She may get the idea of spoon-feeding right off the bat and readily accept unfamiliar flavors and textures, or she may be cautious and need 5 or 10 tries—or even more—with each new experience. Offer the food, and stop right away when she shows she is done—don't play games or persuade. She will do best with eating when you make it clear to her that she doesn't have to eat if she doesn't want to. She will be relaxed and comfortable about experimenting with new foods and learning to eat them. She will be relaxed and comfortable about exploring new flavors and textures when you go by her tempo and take *no* for an answer.

Your four-to-seven month-old starting on solid foods may or may not enjoy letting you spoon-feed her. It's awkward if she doesn't, but doable. Keep offering the spoon at the same time as you thicken up the food with baby cereal, give her piles of it, and let her smear it into her mouth. A friend's determinedly independent 6-month-old granddaughter fed herself semisolid food by putting her mouth down on the highchair tray and sweeping it into her mouth with her hand and arm! Every child is different, so relax and enjoy your own baby's way of learning to eat. Keep offering, don't get pushy, and prepare to be surprised.

The Almost-Toddler

The eight-to-twelve-month-old child, a fascinating and rapidly changing sprite I call the *almost-toddler*, is so taken with being able to feed herself that she eats almost anything. An older baby who is happily eating semisolids from the spoon becomes an almost-toddler when she abruptly refuses to eat unless or until you let her feed herself. Parents generally interpret this uppity behavior as food rejection, but it is really a bid for autonomy. Your almost-toddler wants to do it *herself*, she wants to eat what you eat, and she will refuse to eat unless you let her. She knows *absolutely* that she no longer wants to be fed with a spoon like a baby because she is a little *girl*, not a *baby—so there*! She will do well with three meals a day and snacks between mealtimes that allow her to eat every 2 or 3 hours. Those snacks can be nipple feedings or "big girl" snacks at the table. She will do better nutritionally if you give her table food than if

you give her commercial baby or toddler food.[2] As was the case earlier, your going by information coming from your child to guide feeding makes her feel loved; now, it also lets her feel respected as an individual. Your child will experiment with new food if you give her autonomy; she will not if you don't.

The Toddler Proper

The almost-toddler's eating honeymoon ends at around age 15–18 months when she turns into a toddler proper. At that point, her food intake drops off as she grows more slowly than before, develops mentally enough to become skeptical of new food, and tests limits by refusing to eat meals and then begging for food handouts between meal- and snack-times. You will dig holes for yourself in feeding your toddler—with her enthusiastic assistance—by limiting menus to foods she readily accepts, by playing games to get her to eat, and by leaving out little food dishes for her to graze on when she cruises by. None of it works because it isn't developmentally appropriate. With feeding as in other ways, it is time for the toddler to learn to be part of the family.

Include your toddler in family meals and sit-down snacks at predictable times, let her determine what and how much to eat from what you provide, and don't short-order cook for her or let her panhandle for food or beverages between times—except for water. Don't ask her what she wants to eat—she doesn't know and she isn't mature enough to even think about it. In fact, she is far too busy to know she is even hungry until she collapses, so waiting to feed her until she asks is a big mistake. Plan menus to be considerate of your toddler's limitations with chewing, swallowing, and food acceptance, but don't cater to her likes and dislikes. Time snacks so she can come to meals hungry but not famished and ready to explore the food there.

THE PRESCHOOLER AND SCHOOL-AGE CHILD

The school-age child and even the preschooler is easier than the toddler to have around because she is cooperative and remembers what you tell her to do. Therein lie the pitfalls. Because she admires you and wants to please you, it is possible to shame, motivate, cheerlead, or coerce her into eating what and how much you want her to eat rather than what and how much *she* wants to. Don't do it. It will make her feel bad, both about herself and about eating, undermine her ability to eat the amount she needs to grow appropriately, and spoil her food acceptance and food regulation skills. The preschool or young school-age child pushes herself along to learn and grow, but she learns through her *experience*, not with her *head*. Encouraging the young child to drink her orange juice because it contains vitamin C will not impress her or change her juice-drinking behavior. For more about feeding-dynamics consistent approaches to teaching children about food and nutrition, see appendix H, "Nutrition Education in the Schools."

Because she seems independent and even acts like she doesn't need you anymore, it is all too easy to get casual about parenting the preschool and school-age child. Don't be fooled. She continues to need the structure and support of family meals and structured snacks. With meals as with every other part of life, you are as important as ever and she needs you as much as ever, just in a different way. She needs you to be there, to care about her and to look out for her, to give backup and support, and to show her what and how to learn.

The school-age child works to master her world, including her food world. Provided you give her opportunities to learn and you don't get pushy, she will apply herself to learning to like new food, to learning table manners, and even to doing simple tasks of food preparation. The 12- to 13-year-old begins to think abstractly, which means she can learn basic food-selection principles and apply those principles to deciding what to eat. That allows her to start, ever so gradually, mastering your *what, when,* and *where*

jobs with feeding. Start by letting her manage the timing for her after-school snack ("eat it right after school so you don't spoil your dinner") and pick her snack from choices you make available. If she does well, let her have the privilege of picking out her snack from what you have in the kitchen or with her own money in the quick-stop grocery store. Figure 6.2 gives a guide for your child to use for snack-planning. The same principles can help her plan simple meals. This figure also offers a good basis for a nutrition lesson at the grade school level.

To make yourself an expert so you can advise your child on snack selection, consult chapter 13, "Choosing Food," and appendix G, "Select Foods That Help Regulation."

A young girl I saw buying Snapple and Ho Hos for her snack could have used this list. It was all I could do not to say to her, "Dear, if you would drink milk instead of Snapple or substitute cheese crackers for the Ho Hos you would have a snack with protein, fat, and carbohydrate." Snapple is on the carbohydrate list and cheese crackers are on the first two lists, the same as peanut butter crackers. Since I set out to simplify this list for children rather than complicate, I included muffins and fried snacks on the carbohydrate list, although they are high in fat. Vegetables and vegetable juice are on the carbohydrate list, even though they don't have much. But a relatively high-fat snack of muffins and milk or a low-carbohydrate snack of cheese and tomato juice or celery and peanut butter is likely to be satisfying. Encourage your child to pay attention to which snacks fill her up and keep her going until dinnertime.

FIGURE 6.2 PLANNING A GOOD-TASTING AND SATISFYING SNACK
To taste good and to keep you satisfied until dinner time, a snack needs two or three foods and needs to include protein, fat, and carbohydrate. The first list has protein and fat, the second has carbohydrate. The third has fat. Choose one or more foods from the first two lists; choose from the third list if you want to. Cheese, crackers, and fruit juice work well. So do peanut butter and apple slices. Raw vegetables and dip give carbohydrate and fat. What could you add to give protein?

Protein and fat	**Carbohydrate**	**Fat**
Choose one or more	*Choose one or more*	*Choose if you want*
2 percent or whole milk	Toast or another bread	Dip for raw vegetables
Hard-cooked eggs	Breakfast cereal	Butter or cream cheese for toast
Cheese	Crackers	
Luncheon meat	Cookies, cakes, muffins	
Peanut butter	Fruit juice	
Bean dip	Raw or canned fruit	
Hummus	Popcorn	
	Baked and fried snacks	
	Raw vegetables	
	Vegetable juice	

One of my readers suggested making a chart of snack possibilities and letting the child choose from it. That might work for children in the lower grades. For older school-age children, that strategy doesn't satisfy my goal of beginning to teach children food-selection principles and giving them responsibility for enacting them.

Of course, for your child the best part of any snack is your sitting down and taking an interest in her.

THE ADOLESCENT
Despite their acting like it doesn't matter to them in the slightest, adolescents continue to depend on parents to take leadership with the *what*, *when*, and *where* of feeding. Maintaining the structure of family meals is critical. Adolescents more consistently participate in family meals when parents make meals a priority, use mealtimes for connecting with children, and maintain a positive mealtime atmosphere. As they get older, adolescents increasingly report difficulty finding time for family meals,[3] and adolescents who snack continually tend to skip meals.[4] In the long run, it is critical for the adolescent to learn to manage her time and her snacking to make mealtime a priority. This apparently pays off after children leave home, as young adults who had family meals during adolescence assign importance to mealtime structure and are likely to provide regular meals for themselves and to arrange for social eating occasions. They are also likely to have diets of high nutritional quality.[5]

In the here and now, children who have family meals do better in all ways: nutritionally, socially, emotionally, academically, and with respect to resistance to overweight, dieting behavior, eating disorders, drug and alcohol abuse, and early sexual behavior. Family meals are more instrumental in adolescents' positive outcome than socioeconomic status, family structure (two-parent, one-parent, multigenerational), after-school activities, tutors, or church. But the trend is away from family meals, and as children get older, the incidence of family meals tends to decrease. While half of adolescents eat regular family dinners when they enter the teen years, only a quarter still have family meals as they approach the end of high school. For more, see appendix B, "What the Research Says about Meals."

Your adolescent will become fully independent with managing her eating only after she leaves home. She will be ready. Growing up at your table, she will have gained positive attitudes about eating, she will have developed the meal habit, she will trust herself to go to the table hungry and eat until she is satisfied, and her food acceptance and mealtime skills will allow her to be comfortable with the food that is in the world. In contrast, children do not develop those positive eating attitudes and behaviors in homes where family meals are not a priority or when parents chronically restrict themselves in the name of weight loss. When those children become adolescents and young adults, they enact what they have learned. All too often, they become offhand and casual about providing for themselves, and they put themselves on weight-reduction diets. They become heavier as a result.[6]

The piece that remains is for your adolescent to get ready to take on the discipline of providing for herself with food. She needs to round out her skills with food management. If all has gone well, she has been in the kitchen with you all along—at first unloading the pan cupboard and splashing in the sink, then "helping" by creating a mess, then making a real contribution by doing simple to increasingly complex food preparation tasks. That gives her a huge head start with food management because she knows the rudiments of food preparation and is comfortable in the kitchen. In some families, teenagers cook occasionally or do the shopping. That's great, as long as parents continue to take responsibility for the planning and coordination—and show genuine appreciation for the child's contribution.

During her high school years, support your child's developing food-management skills by increasingly including her in planning, shopping, cooking, and getting meals on the table. Start small and work up. Figure 5.1, "Being Considerate without Catering," on page 48 gives simple guidelines for planning meals that work well for young people just getting started on their own. Think out loud about what you consider when you put together meals. Discuss putting together satisfying and balanced meals on a cafeteria line in the dormitory or in boot camp. Go on a grocery store safari seeking pre-prepared canned, frozen, and fresh foods that make good meal substitutes or meal components. Sit down with your teenager and make a list of 20 fast, easy, and tasty meals that she can make on her own. Point out the grab-and-dump meals and the section "Fast Meals for One" in chapter 9, "How to Keep Cooking." Consider equipment, and identify what your adolescent will need in order to provide for herself. Give her a copy of *Secrets*, and go through it with her. Consider the absolute bottom line of food survival skills, and highlight sections addressing those skills. For instance, highlight the "Keeping Food Safe" section in chapter 11, "Planning to Get You Cooking."

Of course, the adolescent who has gotten into cooking and genuinely enjoys challenging herself in the kitchen will turn up her nose at such stripped-down principles and beginning lessons. Or maybe not. She will be busy when she goes off to whatever comes next, and she will have to cut corners just like the rest of us.

Parent Development

Every stage in feeding is important for parent development as well as for child development. During the infant stages, you learn to respect your child's capability, to set aside your agenda, and to follow your child's lead with feeding. Because trying to feed a toddler any other way simply doesn't work, the toddler stage gives you basic training in giving both the leadership and autonomy of the division of responsibility in feeding and establishing the meals-plus-snacks routine that you will use throughout your child's growing-up years. The preschool and school-age periods remind you how important you continue to be to your increasingly capable child and that it is essential for you to continue taking leadership and giving autonomy with feeding. Until your child leaves home, providing for her by maintaining the division of responsibility in feeding continues to be important. By the time she moves out, you will have lovingly worked yourself out of a job and your child will be equipped to make it in the outside world. She will be able to manage that most important of self cares: being competent with eating.

In short, throughout the growing-up years, to achieve your tasks with both child- and self-development, go by information coming from your child to guide feeding. For fascinating detail about the newborn through preschool stages, see *Child of Mine: Feeding with Love and Good Sense.* For even more fascinating detail about the school-age and adolescent years, see *Your Child's Weight: Helping Without Harming.*

Parents' Feeding Tasks

Now that we have applied the division of responsibility in feeding to stages in development, let's apply it again to the details of who does what with feeding. In order for children to do a good job with eating, parents and other adults have to take leadership with feeding. Leadership tasks include providing regular, predictable, and pleasant meals and snacks, showing your child what it means to grow up with regard to eating, and letting your child develop the body that is right for her. Do your jobs, but stow your agenda. Instead, cultivate an attitude of curiosity.

CHOOSE AND PREPARE FOOD

You are the gatekeeper when it comes to the food that is in your home and on your table. You need to know enough about your child's physical ability to eat and enough about nutrition to offer your child food that is both developmentally and nutritionally appropriate. By *developmentally* I mean that food has to be the right texture and consistency so she can safely and comfortably eat it. By *nutritionally* I mean choosing foods that combine to offer a well-balanced diet.

If you are just getting started with family meals, reread the section, "Work Up to Structure," pages 47 through 48, in chapter 5, "Feed Yourself Faithfully." Eat what you are eating now—just save it for mealtime. Make any changes one at a time and add on foods rather than taking them away. Include foods that contribute protein, fat, and carbohydrate in your meals. Wait until you are fully comfortable with mealtime structure before you consider the more complex menu planning that I outline in figure PIII.1, "The Mother Principle of Meal Planning," on page 91. At that point, you will be ready to consider a wider variety of food.

Whatever your level of meal-management, let your child pick and choose from what is on the table. Don't offer substitutes, don't keep the cereal or peanut butter on the table, and don't let her get up to make something different. Offer everything at the same time, and don't make her eat her vegetables before she can have seconds (or even thirds—fourths) on spaghetti. Don't hide the vegetables *in* the spaghetti. She will cope as long as you let her eat like a child. She will generally eat only two or three food items; she will eat a lot one day and not much the next; she will eat her favorite foods some days but not others; and she will eat no vegetables for weeks then nothing *but* vegetables for more weeks.

PROVIDE REGULARLY SCHEDULED MEALS AND SNACKS

Most children are ready to eat from the family table by the time they are a year old. Once established, the structure of mealtime will support and reassure her. See to it that she is offered three structured meals at reliable times as well as enough sit-down snacks so she gets the opportunity to eat every 2 to 3 hours. For most families, some of those meals and snacks will be at child care or in school. You are still providing when you choose a child care setting where regular, reliable, and structured meals and snacks are a priority.

Make sure your child has planned snacks and that she sits down to eat them. In certified child care centers, those snacks will include two or three foods as well as sources of protein, fat, and carbohydrate. Do the same at home. If the afternoon is long and dinner is late, your child may need two snacks—one with protein, fat, and carbohydrate, and a little pick-me-up an hour so before dinner. Don't just give food or beverage handouts (except for water) when your child begs for them, and don't let her wander around while she eats. Giving in to her random panhandling for food puts her in charge of the menu (your job) and keeps her from working up enough of an appetite to take an interest in meals (her job).

MAKE EATING TIMES PLEASANT

For your child, the most important thing at the table is *you* or another grown-up she trusts. Your child will always do more and dare more with eating if you are there. Even when she is older and seems independent, she benefits from meals with you. If you don't take an interest in eating with her, your child will lose heart, lose interest, and eat poorly. Keep your child company, make easygoing conversation, help her get served, enjoy your own meal, and let her enjoy hers.

Although your being there is important, be a supportive presence and be vigilant about your own behavior. It is way too easy to slip into trying to get children to eat more or less than they want. Eighty-five percent of observed San Francisco parents of kindergarteners tried to get

children to eat more than they did voluntarily. Parents used reasoning, praise, and food rewards; fathers used pressure tactics with boys, and mothers praised girls for eating.[7]

To gain a sense of herself at the same time as she maintains connection with her parents, a child must be given leadership without being controlled and given autonomy without being abandoned. Those parents in the San Francisco study spoiled eating for their children by being controlling. The messages to the children? To have your parents around, you have to let them control you; in order to do it your own way, you have to get away from your parents. If you are careful to observe a division of responsibility with feeding, your child can be with you and be her own person at the same time.

SHOW YOUR CHILD WHAT TO LEARN

Your child learns to like food by being exposed to it, over and over again. She wants to be successful at mealtime. She wants to grow up to eat just like you do and she will learn to eat and enjoy what you eat. It doesn't work—for parents or for children—to limit the menu to what children readily accept, because that takes away their opportunities to learn. It doesn't work to short-order cook for a child. You know how that goes: "Aargh, I don't like that!" "Well, what do you like?" "Peanut butter. Macaroni and cheese. Hot dogs." So you get up and make hot dogs, and your child may or may not eat them—and she loses her opportunity to learn.

Making special food presents its own kind of pressure: "If I make something special for you, you darn well better eat it!" It also lets children dictate the menu, which is not a good idea. You know more than your child does about the food that is in the world. She depends on you to expose her to the foods she needs to master and the skills she needs to learn. If you cater to her, she learns that you don't expect much of her. Let your child grow up to join the family table; don't limit and adapt the family table to suit her.

DON'T LET YOUR CHILD GRAZE

Children graze when they carry around a nursing bottle or tippy-cup of milk or juice or panhandle for snacks. Older children graze when they almost continually eat or drink—whether it be on candy or carrot sticks, soda or milk. Children who graze do poorly with food regulation. Some children who graze eat too much and get too fat; some eat too little and stay too thin. Some graze and still eat and grow just fine. Since you can't predict whether grazing will undermine *your* child's ability to eat the amount she needs, maintain structure.

Children who graze do poorly with food acceptance as well. Grazing children fill up on easy-to-like food handouts and don't learn to eat the more challenging food at meals and snacks. Going to meals hungry but not famished allows your child to take an interest in the food there and increases the likelihood that she will experiment with something new.

Here is where it pinches: In order to keep your child from grazing, *you* will have to give up grazing, as well. Your child will want to eat what, when, and where you do. Sneak if you must, but don't expect her to eat any differently than you do, and don't expect to sneak for long. She is tuned in, and she will soon catch you.

LET YOUR CHILD HAVE THE BODY THAT IS RIGHT FOR HER

This guideline is so important that I essentially put it in twice—once here and once in the section about the child's eating jobs where it says "they will grow predictably." Your job is to feed your child and let her grow. That is not an easy job, because it means you have to keep your nerve and not interfere. Sometimes children grow quickly, sometimes slowly. Some children grow up to be tall, others short, some thin, others fat. Children who grow up to be thin or fat may not necessarily be thin or fat while they are growing up. You don't get to choose, and neither does your child. What you *do* get to do is to help your child have the healthiest body possible, to feel good about that body, and to learn to use her body in the way it works well.

Your small, slender child might not turn out to be a Green Bay Packer; your large, stocky child might not become an Olympic gymnast. But strange turnarounds happen as children grow up, so there is no telling what might happen. But if you try to *make* something happen, you will do damage, and it is highly likely that you will create the very growth pattern you are trying to avoid. There are plenty of opportunities in life besides professional football and championship gymnastics. One part of growing up is for your child and you to come to terms with what she can and can't do.

Your Child's Eating Capabilities

Having done your jobs with feeding, let your child do hers. One of your biggest challenges as a parent is knowing when to let go. Maintaining a division of responsibility in feeding helps you learn when to take leadership and when to let go. If you go to one extreme or the other—if you fail to take leadership on the one hand or fail to give autonomy on the other—your child won't eat as well. My readers think this is a critical point, so I will emphasize it.

> If you become controlling and try to do your child's jobs as well as your own, she won't eat well.
>
> If you are not supportive enough and fail to take leadership with feeding, she won't eat well.

Taking leadership and giving autonomy are both difficult. After you give your child opportunities to learn, you have to slow down, back off, and let her learn. Early on, she will pick up food and drop it, pat some of it into her mouth (and on her cheeks and in her hair), sample the same foods over and over, spit foods out, gag them up, and throw them on the floor. As she gets older, she will eat some foods but not others, eat more than you do or seemingly not enough to keep a bird alive, trade off her bag lunch, use her allowance to buy foods you can't stand, or eat pizza from the a la carte line 8 days in a row—I could go on. Your job is to hang in there with the *what*, *when*, and *where*. To give her the chance to learn, you have to trust that your child will eat what she needs and grow in a way that is right for her.

YOUR CHILD WANTS TO EAT

All children, even the sickest babies, are born with the will to survive and the drive to eat. The drive to eat can be blunted, but it never goes away—and it takes a lot to blunt it. Your child wants to eat because it is an innate drive, because she sees you eating, and because growing up is what she *does*.

If a child seemingly won't eat, I ask, "Why not? What is taking away the child's normal drive to eat?" Often the child is reacting to a pushy parent who tries to get her to eat certain amounts or types of food. In their defense, parents are likely to be pushy if a child has been ill or grows slowly. At the other extreme, sometimes a child eats poorly because she doesn't get enough support: the food isn't right for her, or her parents plop her down with food rather than eating with her. Some children trigger their parents' pushy feeding behavior by being extremely cautious and slow to warm up to new foods. Slow-to-warm-up children aren't very rewarding for parents to feed. It seems to be a natural, if counterproductive, response for parents to get pushy in response to a child's chronic lack of interest in food and unwillingness to eat unfamiliar food. They motivate, play games, encourage, reward, cast about for foods the child *will* eat, or even get rigid and controlling. Whether the pressure is positive or negative, the child eats worse, not better. Like other children, cautious and slow-to-warm-up children need a positive feeding environment, lots of opportunities to learn, and *absolutely no pressure*.

At times, a child undereats because she *can't* eat. A child who was tube-fed early on doesn't even know what eating *is* and certainly doesn't know how to do it. If a child has had uncomfortable procedures done to her mouth, she has learned that anything that happens to her mouth is negative. Other children have problems with nerves or muscles, problems that may first become apparent with feeding. Children who have uncorrected heart defects are so tired and short of breath that they have trouble eating as much as they need. All these children *want* to eat. They just need extra help so they can *do* it. I talk more about helping wary children learn to eat in *Child of Mine: Feeding with Love and Good Sense*, mostly in the toddler and preschooler chapters.

YOUR CHILD KNOWS HOW MUCH TO EAT

Your child was born with internal regulators adapted to her distinctive physical requirements. The large child and the small child, the big eater and the small eater—all know how much to eat. All grow in the often surprising way nature intended. Your child will get hungry, eat, get filled up, and stop eating (even in the middle of a bowl of ice cream). Whether your child needs a lot or a little, she instinctively eats as much as she needs. If you do your job—no more and no less—she will automatically eat the right amount of food to grow and be as active as is right for her. In fact, she faces a whole lifetime of having to regulate her food intake in order to maintain a stable body weight. To do well with that lifetime of food regulation, she needs to be allowed to preserve her sensitivity to her internal sensations of hunger, appetite, and satiety. For more on this topic, see appendix I, "Children and Food Regulation: The Research."

Provided you don't try to control her, your child can even make up for her mistakes in eating. Babies overeat and then spit up a little and eat less the next time. My 8-year-old granddaughter eats little for days at a time, then eats more than you would think she could hold at a given meal. She doesn't think about it or use her willpower. Her instinctive regulators of hunger and fullness take care of it for her.

Children who eat and grow at the extremes make their parents so nervous that they often interfere. It backfires. In our weight-obsessed culture, parents may try to restrict a robust child with a hearty appetite because they assume that enjoying food and eating a lot means she will get fat. It doesn't, and it doesn't work. Parents may try to push food on a small, thin child with a small appetite, assuming she is doing poorly and thinking they should fatten her up a bit. She isn't, and it doesn't work. Children who don't get enough to eat—or fear they won't—become preoccupied with food and are prone to overeat when they get a chance. Children who have food pushed on them become turned off by it and are likely to undereat when they get the chance.

The Girl Who Ate More Than Her Father

In chapter 4, "Eat as Much as You Want," I discussed counterfeit mindful-eating messages—those that give permission and take it away at the same time. Many dietitians and other health professionals tell me they love my work, then they go right back to teaching food plans and portion sizes. A mother recently e-mailed me about her efforts to institute the division of responsibility in feeding her chubby daughter at the same time as she coped with her dietitian's mixed messages. The dietitian had recommended my books, and following my advice, the parents started having family meals and letting the child eat as much as she wanted. The girl had become MUCH LESS (mother's emphasis) preoccupied with food. The parents had been hanging in there, despite their uneasiness and despite the fact that the girl ate "more than my husband." The dietitian "disagreed with letting her [the daughter) eat as much as she wants," reported the mother. She "seemed appalled that she would eat so much." Trusting a child to regulate food intake when she eats and grows at the extremes takes steady nerves and a leap of faith. That dietitian lost her nerve and put on the brakes, and as a consequence, the parents did, too. They went back to restricting their daughter, and their daughter went back to thinking about food all the time and begging for food handouts. As a professional who works with parents, losing one's nerve is not an option for the dietitian.

However, I do know how that dietitian feels. The first time I encouraged parents to use a division of responsibility with a child who was seemingly overeating, I had to white-knuckle it. The child in question was Mark, a toddler who was absolutely preoccupied with food. Mark constantly scavenged and begged for food and had tantrums at mealtimes until he got as much as he wanted to eat. He embarrassed his parents at birthday parties by hanging around the food and not playing with the other children. It emerged that Mark's parents were trying to restrict him to one helping only at mealtime and no snacks between times. I told them: three meals, three snacks, let him eat as much as he wants at those regularly scheduled times, but no food or beverages (except water) between times. At first, Mark ate like there was no tomorrow and his parents feared he would never stop. So did I, but I didn't let on. I acted confident, because I knew that expressing my doubts would undermine their courage and efforts. Then, about 4 or 5 weeks into treatment, the story changed. Mark began eating only a modest amount, leaving food on his plate, and at times he showed little interest in snacks. The proof of the intervention came at a birthday party, where Mark ignored the food and went off to play with the other children.

Since then, I have worked with enough children and parents that my confidence is genuine. Children go through an initial period of eating a lot, but after 4 to 8 weeks, depending on the age of the child, they find their stopping place. If they don't, parents are unconsciously—or consciously—restricting and frightening the child that she won't get enough to eat. Then

the task is finding out where the restriction is coming from and stopping it.

YOUR CHILD WILL EAT THE FOOD YOU EAT

If you eat it, your child will eat it, too. Probably *later* rather than *sooner*, your child *will* eat and enjoy the food you enjoy. The emphasis is on *enjoy*. If you eat it but don't enjoy it, your child won't eat it. Your tuned-in child will note your lack of enthusiasm and think, "That must not be so good, so why should I eat it?" It *is* conceivable that you could put a food on the table and not eat it and *not get pushy*, and your child would learn to like it. Children like canned spaghetti, don't they? Well, all right, some adults do, too!

The handwriting is on the wall. If you want your child to enjoy and therefore eat a variety of food, you have to lead the way. Review chapter 3, "Honor Your Appetite." If you have a too-short list of foods you enjoy, pay particular attention to the last section, "Help Yourself with Food Acceptance."

If you simply cannot *bear* learning to like new food, remember that the goal is helping your child develop food acceptance skills, not getting her to eat certain foods. If she has food acceptance skills, she will learn to like new foods at school lunch, at a friend's table, or when she gets out on her own. Figure 3.2, "Food Acceptance Attitudes and Skills," on page 22, tells you that those skills include being comfortable around unfamiliar food, being matter-of-fact and polite about picking and choosing from available foods, being curious about novel food, and being inclined to experiment with unfamiliar food by looking at it, watching others eat it, and tasting it. Your child will develop good food acceptance skills if you do have meals and you don't get pushy.

YOUR CHILD WILL EAT A VARIETY

Even after your child learns to enjoy a variety of food, she will be inconsistent about what she eats. She won't eat some of everything that is put before her, but only two or three food items. What she eats one day she won't another, because what tastes good to her one day is different from what tastes good another. She may go on a fruit kick one day, breads and grains another, meat another, milk another.

But there is hope. Children tire of even favorite food and eat alternatives. Their erratic food consumption adds up to variety of food, and variety adds up to nutritional adequacy. When I analyze children's diets, I always ask for at least a week of records. (On my better days, I also ask the parent to tell me what they *offer*, as well as what the child eats.) The food record generally looks pretty strange: a bite of this, a cup of that, no vegetables, lots of vegetables. However, I consistently find that the week's intake adds up to a nutritionally adequate diet.

It adds up, that is, if the food is on the table, and the emotional climate at the table is positive. Those two key elements have more to do with a child's getting the nutrients she needs than what she actually eats on any given day. For background and the research, see appendix J, "Children and Food Acceptance: The Research."

YOUR CHILD WILL GROW PREDICTABLY

Your child was born with a blueprint for growth. If you maintain a division of responsibility in feeding, including trusting her to do her part with eating and moving, you don't need to worry about normal growth—it happens.

Most of your child's growth is determined by genetics.[8] She has a natural way of growing that is right for her, and she knows how much she needs to eat to grow that way. As long as your child grows consistently, her size and shape are normal for her, even if her growth plots at the highest or the lowest percentiles.

Consistent growth can mean getting gradually bigger or smaller over time. By age 7 years, your child's weight and height will naturally adjust to reflect some combination of the weights and heights of her two parents. That's normal. But if your child's weight or height abruptly and rapidly shift up or down, it can indicate a problem. If your child's growth accelerates or falters, consult with a health professional who understands feeding dynamics to rule out health, feeding, or parenting problems. To read more about letting your child get the body that is right for her, see my book *Your Child's Weight: Helping Without Harming*.

YOUR CHILD WILL BEHAVE WELL AT THE TABLE

An important part of raising your child is socializing her—helping her to be comfortable when she is in polite company, and teaching her to behave so she feels successful and so that others enjoy having her at the table. Much of

that socializing takes place at the family table. At first, the lessons are basic: Sit on your chair; eat your own food; keep your hands to yourself; don't yell, whine, and cry. Then lessons get more complicated: Use words to ask for what you want, and say "yes, please" and "no, thank you." Lessons after that include: Serve yourself but don't take it all, pass the food to the next person, wait until everyone gets served before you start to eat, take your turn talking. Then you move to the real social niceties: Don't irritate other people by singing, reading, or belching. You get the idea.

At first your child will eat with her fingers and use her plate for a plaything. Later on she will leave her plate on the table and her food on the plate and eat with her fingers. Later still she will use her fingers to push food onto her silverware. By the time she is 10 or 11 years old, she will mostly use utensils. For many years she will make a mess, spill milk, and have trouble estimating how much to serve herself. That is all normal kid behavior. If she makes a mess to get your goat, however, ask her to leave the table. You are teaching her that it is a privilege to be at the table and that to earn that privilege she must behave herself.

Don't intrude on your child's prerogatives with eating. If you try to get her to eat more, less, or different food than she wants, she will behave poorly.

Feeding goes best when you do your jobs with feeding and trust your child to do hers. Your child wants to grow up with respect to eating, the same as with everything else in life. You are the one who knows what growing up is all about. You help her grow up by understanding her developing ability to eat and by offering food she can manage. She is the one with the eating capabilities, and she will retain those capabilities if you maintain the division of responsibility with feeding.

References

1. Satter EM. The feeding relationship. *J Am Diet Assoc.* 1986;86:352-356.
2. Briefel R, Reidy K, Karwe V, Jankowski L, Hendricks K. Toddlers' transition to table foods: impact on nutrient intakes and food patterns. *J Am Diet Assoc.* 2004;104:38-44.

3. Fulkerson JA, Neumark-Sztainer D, Story M. Adolescent and parent views of family meals. *J Am Diet Assoc.* 2006;106:526-32.

4. Savige G, MacFarlane A, Ball K, Worsley A, Crawford D. Snacking behaviours of adolescents and their association with skipping meals. *International Journal of Behavioral Nutrition and Physical Activity.* 2007;4:3.

5. Larson NI, Neumark-Sztainer D, Hannan PJ, Story M. Family meals during adolescence are associated with higher diet quality and healthful meal patterns during young adulthood. *J Am Diet Assoc.* 2007;107:1502-1510.

6. Neumark-Sztainer D, Wall M, Guo J, Story M, Haines J, Eisenberg M. Obesity, disordered eating, and eating disorders in a longitudinal study of adolescents: how do dieters fare 5 years later? *J Am Diet Assoc.* 2006;106:559-568.

7. Orrell-Valente JK, Hill LG, Brechwald WA, Dodge KA, Pettit GS, Bates JE. "Just three more bites": an observational analysis of parents' socialization of children's eating at mealtime. *Appetite.* 2007; 48:37-45.

8. Wardle J, Carnell S, Haworth CM, Plomin R. Evidence for a strong genetic influence on childhood adiposity despite the force of the obesogenic environment. *Am J Clin Nutr.* 2008;87:398-404.

Chapter
7
Stuff to Know to Have Family Meals

With feeding your child as with feeding yourself, the *how* of feeding is far more critical than the *what* or the *how much*. If you get the *how* right, the *what* and *how much* will fall into place.

What work does this chapter need to do? In part I, "How to Eat," I addressed how you can help yourself become competent with eating. In chapter 6, "The Feeding Relationship," I covered helping children to grow up to be good eaters by maintaining the division of responsibility in feeding throughout the growing-up years. In the cooking and planning chapters and in chapter 13, "Choosing Food," I will go into detail about food, food management, and nutrition.

That leaves for this chapter an intriguing grab-bag of *stuff you need to know in order to have family meals.* I have already said that there are two main—and interrelated—parts to doing a good job with feeding your child: taking leadership and giving autonomy. This chapter addresses both parts in more detail. Relative to giving autonomy, I discuss how to establish and maintain pleasant and good-natured mealtimes, how to build your child's positive mealtime behavior, how to address *negative* mealtime behavior, and how to tell the difference. Then, I give you some additional tips on taking leadership with food management: how to orchestrate snacks, how to make wise use of planned substances, and how to manage family meals in restaurants. However, before we get started, I consider it essential to take a short detour to protect you from interference.

Don't Be Spooked by Nutritional Hand-Wringing

Fueled by the hysteria about child overweight, there are far too many "advisors" who can trigger your concern about the *what* and the *how much*. Your own admirable desire to do a good job with parenting makes you easy prey for the shoulds and oughts with respect to feeding, whether those shoulds and oughts come from your advisors or from your inner food cop. I work hard in *Secrets* to encourage you to enjoy food. But along with being a parent comes guilt, and that guilt can send you back to feeling anxious and unsure about the food you choose for your child. Your food guilt will be activated by implied and outright criticism about the consequences your supposedly poor nutritional behavior will have on your child. To understand what I mean, pay attention to your feelings as you read the following excerpt from a study on parents' overweight-prevention behaviors.

Parents in focus groups reported the main barriers to their preschoolers' healthy eating to be 1) Not having enough time to prepare healthy food; 2) Parents disliking the taste, appearance and smell of healthy foods; and 3) Parents making unhealthy food choices readily available to their preschoolers.[1]

Does that make you feel guilty? The statements are made by parents criticizing themselves about the foods they choose for their children. Parents know the food rules and scold themselves for falling short. You recognize the bind those parents are in. They schlep their children around to physical activities at least in part because they want to prevent child overweight. But being on the go leaves them with what they feel is too little time to prepare healthy meals. "The most common unhealthy choices to which the parents referred," observed the study authors, "were fast-food restaurants."[1]

A-ha! That will get your guilt going if nothing else does! Such statements make me angry on your behalf. How does it make you feel to have your food choices condemned as being unhealthy? What does it do to your eating attitudes and behaviors? If you feel your Big Mac or your Whopper and your French fries are bad for you and your child, will you treat them with respect? What will you teach your child about this perfectly good food that you paid for with your perfectly good money? How capable will you be of enacting the division of responsibility in feeding when you offer your child food you consider to be inferior? Will you teach him to treat his food with respect? Will you tune in and enjoy your food and in the process teach your child to do the same? Will you let him matter-of-factly eat French fries until he gets full, will you nag him to slow down or leave some, or will you not order them in the first place?

If you nag, you have company: Studies show that parents provide high-fat food and then restrict the amounts their children eat, whereupon children's preference for high-fat food increases. I assume that parents restrict the high-fat food because they feel guilty about letting their child eat it. Their feelings of guilt and their restrictive behavior teach the child that high-fat food is forbidden fruit, and that makes it even more enticing. As a consequence, the child is likely to eat in a hurried, sneaky, or defiant fashion and consume more than he would otherwise. It's the principle of restraint that we have bumped into again and again: Restricting food intake makes people eat more, not less. By the way, unless I give you references, the principles I address in this chapter are based on studies cited in either appendix J, "Children and Food Acceptance: The

Research," or appendix I, "Children and Food Regulation: The Research."

SUGAR AND FAT DON'T CAUSE OVEREATING

Back to the article that got me so riled up. A few parents pointed out that thinking ahead was the key to doing it all: "Constantly planning, preparing meals, and keeping a well-stocked refrigerator enabled those parents to manage both healthy eating and physical activities for their preschoolers."[1] That's great, but why not replace the word "healthy" with a less loaded term, such as "enjoyable" or "satisfying"? Insisting on "healthy eating" raises the bar—it makes getting a meal on the table seem difficult and dreary.

Nutrition professionals are fond of saying "all foods can fit in a healthy diet." Do you believe it? Or do you assume there is a catch, such as don't-eat-so-much, don't-eat-it-so-often, or make-up-for-it-later? Well, in the nutrition world, there *is* a catch. Here is a line from an American Dietetic Association position statement: "All foods can fit within this [overall pattern of food intake], if consumed in moderation with appropriate portion size and combined with regular physical activity."[2] This is an example the counterfeit permission I talked about in the section, "Beware of Counterfeits," pages 39 through 40, in chapter 4, "Eat as Much as You Want." Giving counterfeit permission is based on the fear that, given *true* permission to eat, you will take license to eat what you want and as much as you want.

Well, so what? The fact of the matter is that ecSatter *supports* your deliberately eating what you want and as much as you want. Out of such permission and discipline grow order and predictability, not gluttony and nutritional anarchy.

Back to the article about the focus groups. The authors quite rightly point out that parents tend to have foods in the house that they enjoy and that children get the repeated exposure they need to learn to like those foods. So far so good. But the authors spoil it all with the next sentence. "Unfortunately, sugar and fat are currently the most familiar and preferred foods in childhood."[1] Well of *course* they are! Every child is born with a sweet tooth. Young children instinctively prefer fat because they need the calories and because high-fat foods taste good. Because children's stomachs are small and their energy needs high, they need some foods that are concentrated in calories in order to get enough to eat. They automatically seek out high-calorie foods, those containing sugar and fat, when their calorie needs are particularly high. However, preferring fat or sugar doesn't cause overeating.

Children and other people who have structure and support for eating and whose internal regulators are intact can get full without overeating when they are offered sugary and fatty foods, the same as they do when they are offered other foods. But if sugary and fatty foods are forbidden and purged from the family food supply, children will overeat on them when they get a chance and be fatter than children whose parents are more matter-of-fact about including them in meals and snacks.

Once again, having outlined the dilemma, we arrive at the heart of the matter.

The logic of the unfortunate authors whose article I am getting all wrathy about is the same as that of almost every other author on child overweight: that eating the right food and avoiding the wrong food will prevent child overweight. This is simply not true. But it is such a destructive and pervasive idea that I highlight the following statement:

> There is absolutely no evidence to back up the idea that eating the right food and avoiding the wrong food will prevent child overweight.
>
> In fact, evidence shows that children who are restricted in that fashion eat more, not less.
>
> Teenagers who strive for weight reduction by eating the "right" food and avoiding the "wrong" food get heavier, not thinner.

Roughly three-quarters of teenagers try to restrict their food intake to lose weight. Even those who use "healthful" methods—those who try to eat the "right foods" and avoid the "wrong food"—get heavier, not thinner. Years later they have gained just as much excessive weight as teenagers who diet using extreme methods. Teenagers who don't diet don't gain too much weight.

MEALS ARE THE BOTTOM LINE
Feel guilty if you must, but at least feel guilty about the right thing. If you have children, you absolutely *have* to feed them three meals and anywhere from one to three snacks a day. *Anything less amounts to neglect.*

Will you be more likely to discharge your responsibility to your child if you cut yourself some nutritional slack, or if you insist that every meal be a nutritional masterpiece? Getting meals on the table is an enormous and unrelenting labor of love. You will be most likely to do that unending and essential job if you find your food richly rewarding to plan, prepare, provide, and eat. Snootiness about food is counterproductive. It makes it hard for all of us—for young parents, in particular, because they are generally so strapped for time and money—to be consistent and reliable about eating and feeding. Moreover, you, not your child, get to choose food you enjoy. You are the parent; you know the most about the food that is in the world. Your child will learn to eat the food you eat. When he grows up, he gets to choose.

That's the end of my rant, except for the mopping-up. I have said some things that need to be clarified.

A rule of thumb for protecting yourself against negative advice:
It is good advice if it supports your trust in yourself and your child. It is bad advice if it takes that trust away.

Attitude
If you and your child sit down together and eat your Whoppers and fries with a glad heart, it will be a fine meal. On the other hand, if you whip through the drive-through and toss dinner-in-a-bag into the back seat, it will not.

Activity
Organized activity for children is fun and great for socializing, but you do not have to haul your child around to such activities to encourage him to move his body. You do have to keep control of the television set. Restricting television increases children's activity more than trying to get them to be active.[3]

Priorities
In terms of supporting your child's overall social and emotional welfare, family meals are more important than organized activities. Thinking that everything else is more important than family dinner is the same as thinking everything else is more important that *you*. Your child knows better: He knows that you are most important. Children treasure dependable time

with their parents. Your making meals reminds your child again and again that you make him a priority and that you want to give him your undivided attention.

Overweight

Maintaining the division of responsibility in feeding will allow you to raise your child to have the body that is right for him. If your child gets the idea that his weight is unsatisfactory to you, it will make him feel bad in all ways: not smart, not physically capable, and not worthwhile. No matter your child's size and shape, he can feel good about himself if you feel good about him and do a good job of raising him. Help him feel good about his body and raise him to have good character, common sense, effective ways of responding to feelings, problem-solving skills, and the ability to get along with others. Of course, to do all that, you must stop disrespecting your own size and shape. It is a tall order, but worth it! To understand the issue of child overweight from the perspective of good parenting and positive feeding, read *Your Child's Weight: Helping Without Harming*. For the key concepts, go to www.EllynSatter.com and search for "Child overweight."

You Have to Have Meals

Consider yourself vaccinated. Now to the topic at hand: orchestrating family meals. Meals make you a family. Meals reassure your child he will be fed. Going to the table hungry and eating until he is satisfied is critical to your child's eating the amount of food he needs to grow well. Meals help your child learn to like new food by giving a setting where he can be exposed to those foods again and again without pressure to eat them. Meals give your child emotional reassurance: access to you, structure, and limits.

As I have told you before, children who have family meals do better in all ways: nutritionally, socially, emotionally, academically and, with respect to resistance to overweight, dieting behavior, eating disorders, drug and alcohol abuse, and early sexual activity. Family meals have more to do with adolescents' positive outcome than socioeconomic status, family structure (two-parent, one-parent, multigenerational), after-school activities, tutors, or church. For more on that, see appendix B, "What the Research Says about Meals."

Meals provide the backbone for family life by giving a reliable context for the work of the family: nurturing children, helping individual growth, and easing relationships with the outside world. The day-in, day-out routine of structured, sit-down family meals and snacks reassures children that they are loved and that they will be provided for. Children are a captive audience who *absolutely* depend on us to provide for them. They feel afraid when parents are casual about feeding them or don't let them have enough to eat.

It is difficult for us to know—or remember—what a child's absolute dependence on grown-ups feels like. To get a sense for that childhood dilemma, consider this story told by an experienced outfitter who equipped groups to whitewater raft through the Grand Canyon. "It's hard for our guests," he observed, "because for at least a week, maybe two, they are entirely dependent on us. We used to get a lot of whining and worrying from them—had we thought of this or that, what if this or that happened. We also had a lot of feeding frenzies. They ate as if every meal were their last. Finally, we hit on the solution. Now, the first night out, we make this enormous, delicious meal. We urge seconds and thirds, and keep urging until everyone protests they have had enough. Then, in full sight of everyone, we bury the leftovers. After that," he grinned, "they are fine. Not nearly so much whining or worrying, and no more food frenzies."

The message was clear: We will take care of you. Not only do we have enough, we have *more* than enough. In providing the guests with elaborate reassurance about their food, he provided them with reassurance that they would be provided for. Think about it. That story is about *adults* who know they will get off that river in a week or two. What must it be like for a child, who anticipates being that dependent forever?

MEALS SUPPORT GOOD PARENTING

Children do best—with eating and in every other way—when they are given both leadership and autonomy: love, structure, opportunities to learn, guidelines for behavior, and choices within these safe boundaries. This is the authoritative approach to parenting. Children whose parents give both leadership and autonomy are most likely to become successful, happy with themselves, and generous with others. Children whose parents are overly strict—who give leadership without autonomy—are likely to be obedient but unhappy; those of permissive parents—those who give autonomy-without taking leadership—are likely to feel insecure and lack self control.[4,5] Remarkably, children of authoritative parents grow appropriately, whereas children of overly strict mothers were nearly five times as likely to be overweight as those of authoritative mothers, and those of permissive or neglectful mothers were at nearly three times the risk.[6]

Ellyn Satter's Division of Responsibility in Feeding (see figure 6.1 on page 58 is an *authoritative* approach to parenting. Authoritative parenting with respect to food demands that you take responsibility for the *what*, *when*, and *where* of feeding and turn over to your child the *whether* and *how much* of eating. The family meal is an integral part of the division of responsibility in feeding. The parent who gives leadership and autonomy says, "It's dinnertime. Here's what we have; you may eat or not eat. No more until snack time." The overly strict parent says, "Eat it or else. Clean up your plate." The permissive parent says, "What do you want to eat? When do you want it?" The neglectful parent says, "Don't bother me. Get it yourself."

The pattern for family meals is set during the toddler stage, when a child learns to participate in the meals-plus-snacks routine of the family—or not. Like other developmental tasks, if you miss the window of opportunity, it is harder to achieve later on. Getting your preschooler or school-age child back to the family table is possible—but difficult. Getting your teenager back is possible—but only if he sees the need and is willing to be there.

Your taking leadership with feeding continues to be important throughout the growing-up years. Your school-age child will work up to getting his own snack when he comes home from school and will experiment at friends' homes with foods you don't purchase or prepare. Your teen will eat what he wants for lunch, snack where and on what he wants, and eat at friends' homes. But he will also cooperate when you say, "Get your snack early so you don't spoil your dinner." Even if he complains he is the only one in his group expected home for dinner, do not be deterred. His complaining is his way of seeking your support—of finding out if you really mean it. If your dinners are pleasant and offer a way for your family to connect, your teen will want to be there. His friends will secretly envy him, and they may

even show up for dinner! In fact, you might want to invite them!

How to Have Meals

If you are not having rewarding family meals, you can get them back. Some years ago, Oprah Winfrey conducted a Family Dinner Experiment. Five families volunteered to eat dinner together as a family every night for a month. At first, sharing meals was a chore. But by the end of the month, the families found their time together to be so rewarding that they planned to continue having family dinners. The greatest surprise to the parents was the reaction of their children. They treasured the dependable time with their parents. Not only do parents want to feel attached to their children, children want it, too.

ADDRESS YOUR ATTITUDE
It's a matter of priorities. If you want family meals and are convinced that they are important, you will find a way to have them. In *Secrets*, I bend over backwards to make cooking and eating as realistic and rewarding as possible. Everyone in the family contributes to pleasant, relaxed, and low-key mealtimes by behaving nicely. Being included in family meals is a privilege that everyone *earns* through positive behavior.

It's still a lot of work. In order for you to keep up the day-in-day-out commitment of family meals, those meals have to be richly rewarding for you to plan, prepare, and eat.

If your attitude is that meals are important, your child will know it, and he will do better because he knows he can depend on you to look out for him. Your attitude that meals are important is identical to your attitude that *you* are important. You *are* important, and your importance extends *way* beyond being transportation and a checkbook. Your child will do better when he spends time with you and when he has a sense of family. Key to that connection is the family meal.

ADDRESS INTERFERENCE
I realize it is not easy to have family meals. There is so much interference. Workdays and commutes are long. Events get scheduled at family dinnertimes. To make matters worse, advertising makes it seem that family meals are unimportant. Instead of breakfast, children on

television are handed a high-energy bar on their way out of the house. Frozen, microwavable "meals for kids" with pictures of children doing the preparation and sitting down to eat by themselves assure us that children can take care of feeding themselves. Prepackaged food and fast foods are readily available. Children can take some money and buy dinner for themselves. It all makes it seem as though family meals are a thing of the past.

Parents know better. A Food Marketing Institute–Better Homes and Gardens survey indicates that parents' commitment to dinner is strong. When asked why they believe family dinners are important, parents share their conviction that eating meals together strengthens family ties and unity and that children who have family dinners eat a more healthful diet. They feel that eating together gives important opportunities for family communication and promotes a better family atmosphere, including giving a sense of stability and togetherness. Those parents have the right idea. In my experience, parents don't need to be persuaded that family meals are important. What they need is help figuring out how to get those meals to happen. For more information, see appendix B, "What the Research Says about Meals."

BE REALISTIC, AND STREAMLINE
While I show and tell you everything I can think of to make family meal planning and preparation as streamlined as possible, it is still a lot of work. You will still feel you spend most of your life in the grocery store or the kitchen. There is simply no way around it. As your child gets older and doesn't require a food infusion every 2 or 3 hours, it will get better. If you make the early investment in time, mess, and aggravation to encourage other family members to help in the kitchen, eventually their contribution will turn into genuine help that will lighten your load. But having family meals still requires vigilance: continually making them a priority and continually orchestrating them. If it *seems* hard, that's because it *is* hard.

Nutrition is important, but be realistic about your nutritional standards. Review the section, "Work Up to Structure," pages 47 through 48 in chapter 5, "Feed Yourself Faithfully." As I advised you there, build the meal habit by first getting the structure of meals well in place using the foods you currently eat.

Respect and enjoy your food, no matter what it is. The purpose of eating is to sustain life. To keep up the day-in-day-out of family meals, have food *you* find richly rewarding to plan, prepare, provide, and eat. It's what you like— don't apologize for it. Emphasize enjoyable meals, and nutrition will fall into place. With feeding your child as with feeding yourself, put pleasure and self-trust first. Don't get me wrong. I am not saying that good nutrition is unimportant. On the contrary, I think good nutrition is very important. However, *nowhere* do I tell you what to eat, and nowhere do I give you a list of foods to avoid. From my previous experience, I know that such directives would do way more harm than good with respect to both feeding yourself and feeding your child.

Include protein, fat, and carbohydrate so your meals are immediately satisfying and stay with you a while. Once your meal habit is well in place, expand slowly on the foods you regularly eat. Then cautiously organize your menu-planning, taking into account eaters' limitations with chewing, swallowing, and food acceptance without limiting menus to foods they readily accept. Work toward including the food groups—protein, breads and cereals, vegetables and fruit, milk—but take it easy. Continue to have the foods you like, add on rather than taking away, and make only one change at a time. The point is to put together meals that are accessible and enjoyable enough so the juice is worth the squeeze.

Build Positive Mealtime Behavior

As the Winfrey experiment showed, not only do parents want to feel attached to their children, children want it, too. Children feel attached to parents and siblings when family meals are positive and rewarding—when everyone gets a chance to talk and listen, to share news of the day, and to have fun making conversation that is of interest to everyone. To preserve family meals as a source of *emotional* as well as *nutritional* support, show children how to behave, avoid lecturing and haranguing, and avoid being controlling about what and how much *anyone* eats.

It is a meal when you and your family sit down together, facing one other, and share time and attention as well as food. You can sit at the kitchen table, at a table in a fast-food restaurant, or around a blanket on the floor. It is *not* a meal if the TV is on, if people are reading, if you have fights at the table, or if you feed your child rather than eating with him.

What happens at a rewarding meal? You connect, check in, talk, and listen. Your child gets his share of attention, but not all of it. Take an interest in your child—it is the best thing you can do for him. Ask specific questions, and *listen* when he answers: "Who did you see today?" "What word did you study today?" "What did you have to eat for lunch today?" Then ask for more detail. Better yet, be alert for openings and ask questions instead of giving answers: "What do you think of that?" "How do you feel about that?" "Why do you think he did that?" "Tell me more about that," isn't a question, but it is a wonderful invitation that tells your child you take an interest.

Don't hesitate to talk as well as listen, but try to make mealtime conversation reasonably accessible to everyone. In her book *The Surprising Power of Family Meals*, Marion Weinstein points out that children love hearing family stories, and the more they know about their families, the more securely attached they feel and the more resilient they are in coping. Each time we have chicken, my granddaughters remind me of a family story about my cousin Everett who could eat fried chicken with his fingers without getting them greasy. I am not sure if that story has a moral—maybe it is that everyone is good at something.

PLAN MEALS TO ALLOW YOUR CHILD TO BE SUCCESSFUL

Children want to be successful and they want to learn. To make both possible, match familiar food with unfamiliar, favorite with not-so-favorite. Always put at least one food on the table that your child generally enjoys, such as bread. In fact, always put out bread. Your child can eat bread if all else fails. The familiar, accepted food reassures your child that he can be successful with the meal. The unfamiliar, not-so-favorite food gives him opportunities to learn. Your child will, of course, eat what's familiar and favorite. He may eat four or five slices of bread for eight dinners in a row. Have faith. He will tire of even his favorite food and be braver about sneaking up on new food and learning to like it if he knows he has something he likes to fall back on.

Go to some trouble to make food taste good, and do use fat in your cooking. Once your child has been introduced one by one to a variety of foods and textures, don't be afraid to experiment with spices, mixtures, and sauces. Children like interesting food, even if it is a little challenging at first. So-called ethnic food is somebody else's standard fare, and their children learn to like it.

Don't limit menus to food your child readily accepts, but don't do sadistic menu planning, either. A sadistic meal would be something like liver, boiled potatoes, and cooked cabbage. Assuming you like liver yourself, a child-friendly menu featuring liver would include bread and might substitute corn for cabbage. Cabbage-family vegetables like cauliflower and broccoli often taste bitter to children. Mashing the potatoes with milk and butter or cream would help, because children can generally manage soft and creamy foods better than dry, hard foods. Serving fried onions and bacon along with the liver will tone down the flavor.

Most important of all, absolutely do not insist that your child eat the liver—or anything else that is on the table. My children eventually learned to like liver, although for a long time they ate only the bacon. Liver is such a strong-smelling, strong-flavored, strange-textured food that your child might not ever learn to like it. If that's that case, serving liver will give him practice with controlling his revulsion and saying politely, "no, thank you." You don't have to make him eat, but you do have to teach him to behave in polite company.

TRUST YOUR CHILD TO DO HIS PART

I told you in chapter 3, "Honor Your Appetite," that from the perspective of eating competence, the key to nutritional excellence is variety growing out of genuine food enjoyment. Preserve your child's food acceptance skills. Observe and accept how he sneaks up on new food and learns to like it. Don't get pushy. Getting pushy will spoil the meal and undermine his food acceptance skills.

Give your child plenty of opportunities to learn to like new food. Adults typically have a food only three times before they decide they don't like it. That's not enough. Your child needs more opportunities to learn, and so do you.

Everyone is entitled to food likes and dislikes, and some food won't appeal to your child or to you. Trust that both you and your child would eat it if you could. If you are the cook, you will be inclined to make foods you like. That is only fair. If you like a reasonable variety of food, you are in good shape. But if you have a short list of liked foods and a far longer list of disliked foods, you have work to do. Perhaps your partner will cook and you can pick and choose from what is available until you learn to like a greater variety of food. If you mind your manners and don't criticize or complain, your children will do their learning from watching your partner eat.

Prepare to be surprised. Two-year-old Clyde was a patient of Pam Estes, a colleague who works with special-needs children. Clyde ate few foods and ate so poorly at meals that his mother, Jennifer, fed him at the coffee table in front of the TV and left a supply of food for him in a low cupboard so he could help himself. Jennifer didn't want to force Clyde to eat because she was forced when she was a child and she knew how miserable that felt. But Clyde's list of acceptable foods got shorter and shorter. Under Pam's guidance, Jennifer established a division of responsibility in feeding. Jennifer moved all eating to the kitchen table. For each meal and snack, Jennifer chose one of Clyde's favorite foods as well as other foods from her own short list. And she reassured him: "You don't have to eat anything you don't want to." Clyde learned to behave nicely at meals and ever-so-gradually began to experiment with new food. Before long, he mastered Jennifer's list. To provide for Clyde, Jennifer began preparing new foods and cautiously trying them. And Clyde, by this time almost 3 years old, reassured her, "It's okay, Mommy, you don't have to eat it."

Trust your child to know how much he needs to eat. Some meals or some days or some weeks your child will eat a lot; other times not so much. Some children need to eat more than others, even if they look and act the same. Some girls need to eat more than some boys, and some boys and girls eat more than their fathers do. Eating a lot doesn't mean that your child will grow up to be too fat. Eating a little doesn't mean that your child will grow up to be too thin. Don't try to get your child to eat more or less than he wants or you will spoil family meals.

Address Negative Mealtime Behavior

Just because you are on the side of the angels in maintaining the division of responsibility in feeding does not mean that your child will enthusiastically get with the program. Parents often cross the lines of the division of responsi-bility in feeding because their child's eating behavior triggers controlling or permissive feeding behavior.

Figure 7.1 on the next page gives examples of moves (your child's) and countermoves (yours) in feeding. The moves start with those typical of the young child and work up to those typical of school-age children and adolescents. Your child's moves entice you across the lines of the division of responsibility in feeding. Your coun-termoves keep you doing your jobs and resist-ing the temptation, if not the outright invitation, to do his jobs. Your child is not being naughty. He is just clarifying the rules and—oh, yes—trying for control. That's what children do and how they learn. Children always try for control—it is part of growing up.

Remember, *your* job is feeding; his is eating. All the little skirmishes matter because they add up to the big picture in parenting. If you consistently deal with the small things, you won't have to deal with the big things. Struggles for control that you don't resolve when your child is young will be there in spades when he is a teenager.

If your child is hungry and can find some-thing on the table that he likes well enough to eat, he will pay attention to his eating. When he starts to get full, his attention will begin to wander. When he *is* full, he will lose all interest in food and will want to get down. If you keep him there after he is full, he will misbehave.

Many times parents keep children at the table after they are finished in hopes that they will eat a few more bites. Children behave poorly, parents wheedle them to eat and are upset when they don't, children put up a fuss but still feel bad about not pleasing their parents, and nobody has fun. When I ask them why they don't just let their child run off and play, par-ents say, "If he doesn't eat, he will be right back, begging for snacks."

"Ah," I say. "That is a separate problem. The solution to *that* is the *planned snack.*" We will get to that in just a moment.

Accept Normal Child Eating Behavior

If you are like most parents, you want your child to eat more fruits and vegetables, to drink his milk, and to eat some of everything that is put in front of him. He will and he does. But he

FIGURE 7.1 MEALTIME MOVES AND COUNTERMOVES

Your Child's Move	Your Countermove
He says, "I'm not hungry."	You say, "You don't have to eat; just sit with us for a while."
He is too worked up and busy to eat.	Spend a few minutes with him reading a book or washing hands.
He can't take time to eat.	Arrange for him to be hungry by not letting him graze for food.
He is too hungry to wait for meals.	Have sit-down snacks between meals.
He is too messy; he uses his fingers to eat.	Grin and bear it, cover the floor. Observe his concentration and creativity.
He doesn't want to stay at the table until you finish eating.	Let him down when he gets full. He will stay at the table longer as he gets older and learns to enjoy conversation.
He is naughty or otherwise disruptive at the table.	Let him down. He is full or he would eat—and behave!
He comes back right after the meal, begging for a food handout.	Don't give him food until snack time. Ignore his tantrums.
He gets down, but wants your attention, to sit on your lap, to eat off your plate.	Pat him on the head and send him away. Teach him to play quietly while you eat.
He doesn't eat "enough" at mealtime.	Only he knows how much is enough. Don't let him graze between times for food or beverages, except water. Plan a snack for a specific time and stick to it.
He says, "Can I get the peanut butter? I can put peanut butter on my bread."	You say, "No, that's like making a separate meal. You don't have to eat anything if you don't want to, but you do have to settle for what is on the table."
He wants to make something different: "Why isn't that all right? You don't have to do it!"	"Because part of family meals is sharing the same food. You don't have to eat anything if you don't want to…."
"Why not?"	"Because those are the rules."
"Why do I have to be home in time for dinner? How about if I just warm up what you had when I get home?"	"Dinner is more about family than about food. You are an important part of the family."

does it in quirky ways apparent only to the educated eye. To most parents, it all looks like food rejection. Does this sound like your child?

- He looks at the food and doesn't want it on his plate.
- He watches you eat it but doesn't eat it himself.
- Sometimes he allows the serving dish by his plate.
- He wants a small amount on his plate—but doesn't eat it.
- After many meals, he tastes it—then takes it back out again—and again.
- After many tastes and take-outs, he swallows. That means he likes it!

- After that, he likes it, and eats it—sometimes.
- Even if he likes everything on the table, he doesn't eat some of everything that is put before him.
- He eats one or two or three foods.
- Another meal or another day, he eats a different set of one or two or three foods.

All of these are normal child eating behaviors. If your list includes unacceptable mealtime behaviors such as "whines and cries," "refuses to eat," "complains and says 'yuck,'" or "begs for different foods," you are crossing the lines of the division of responsibility in feeding. Children behave poorly when they are pressured.

The key word to describe children's eating is erratic—or *picky*, if you will. Children's normal pickiness is discouraging for parents, who interpret the whole routine as food rejection. It's not. It's a child's way of sneaking up on new food and learning to like it. Research says that it takes children 10–20 neutral exposures before they eat a food. *Neutral exposure* means it shows up on the table again and again, with no pushing or prodding, no persuading or cheerleading, no bribes or nutrition lessons, and no little lectures about starving children *anywhere*. Elizabeth Jackson, reviewer and mother of three nearly grown children, recalls that in the entire 7 years between ages 3 and 10, one of her sons wouldn't allow tomato sauce on his spaghetti. It was the same homemade sauce that he happily ate on his pizza. Reviewer Pam Estes tells of a mother who actually *counted* her number of offerings. After a while, she called Pam. "It's been 20 tries," she reported, "and she still hasn't tasted it. What do I do now?" "I don't know," confessed Pam. "But if you like it, keep having it." Months later, the mother called again. "Thirty-six," she announced. Pam's answer was exactly right. I hope that after running her experiment, the mother stopped counting. For cautious children, it takes years of neutral food exposures, but eventually they learn to eat most foods.

DON'T GET ANTSY
They learn, that is, as long as parents provide both leadership and autonomy with feeding. Parents who can't see their child's molasses-in-January progress get pushy. Those parents raise finicky children. As defined by, well, *me*, picky is okay, but finicky is not. Finicky is when the child eats from a short list of foods that are almost always easy to like, such as sweets, fruit juice, peanut butter, chicken nuggets, and French fries. Children's finickiness is caused by one or both of two feeding behaviors: too few opportunities to learn and pressure. Limiting the menu to foods children readily accept gives them too few opportunities to learn. Trying to hurry things along by over-encouraging, by mandating "no-thank-you bites," or by downright insisting the child eat puts on pressure.

A no-thank-you bite is when you insist that your child taste everything that is on the table. I don't allow no-thank-you bites at my table because children who are forced to taste can't help saying "yuck" and rejecting whatever it is, and I can't help glaring at their parents. Trying

to hurry up food acceptance slows it down. Children who are rushed and pressured are *less* likely to learn to like new food, not more.

Pressured children are also likely to lose their food acceptance skills. As I have said before, your child's food acceptance skills are more important than his eating any particular food on any particular day. Those skills include being comfortable around unfamiliar food, being matter-of-fact and polite about picking and choosing from available foods, being curious about novel food, and being inclined to experiment with it by looking at it, watching others eat it, and tasting it. Your child will develop good food-acceptance skills if you do have meals and you don't get pushy.

Here are some additional don't-get-antsy guidelines:
- Don't hold your breath waiting for your child to eat certain foods. It can take years.
- Don't limit the menu to foods your child readily accepts. You will be bored.
- Don't try to predict what your child will eat. You will go berserk trying to outguess him.
- Don't be invested in getting him to eat. Find something else to feel good about, such as getting a meal on the table.
- Don't run out of food. To be sure everyone gets enough to eat, make enough to have leftovers. Having only enough steak or strawberries to go around once is fine, but have plenty of potatoes to fill up on.
- Don't say "You must eat this before you can eat that." Your child will say, "How many bites?" and you won't know.

The toddler and preschooler chapters in *Child of Mine: Feeding with Love and Good Sense* tell more of the fascinating and often hilarious stories of having young children at the table.

Orchestrate Snacks

Planned sit-down snacks are the ace in the hole of the beleaguered parent. Notice the key words: *planned* and *sit-down*. Planned snacks are not food handouts. In fact, you give planned snacks *instead* of letting your child graze for food and beverages between times. It won't hurt your child to go hungry for 2 or 3 hours until snack time. However, waiting four to six hours until the next meal is way too long for both of you. Keep the snack from spoiling meals by having it 2 or 3 hours after the previous meal and 2 or 3 hours before the next one. That will give your child time to get hungry for the next meal.

As I said earlier, a snack is not a treat—it is a little meal. Include protein, fat, carbohydrate, and maybe some fruit or a vegetable. A good snack might be cookies and milk; apples and peanut butter; crackers, cheese, and fruit juice; or cereal and milk. Snacks help make up for what is missing the rest of the day, so if you had lunch at a fast-food place, include fruit or vegetables in the afternoon snack.

Do not use snacks to put leverage on your child to eat at mealtime, as in "If you want your snack, you had better eat your dinner," or "Since you didn't eat dinner, you can't have a snack." No, no, no! A snack just *is*. It is not a reward or a punishment for *anything*. I use dinner in my examples because it is a bit of a setup for both parents and children. Young children often don't eat much at dinner. They have been eating all day and the dinner menu tends to feature more grown-up food. Parents go to trouble to prepare dinner, want their child to eat it, and may get pushy. Make bedtime snack enjoyable (such as toast or cereal and milk) but not glamorous (don't save dessert for snack), and let your child have snack whether or not he ate much for dinner.

YES, I REALLY MEAN *PLANNED* SNACKS
Consider this scenario. Your child gets up from the table after eating little or nothing and is back 5 minutes later, begging. Many parents say, "Why didn't you eat more? See what I told you—you didn't eat enough and now you are hungry. Oh, all right, what do you want? But next time you have to eat!" Now, what self-respecting child wouldn't be willing to put up with a little aggravation in order to get his way? Reasoning and explaining don't work, either. He won't understand, he won't be persuaded, and he will still want what he wants.

Instead, say, "The meal is over, but snack is coming soon. You can eat then." Then stick to what you say. If he is like most toddlers who are learning that *no* means *no,* he will pitch a fit. Step over him. When he gets done yelling and kicking, the answer is still *no.* After 2 or 3 days he will learn to tend to business when it is time to eat.

"Isn't that a little harsh?" parents ask. "After all, he is *so* little and it *is* only one little cookie. Why make such a big deal over it? What if I offered him whole-wheat crackers instead?"

Sorry, it *is* a big deal. *Your child depends on you to set the limit.* This is not a power trip on your part. If you give in to his food-begging, the list of foods he likes will become shorter and shorter, and his behavior at meals will get worse and worse. When he begs, he doesn't beg for broccoli. He begs for juice and crackers and cookies and candy and potato chips and all the easy-to-like food he has already mastered. He will fill up on those familiar foods and won't be interested in experimenting with new food at mealtime. Most importantly, with food panhandling as in all other ways, it scares your child to get the upper hand with you.

Also consider that in these skirmishes you are building your child's eating attitudes and behaviors for a lifetime. Australian studies show that adolescents who snack on the run, on the way to or from school, all day long, or in the middle of the night are more likely to skip meals than are adolescents who don't snack at these times.[7]

OLDER CHILDREN USE SNACKS FOR LEARNING
As children get older, they take more responsibility for choosing their snacks. A late-school-age child can use figure 6.2, "Planning a Good-Tasting and Satisfying Snack," on page 62, as a guide for snack planning. But even when your child puts together his snack for himself, the schedule doesn't change. "Eat your snack by four o'clock so you don't spoil your dinner" is a legitimate, doing-your-own-job-with-the-division-of-responsibility guideline for a school-age child or teenager. Of course, the timeline depends on your child's school schedule and your family dinnertime.

If your child doesn't take responsibility, consider your parenting. A mother approached me after a presentation complaining that now that her school-age daughter had a bike and money she was buying her own snacks—stopping at the convenience store to get ice cream and other goodies. I told her she couldn't control what her daughter purchased with her own money. However, she could give her a guideline: "Eat your snack by four o'clock so you don't spoil your dinner." What would make her daughter do that, she wanted to know, when she wasn't there to enforce it? Your *authority*, I responded. Your daughter loves you and wants to please you. That is a reasonable limit and you have told her why. She will do what you say if you expect her to.

"But she eats all that high-calorie food that I won't allow in the house!" she finally blurted out, exasperated. I just wasn't getting it! Surely *now* I would tell her what to do! "The only solution for that is to allow those foods in the house!" I told her. "Kids whose parents restrict high-calorie treat foods overeat on them when they get a chance." The mother was sorely disappointed in me. She wanted me to tell her *what*, and I persisted in telling her *how*.

Make Wise Use of Controlled Substances

Controlled substances are the "forbidden foods" in some households—high-fat, high-sugar, and therefore high-calorie foods such as cookies, candy, cake, and chips. How do you manage those foods so *your* child doesn't sneak off to eat them? Purging controlled substances from your menus sets your child up to overeat on them when he gets a chance and increases the likelihood of his gaining too much weight. Make controlled substances a routine part of family meals and snacks. Put potato chips on the table once or twice a week—or more—with the sandwiches. Have a large enough bowl so there are chips left over at the end of the meal. That way, you can be sure everyone has had enough. If chips have been a controlled substance, at first your child will eat a lot of chips and virtually nothing else. After a few meals, the newness will wear off and he will go back to eating his sandwiches and not so many chips.

Offer cookies and milk for occasional snacks—once a week, twice a week—in the long run it won't matter. Put out a big plate of cookies—enough so there are some left over. Your child needs an opportunity to eat as many cookies and others sweets as he wants. At first he may eat a lot, but soon, the newness will wear off and he won't eat so many. Consider making cookies nutritious—peanut butter or oatmeal chocolate chip cookies, chocolate with nuts. While you can nudge the fat and sugar down a bit with too-rich and too-sweet recipes, don't cheat by making cookies low-fat or low-sugar. They won't taste good and your child won't trust you.

Manage desserts by putting a single serving at each person's plate when you set the table. Let your child eat dessert when he wants to—before, during, or after the meal. Don't give seconds. Because desserts have an unfair advantage over vegetables and other nutritious mealtime food, this rule deliberately violates the division of responsibility in feeding. With a new sweet, you get one-trial learning. With new vegetables and other meal-type foods, it takes many exposures. Making desserts available in unlimited quantities takes away the motivation to learn to like new foods. It is all right to offer unlimited cookies at snack time because the cookies aren't competing with other nutritious food.

Treat candy the same as you do other sweets: Offer it for the occasional snack or dessert. Despite what most people think, studies show sugar does not affect children's behavior or cognitive performance.[8] But allowing children to eat candy and other sugary foods instead of meals and snacks amounts to neglect, and neglected children behave poorly. For more suggestions, see the discussion of Halloween candy in figure 7.2.

FIGURE 7.2 THE STICKY TOPIC OF HALLOWEEN CANDY

Halloween candy presents an opportunity for your child to learn to manage sweets and to keep sweets in proportion to the other food he eats. Work toward having him be able to manage his own stash. In order for him to learn, you will have to keep your interference to a minimum. When he comes home from trick-or-treating, let him lay out his booty, gloat over it, sort it and eat as much of it as he wants. Let him do the same the next day. Then have him put it away and relegate it to mealtime and snack time: a couple of small pieces at meals for dessert and as much as he wants for snack time. Offer milk with the candy, and you have a chance at good nutrition.

If he can follow the rules, your child gets to keep control of the stash. Otherwise, you do it, on the assumption that as soon as he can manage it, he gets to keep it.

CONTROLLED SUBSTANCES IN THE SCHOOLS

Hysteria about preventing child obesity has created a school nutrition environment that emphasizes avoiding and restricting rather than providing and nurturing. State and local school districts have gone dashing off after the *what* of feeding, giving little or no attention to the *how*. Across the country, school wellness committees have purged school cafeterias, vending machines, and classrooms of anything that approximates controlled substances: high-fat, high-sugar foods and beverages. Given this preoccupation with restricting the calorically concentrated food that children depend on to get enough to eat, young children especially may have difficulty getting filled up at school.

In my view, our first responsibility with respect to feeding children—at school or anywhere else—is nurturing them: providing them with the nutrients and energy they need to be physically, emotionally, socially, and mentally healthy, and reassuring them that we will take care of them. In order for children to learn well, they must be fed. Making slimming children down the priority of school wellness programs represents misplaced priorities. I would be far happier if wellness committees would address good parenting with food by scheduling meals at regular times when children are hungry—not too early or too late, which is commonly done in order to get everyone through the cafeteria. Just like at home, such good parenting would involve controlling children's access to food so they can go to lunch hungry and ready to eat.

I would appreciate it if school nutrition curriculums emphasized giving children experience with food rather than teaching them lessons about nutrition. Such curriculums would wait until children are intellectually ready, at 12 to 13 years old, to learn the basic food groups and food composition. They can apply that information to snack planning, a part of the food context that is appropriate for them to begin learning to manage. An example would be my little crib sheet in figure 6.2, "Planning a Good-Tasting and Satisfying Snack," on page 62. When they get into high school, they can apply their knowledge about food groups and food composition to meal planning.

My dream curriculum would *never* teach children what to eat, how much to eat, how many servings to have from each of the food groups, what portion sizes to use, and how to limit fat, salt, and sugar. In appendix H, "Nutrition Education in the Schools," I outline principles and strategies that are consistent with the principles of eating competence and feeding dynamics.

But wishing won't make it so. In the meantime, help your child cope with a nutritionally austere school environment by compensating at home. See that he gets enough to eat to get through the day by offering him a good breakfast that contains protein, fat, and carbohydrate. Provide him with a substantial after-school snack that does the same. If controlled substances have been deemed forbidden food at school, guard against your child's developing a heightened appetite for them by being particularly careful to make them a routine part of family meals and snacks.

Be Strategic About Restaurant Food

Seventy percent of families eat out at least once a week. If you can afford it, eating out is a way of having a pleasant and relaxed family meal time. Keep in mind that the first priority is *having* a meal. The second is the *nutritional quality* of the meal—but you can have both. If you eat out rarely, you can afford to throw nutritional considerations to the winds and let your child order only what he likes. If you eat out a lot, it's worth setting up some simple guidelines to help him balance things out.

My suggestions in figure 7.3 on the next page are prescriptive, and here's why. When your child chooses what he wants to eat in a restaurant, he takes over your job of meal planning. As a result, he needs guidelines for choosing what to eat.

Orchestrating family meals requires effort, discipline, leadership, and commitment. The sustained effort of having regular family meals may involve considerable learning and change for you. The discipline is positive and achievable, and joyful rewards are built right in, but it is discipline nonetheless. Take it easy on yourself. Emphasize providing and food-seeking, not depriving and avoidance. Remember how important those meals are as a reliable way for your family to connect. Don't try to change everything at once. Set your priorities, be realistic about what you can do, and acquire new skills and discipline slowly over time. Eventually you will have put together your own personal, useful, and agreeable way of having family meals.

FIGURE 7.3 CHOOSING FOOD IN RESTAURANTS

- Try for three different food groups. This happens automatically anyway. A hamburger and a bun with French fries qualifies, as does pizza (crust, cheese, and topping). A salad, bread, and milk works, as does a taco (tortilla, meat, and vegetables).

- Limit sweets to one per meal. If your child has a milkshake or soda for his beverage, that counts as his sweet. However, if he chooses milk or water, he can still have dessert.

- Keep fried foods down to one per meal. For example, if your child has French fries and a hamburger, a fried pie for dessert will add up to too many fried foods. To have the fried pie, he would have to skip the French fries, and in order to fill up, he might need a second hamburger. Grilled foods such as hamburgers don't count as fried foods because they are relatively low in fat compared with French fries, chicken nuggets, and fish sandwiches, which are starchy and deep-fried. The starch soaks up more fat.

- Keep dessert portions child-size, just as you would at home. That might mean splitting a dessert with someone else at the table, or ordering a sundae rather than a banana split.

- Don't feel obligated to order from children's menus, which are typically limited. Instead, consider the appetizers or a la carte menu. Split meals, or plan to take some home from an adult portion.

- Lay out cost limits ahead of time, then let your older child cope. Order bread and let him fill up on that if he doesn't like what he ordered.

- Expect and enforce positive mealtime behavior. You owe it to the other diners.

References

1. Tucker P, Irwin JD, He M, Bouck LM, Pollett G. Preschoolers' dietary behaviours: parents' perspectives. *Can J Diet Pract Res.* 2006;67:67-71.
2. Nitzke S, Freeland-Graves J. Position of the American Dietetic Association: total diet approach to communicating food and nutrition information. *J Am Diet Assoc.* 2007;107:1224-1232.
3. Epstein L, Paluch R, Consalvi A, Riordan K, Scholl T. Effects of manipulating sedentary behavior on physical activity and food intake. *J Pediatr.* 2002;140:334-339.
4. Baumrind D. Current patterns of parental authority. *Developmental Psychology Monograph.* 1971;4(1 pt.2):1-103.
5. Elder GH. Structural variations in the childrearing relationship. *Sociometry.* 1962;25:241-262.
6. Rhee KE, Lumeng JC, Appugliese DP, Kaciroti N, Bradley RH. Parenting styles and overweight status in first grade. *Pediatrics.* 2006;117:2047-2054.
7. Savige G, MacFarlane A, Ball K, Worsley A, Crawford D. Snacking behaviours of adolescents and their association with skipping meals. *International Journal of Behavioral Nutrition and Physical Activity.* 2007;4:3.
8. Bellisle F. Effects of diet on behaviour and cognition in children. *Br J Nutr.* 2004;92 (suppl 2):S227-2232.

Part
II

Epilogue

If you are lucky, you are learning about positive feeding dynamics when your child is an infant. That will allow you to start off on the right foot by establishing and maintaining a division of responsibility in feeding from the first and by feeding in a way that is positive and gratifying for both you and your child. As a result, your child will gradually develop the eating capabilities discussed in chapter 6, "The Feeding Relationship."

On the other hand, feeding may be painful and problematic for you. If you have been controlling the *how much* or *whether* of your child's eating (or trying to), your child will let you (or let you try) and then intuitively find ways of getting around you. If you have been trying to get your child to eat more, less, or different food than she wants, you likely have unpleasant mealtimes full of struggle and strife. At the other extreme, if you haven't taken responsibility for the *what*, *when*, and *where* of feeding and instead have had an open-kitchen policy, your child is likely a grazer and a grabber, eating only the least-challenging food and taking little interest in meals or in learning to like unfamiliar food.

During preadolescence, children internalize what parents have taught them and begin to do to themselves what has been done to them. Preadolescents and adolescents are casual about feeding themselves if that is the way they have been raised. They diet if they have been dieted; they are slavishly puritanical about eating if that is the way they have been raised. (On the other hand, they may be slavishly defiant.)

Making Repairs

If you have been crossing the lines of the division of responsibility and getting into struggles about feeding, you have some repair work to do. But not to worry—we all make mistakes. The name of the game with raising children is to give it your best effort, find out if it works, and then tinker with it. Children have a wonderful way of changing if their parents change—provided their parents *really* change and *stay* changed. The younger children are, the more quickly they change.

HAVE A TALK ABOUT CHANGE

If your child is a preschooler or older, tell her there is a change coming, tell her what that change is going to be, and tell her why. You might say, "You know, I have been trying to get you to _____ (eat your vegetables, eat less, use your silverware all the time, *put your feeding error here*). It seems like it hasn't worked. You don't like it, and I don't like fighting with you about it. So, from now on, here is what I am going to do. I am going to put the food on the table, and I am going to leave it up to you to decide what and how much to eat from what's on the table. What do you think of that?"

Now, chances are your child will like the sound of this quite a lot. "Does that mean I can have all the dessert I want?" she will ask. "No." (The answer *is* no.) "But I will put your serving of dessert by your plate and you may eat it when you want to."

Wow! Cool! What kid wouldn't like that? Well, wait, there's more. So you go on. "Now, part of the reason I nag you to eat at mealtime is so you don't keep snacking all the time. So the snacks are going to change, too. From now on, instead of letting you eat whenever you want, we will have special snack times. We'll talk about foods you like and foods I am comfortable giving you. I'll keep track of snack time and put the snacks on the table for you just like it's a meal. And just like at mealtime, you can eat what you like and as much or as little as you like from what is on the table. What do you think of that?"

Younger children may not have much to offer at this point. They may think of a few things they want for snacks, and you can negotiate about that. Keep in mind that "snack" doesn't mean "treat"; it means "little meal." If your child has been grazing to get treats, simply incorporate those treats into your planned meals and snacks. Have potato chips or Flamin' Hot Cheetos with the lunchtime sandwiches or offer cookies or snack cakes and milk for snacks. (Read the label—the Cheetos are made with enriched flour, and the cakes and cookies probably are, too.) Otherwise, your changes will be more negative than positive, and you will get a lot of unnecessary resistance.

Older children may have thoughtful contributions to make. A 12-year-old and her parents agreed on set snack times and that she could get her snack herself, choosing from a list of foods that were acceptable to all parties. The next week, the parents complained that she loaded up on food just before dinner. I asked why. "Well," she responded, "the reason I eat so much before dinner is because we always have something I don't like at dinner, like roast beef, and then they make me eat it." Her parents saw her point. They agreed to lay off the strong-arm feeding, and she agreed to get her snack out of the way by 4:00 so she could be hungry for dinner. The next time they had roast beef she surprised them by trying a little. It is impressive what kids will do if they feel their parents respect how they feel and what they have to say.

PREPARE TO BE THE ENFORCER

Just because you and your child have agreed on a plan of action doesn't mean instituting it will be trouble-free. Like grown-ups, children can be enthusiastic about setting up rules but less than enthusiastic about enacting them. Your child will want to bend the rules. Reasoning with her and reminding her she helped make them won't help. You have to be the enforcer.

Clearly, discussion with younger children about enacting a new plan is mostly nonverbal. Do tell your toddler in simple words about meals and snacks; she is likely to understand more than you think. But the primary way you communicate with her is by enforcing the plan. You will "tell" your toddler about the division of responsibility by having pretty set times for meals and sit-down snacks, by letting her eat as much as she wants at those times, and by eliminating her between-time food and beverage handouts (except for water), even when she begs. Your toddler may "tell" you about her displeasure by having tantrums when she doesn't get handouts. You will answer back that you mean what you say by stepping over her while she rages.

Your child will change relatively quickly if you change and stay changed. Toddlers take 3 or 4 days to change if you weather the storm and are consistent with setting limits. Preschoolers change within 2 or 3 weeks; school-age children take about twice as long. Older children need more time to trust that their parents mean what they say and won't go back to the old ways. Teenagers change if they see the merit of what you propose and are willing to make family meal participation a priority. If you waffle and slip and give in sometimes, it will take longer.

Once you change, you have to stay changed or the old behaviors will come right back. After 3 or 4 months, continuing will get lots easier. The new behavior will feel familiar and you will be reaping the rewards of having pleasant mealtimes where your child does well with eating.

KNOW THINGS WILL GET WORSE AT FIRST

If you decide to change the way you handle feeding, be advised that your child's eating will become more extreme before it reverts to "normal." Your food-restricted child will eat lots more for a while. Your vegetable-coerced child will take a long vacation from vegetables. Your food-pressured child will eat very small amounts for a while. One mother, a dietitian, told me that after she decided to stop forcing her school-age sons to eat their vegetables and drink their milk (and having fights about eating), it took more than 6 months before the children started experimenting with them. At first, all they consumed was meat and bread. As you can imagine, seeing her children not eat vegetables or drink milk made that dietitian mother pretty nervous. In fact, it may have taken the boys longer than usual to start experimenting because they sensed her nervousness. Kids are perceptive—her sons knew how important it was to her that they eat well, so they needed plenty of time to trust that she wouldn't go back to pressuring them.

If Things Don't Get Better

If your child's eating doesn't get any better after a few weeks, consider the possibility that you aren't quite getting it. Review the discussion in chapter 7, "Stuff to Know to Have Family Meals," to be sure you are using effective strategies for establishing and maintaining pleasant and good-natured mealtimes, resisting being drawn across the line of division of responsibility in feeding, building your child's positive mealtime behavior, addressing *negative* mealtime behavior, and knowing the difference between normal and negative child eating behavior. Also follow the advice in chapter 7 to be sure you are using positive strategies for orchestrating snacks, making wise use of controlled substances, and managing family meals in restaurants.

CHECK YOURSELF FOR FEEDING ERRORS
Consider the possibility that you are being restrictive or pushy without realizing it. Both tendencies are subtle, pervasive, and difficult to dislodge. Identifying the glitch can take some real detective work. Carefully review chapter 6, "The Feeding Relationship," to look for clues as to whether you are failing to do your jobs with feeding or intruding on your child's prerogatives with eating. It can be something as subtle as holding your breath when you pass second helpings to your large or enthusiastically eating child or as obvious as being inconsistent about structure. Two of my small patients continued to eat poorly, even though their parents insisted they weren't pressuring them to eat. It finally emerged that the father cared deeply about table manners. He continually insisted that his 3- and 5-year-old sons neatly use their silverware and napkins. It appeared the boys were so overwhelmed by his unrealistic expectations that they weren't able to eat. In *How to Get Your Kid to Eat … But Not Too Much* I go into more detail about how to solve childhood feeding problems.

A LEAP OF FAITH AND STEADY NERVES
Weather the storms, keep your courage, and don't revert to your old patterns. Trusting that your child's eating will improve takes a leap of faith and steady nerves. You may need to consult with a feeding specialist who *truly* understands and accepts the division of responsibility in feeding to plan your strategy, detect your negative behaviors, and maintain your courage and commitment. Changing the way you *feed* may require changing the way you *eat*. You can only take your child as far as you have gone yourself. To be confident that your child will sneak up on new food and learn to like it, you first have to develop your own food acceptance skills. To trust that your child will regulate her food intake based on her hunger, appetite, and satiety, you first need to have experienced that for yourself. Do it if you need to. Helping your child become a good eater is *that* important.

Part
III
HOW TO COOK

Prologue

In previous parts I encouraged you to celebrate eating and take good care of yourself and your child with food. Now we move on to extending and supporting that celebration and caring with food management. Our task is to translate the positive principles of eating and feeding into food preparation. Unless you have unlimited resources, in order to celebrate eating and take good care of yourself with food, you have to cook—and keep on cooking. In order for you to keep it up, it has to be rewarding, and you need to feel successful at it. As we found in our research, feeling comfortable with cooking, and even enjoying it, can increase your overall eating competence.[1]

This part is a food-management primer—an instructional manual about planning and preparing family meals as well as including children in the kitchen and at the table. *Secrets* is written to convey the message, "You can do this," and to help you begin to learn your way in the kitchen.

Secrets Teaches Food Management

I chose every one of the recipes in this book to teach you something about food, nutrition, or cooking. More importantly, I chose every recipe because I like to eat it, and most other people do, too. I used many of the recipes when I was raising my own family, and my children still make them. They are easy, they use familiar foods, and they can be assembled and cooked in 20 to 30 minutes. Because some are cooked in the oven, others in the slow cooker, and still others simmered on the stove, they may take longer to cook in some cases, but your actual *production* time is low. To help you with longer-term planning, the recipes in all three chapters have been combined into a cycle menu in the planning chapter.

In chapter 8, "How to Get Cooking," and chapter 9, "How to Keep Cooking," I plan every main-dish recipe into a meal. Then I go on to give you fast tips about the recipe, list jobs you can do the night before, and give suggestions for presenting the food to make it attractive. Then I address the children—both in the kitchen and at the table—with suggestions for involving your children in food preparation and adapting the meal for children.

Chapter 10, "Enjoy Vegetables and Fruits," reminds you that enjoyment is a far better reason than nutritional obligation for eating your broccoli or zucchini. Chapter 11, "Planning to Get You Cooking," emphasizes using planning as its own reward in making cooking and eating enjoyable. Chapter 12, "Shopping to Get You Cooking," shows you how to streamline, as much as you can, your efforts to keep groceries in the house.

I have chosen recipes to help you learn food skills and strategies so you can be successful with the everyday challenge—and reward—of getting meals on the table. Many of the recipes have figures that give more detail about the food—how to purchase, how to handle, how not to worry. I find food fascinating and the science of food even more so. Knowing the basic principles of cooking and why certain things work and others don't can give you the satisfaction of knowing what to do and, more than that, why you're doing it.

At the end of many of the recipes, I suggest variations. Check those out, because the simple changes will vastly expand your recipe repertoire without complicating your cooking life. To remind you that they are there, the variations are bolded, indexed, and listed in the recipe list. I also hope that the variations spark some ideas and that you'll feel comfortable expanding on them.

Increase Your Efficiency

To help manage daily time constraints and competing priorities, think before you cook. Read through the recipes, make up your mind about your menu, do the night-before jobs, and plan your sequence of cooking times.

Think about cleanliness. Keep an orderly space by cleaning up as you go along. Keep a bowl of hot sudsy water handy to wash your utensils.

Think about putting other people to work. Coordinate and supervise while they cook.

Think about PPMs—pre-prepared meals—by using extras from dinner for lunch the next day and by doubling recipes and freezing half.

Think about the future. Letting your young child play in the kitchen and admiring odd-looking food prepared by awkward little fingers will produce an older child who is hooked on cooking and can make a real contribution.

Think about food safety. Wash your hands thoroughly and often, and teach your children to do the same. Keep hot food hot (above 140 degrees F—simmering or hot eating temperature) and cold food cold (40 degrees F or below—refrigerator temperature). Discard food held at room temperature for 2 hours or more.

The Mother Principle

Figure PIII.1 on the next page outlines the Mother Principle of meal planning. I planned the recipes and menus in these chapters with these principles in mind. I am using the term "mother" as an honorary title to denote the person who takes primary responsibility for nurturing with food. That person could be a father

or a grandparent as well as a mother. The Mother Principle combines nutrition principles with feeding dynamics and eating competence principles. The Mother Principle gives you the same guidance as in figure 5.1, "Being Considerate without Catering," on page 48, but in more detail.

APPLYING THE MOTHER PRINCIPLE
I realize the list adds up, but settle down, we can do this. Let's start by planning a meal that includes all the food groups as well as includes four or five foods or more. Consider our first menu: tuna noodle casserole, poppy seed coleslaw, celery sticks and dill pickles, bread, butter, and milk. Now let's do the count: protein (tuna), two starches (noodles and bread), two vegetables (cabbage, celery, and cucumbers), and milk. That's six. I counted celery and cucumbers together as one because you usually don't eat that much of the crudités. Oh, and butter. That's seven. Then if you count the cream cheese, that's eight, and why not count the jam? That's nine.

If someone in your family is skeptical about the tuna and you feel like going to the trouble, flake the tuna, heat it up with the mushroom soup and milk to make a sauce, and serve the sauce in one dish and the noodles in another. If you don't feel like it, don't worry. There are plenty of other foods to eat. Sometimes one person gets lucky, sometimes another.

The Mother Principle also says, "to give your child the fat he needs without overloading your menus with fat, include high-, moderate-, and low-fat foods." Let's again examine our menu. The tuna noodle casserole and coleslaw are moderate in fat; the celery sticks, dill pickles, and bread are low in fat; and the butter and cream cheese are high in fat. If you offer whole milk, you will have three high-fat foods. That's just fine. Trust your child to eat as much or a little fat as he needs. Chapter 13, "Choosing Food," discusses nutrition and food composition in more detail.

Put pleasure first. The Mother Principle incorporates pleasure, but the element of planning might spook you into forgetting it. *You might eat dreary food in order to satisfy your nutritional requirements, but your child won't,* even if you tell him it is good for him. You will tire of foisting dreary food on your child, and you just might give up on family meals altogether.

FIGURE PIII.1 THE MOTHER PRINCIPLE OF MEAL PLANNING

Plan meals that include all the food groups: meat or other protein, grains, fruits and vegetables, and dairy. Round out your meals with spreads and sauces and with dessert, if you wish. Offer four or five foods. Let your child (and yourself) choose what and how much to eat from what is on the table. Here are the kinds of foods to put on the table:

- **Protein source.** Meat, poultry, fish, dry beans, eggs, or nuts. If you have cereal and milk for breakfast, milk can be the protein. Cheese, like milk, gives protein and also calcium so it can do double duty.

- **Two grains or starchy foods.** Include two foods from this list. Every culture has a certain starchy food that *has* to show up on the table, such as rice, spaghetti, grits, potatoes, or plantain. Children and other people can generally eat bread and other starchy foods if all else fails. Potatoes aren't a grain, but they are starchy and easy to like. Make the second starchy food bread, and put it on the table with every meal. Your bread can be anything made with grain, such as regular sliced bread, tortillas, biscuits, cornbread, oatmeal bread, chapattis, fry-bread, or bagels.

- **Fruit or vegetable or both.** Canned, frozen, or fresh fruits and vegetables are all okay. Try raw vegetables with a dip, put a dab of butter or some cheese sauce on vegetables to perk them up, or toss frozen vegetables into the soup. Corn, potatoes, and lima beans are starchy, so you get a twofer—they count as a choice from two lists. In fact, lima beans also have a lot of protein, so there you get a *three*fer. However, the fewer choices you put on the table, the greater the likelihood the meal will defeat inexperienced eaters.

- **Dairy.** Use whole milk for children under age 2 years. After that, only switch to lower fat milk if everyone likes it, drinks it well, and has another reliable fat source. You depend on milk for calcium and vitamin D, so if you substitute a soy or rice milk, compare the label to be sure it gives the same amount of protein, calcium, and vitamin D as cow's milk and keep in mind the product is likely to be low in fat. Milk and other dairy products are a twofer because they give protein *and* calcium. At breakfast, milk can do double duty as both a protein and a calcium source and the fruit/vegetable can be orange juice.

- **Butter, margarine, dressings, sauces.** Offer regular (not diet, low-calorie or fat-free) salad dressing, vegetable dip, or gravy. These fatty foods make foods taste better. Children depend on fat with the meal to get the calories they need. Let children eat as much or as little fat as they want. To give your child the fat he needs without overloading your menus with fat, include high-, moderate-, and low-fat foods.

You offer the food, your child eats—or doesn't. Help him be successful by matching familiar with unfamiliar food, favorite with not-so-favorite. Don't make more or different food. Don't make him eat some of everything on the table. He may just drink milk and eat bread. That is all right. At another meal he will eat more or different food choices.

Children in the Kitchen

Your child will grow up enjoying cooking, and it will hold no terrors for him when he is grown, if you let him share cooking chores with you. Many of the recipes in this book have suggestions for involving children. When your child is young, your task is to find chores for him that are safe and interesting and that don't slow you down too much. A toddler can happily play in water in the sink, with mixing cups and spoons, or he can more or less wash durable vegetables like potatoes, carrots, and celery. A pan of rice for measuring and pouring is good for a few minutes of entertainment.

As your child gets older, he will become more and more helpful. An older child can assemble simple recipes, if you help with the hot dishes and sharp knives. I have written the recipes simply, but you might want to simplify them further for a child by making note of which pan or bowls to use. For a child who does not read, adapt written directions by drawing pictures of the ingredients. To get an idea of how to do this, see Mollie Katzen's book *Pretend Soup and Other Real Recipes* or use some recipes from Katzen's book. Older children can do most of the tasks for simple recipes and you can be the assistant.

Of course, a child can set the table. At age 16 months, Sebastian, our office toddler, is most territorial about *his* job of putting the glasses on the table. Your child might enjoy setting the table, and it is helpful, but don't get in a rut. To keep cooking interesting to your child, share the cooking jobs. Even when your child becomes adept in the kitchen, however, don't wander off.

For children, the main attraction of cooking is being with *you*. If you run out of jobs to do for tonight's dinner, keep yourself in the kitchen by starting on the next day's meal. Read the suggestions for the night before and work ahead.

Make sure you have equipment that will make your child's participation in meal preparation safe and fun. Children need sturdy stools to stand on. I like the little two-step folding ladders that have the waist-high, overarching handles because they give children something to hang on to. Sebastian drags a chair into the kitchen to join his parents with cooking. Children need aprons. Consider cutting the arms out of a big old shirt, then button it on backward. Or check out the hardware store for the little full-length carpenter aprons. If you tie a knot in the string that goes behind the neck, it converts easily to child size.

Children at the Table

With most of the recipes, and the menus accompanying them, I have made suggestions for adapting meals for children. Being considerate in the ways I suggest is not short-order cooking. It is just setting up the menu to help your child to be successful. If the dish seems a little strange, like Mostaccioli with Spinach and Feta, it will help your child to have something familiar on the table that he knows he can manage, like corn. Remember, your child doesn't have to eat everything that is served; he can pick and choose from what you have made available. If a dish is complex, like Marinated Chicken Stir-Fry, I suggest making some minor modifications to serve some of the parts separately. After a child masters the parts, he will be ready to start learning to like the whole.

For the learning eater at the table, we have to be careful about the shape and texture of food and about detecting food sensitivities and allergies. A young child could choke on whole, raw vegetables like carrots or celery, or on some crisp-tender cooked vegetables, such as carrots again, or broccoli. You might cook a few vegetables a little longer for your youngest eater, or give him the more tender ones, like zucchini. Before you give the beginning eater a mixed dish, try to introduce him to all the components separately. That way, if he has an allergic response, you won't have to guess about what caused the reaction.

Sometimes I suggest dessert, and sometimes I don't. You don't have to have dessert; you don't have to avoid it. I have used dessert to make a meal more enjoyable and filling and to make a nutritional contribution. Many desserts have fruit; many have milk as well. When serving dessert to a young child, it works best to put a single helping of dessert at each plate and let him eat it when he wants to—first, last, or during. Don't give seconds on dessert. Putting dessert on the table keeps it from being something that you hold out to reward your child for eating his vegetables. When your child is older and has mastered his food acceptance skills, you can go back to the traditional method of offering dessert at the end of the meal.

Taste Comes First

I hope that dealing with food and cooking so concretely will help you settle down and stop worrying so much about fat, nutrition, food safety, the environment, and who-knows-what-else that you can't get a meal on the table. To help you relax about those worries, I will help you find the middle ground. In order for food to taste good, you have to use some salt and fat in preparing it. You don't, however, have to throw away all controls and let the sky be the limit. You will discover an in-between, where you use fat and salt but don't overload your food—or yourself—with it. Be moderate, but do *not* filter out the essence of good taste by strictly limiting fat and salt. These recipes will help you know what is moderate—not too much and not too little.

SALT

My menus contribute to an average sodium intake of 3,000–4,000 milligrams per day—a moderate amount. My standard is 1/4 teaspoon of salt (525 milligrams of sodium) per cup of food (or broth, or water for cooking pasta or vegetables). To reduce sodium to the 2,300-milligram therapeutic level recommended by the Dietary Guidelines, leave out the salt in the recipes, choose salt-free soups, avoid cured meats, and use frozen or fresh vegetables instead of canned. And see a registered dietitian.

FAT

My recipes have about 1 to 2 teaspoons of fat per helping. I follow my own advice about including low-, moderate-, and high-fat foods in meals and varying fat sources. I use butter, olive oil, and a variety of vegetable oils. I recommend olive oil when a recipe benefits from the flavor. Use the better-tasting virgin olive oil for dressings and sautéing and the more heat-resistant "refined" or "pure" olive oil for frying. To find the virgin olive oil that is right for you, have a tasting party.

I have said this before—more than once—but it is worth repeating: If you are going to go to all the trouble of keeping up the day-to-day routine of family meals, those meals have to be richly rewarding for you to plan, prepare, and eat. The juice absolutely and positively has *got* to be worth the squeeze. Otherwise, your energy will run out, you will drift away from your best intentions, and you will go back to grabbing, eating on the run, and feeling dissatisfied and guilty. When the joy goes out of eating, nutrition suffers.

References

1. Lohse B, Satter E, Horacek T, Gebreselassie T, Oakland MJ. Measuring Eating Competence: psychometric properties and validity of the ecSatter Inventory. *J Nutr Educ Behav.* 2007;39 (suppl):S154-S166.

Chapter
8
How to Get Cooking

Approach your cooking with the anticipation of pleasure, respect for the food, a clean kitchen, an organized mind, and flexible expectations. This chapter and the five that follow will help you build a foundation for being a good, fast, efficient, and wholesome cook. In previous chapters, I encouraged you to celebrate eating and take good care of yourself with food. Now, dish by dish, I bless the food. It is remarkable how discussing actual food says, "Yes, I really mean it. You may eat that—and that—and that."

I assume you don't know much about food preparation. I have chosen good-tasting 20- to 30-minute recipes and menus to teach you about a variety of foods and a variety of cooking methods using minimal cooking equipment. I have followed the Mother Principle that I outlined in Prologue III, "How to Cook," to plan menus that allow variety and exploration but are considerate of inexperienced eaters.

We will start with success and build on it. There is much to learn, and developing cooking intuition takes time. Working off the principle that you will benefit from learning to walk before you can enjoy running, this chapter starts out easiest and ends up easy. The next

chapter, "How to Keep Cooking," has recipes that are equally timesaving, have a few more steps, and may be a bit more interesting. Wait to prepare those recipes until you have had some success with the simpler ones in this chapter.

These are dinner recipes that make about six servings and that use standard cans, boxes, and bottles of ingredients. Since serving size is relative, you may find that you have to increase or decrease the recipe size to provide for your family. Keep your own little recipe history. Make notes in the margins about cooking times, oven temperatures—anything you think will help you the next time you make the recipe.

Because I want this cooking lesson to be brief and accessible, I haven't given guidelines for breakfast or lunch. However, you can provide very well for your lunches by eating leftovers; you can even double a recipe and have the extra for lunch. In chapter 10, "Enjoy Vegetables and Fruits," I suggest serving pumpkin or apple custard for breakfast. Breakfast is often a simple meal, and that's fine—the important thing is *having* it. Your child will eat breakfast well if you do.

Now let's have some fun learning how to cook!

Tuna Noodle Casserole

I am starting with tuna noodle casserole to make a point, and it is this: *Do not be a food snob!* This dish tastes great, is easy to make, and uses ingredients you can keep on hand. Like many other cooks, I started out learning to cook from a recipe book called *Take a Can of Soup*. You can mix canned soup with almost anything and turn it into dinner! Today, in addition to being just too, *too* ordinary, cooking with canned soup has fallen into disfavor because of the high salt and presumed high fat content. However, diluted in the recipes we use here, the amount of sodium or fat per serving is reasonable. Once again, eating dinner is far more important than avoiding salt and fat.

INGREDIENTS

1/2 lb dry packaged noodles (either wide or narrow)
7-oz can water-packed tuna
10 1/2-oz can cream of mushroom soup
1/2 cup milk
10-oz package frozen peas

MENU

Tuna noodle casserole
Poppy seed coleslaw (page 155)
Celery sticks, dill pickles
Crusty bread for something to chew: try toasted or
*   plain bagels, English muffins, or French bread*
Butter
Milk
Bread with cream cheese and jam for dessert

METHOD

Summary: Boil and drain noodles, mix them with tuna, canned soup, milk, and peas, and then gently heat.

Fill a 4 1/2-quart pan about half to two-thirds full of water, add 1 teaspoon salt per quart of water, and bring to a rapid boil. Add *1/2 pound dry packaged noodles* and boil until al dente (see figure 8.1 on the next page).

Meanwhile, open a *7-ounce can water-packed tuna*, drain it, and break the tuna into flakes with a fork. Mix with a *10 1/2-ounce can cream of mushroom soup* and *1/2 cup milk.*

Then open a *10-ounce package frozen peas* and empty it into a colander. When the noodles are done, drain them through the peas in the colander to thaw the peas and warm them up.

Combine everything: Put the noodles and peas into the noodle pan and add the tuna-soup-milk mixture.

Turn the heat on medium low and warm the whole thing up, stirring occasionally until everything is hot.

RECIPE NOTES

Fast tip: Warm the mushroom soup up ahead of time in the microwave or a pan to save stirring and reheating time and keep from breaking apart and overcooking the noodles.

The night before: Review the recipes for the whole menu; find all the ingredients, menu items, and equipment, and put them where they will be handy.

Added touch: Add any or all of the following vegetables or herbs:
*   2 to 4 Tbsp dried onion flakes*
*   1 to 2 Tbsp dried parsley flakes*
*   4-oz can mushroom stems and pieces, drained*
*   1/4 cup chopped green or black olives*

If you want to substitute fresh herbs for dried herbs in a recipe, use about three times more. Dried herbs are potent, and too much can ruin the dish. As a rule of thumb, one teaspoon of dried herb equals one tablespoon fresh herb.

Involving your children: For this meal, a preschooler can cut up the dill pickles and olives with a plastic picnic knife; she can also open the peas and pour them into the colander.

If you help with draining the hot noodles, an older child can make this all by herself!

Adapting this meal for children: This meal is kid-friendly. It is all right to serve tuna noodle casserole to children who are just getting started with table food, as long as they have been previously exposed to all of the ingredients. For them, cut the noodles quite finely, mix in enough sauce to make it moist, and let them eat with their fingers. Keep in mind that a finger food is anything that sticks together long enough to get from dish to mouth. Even preschoolers and younger school-age children make use of this technique. Often they eat with their fork or spoon—but load it with their fingers. So relax. For a young child who might have trouble chewing the celery and dill pickles, open a can of mandarin oranges. Plain bread or toast will also be easier for a toddler to chew than bagels.

The bread with cream cheese and jam makes a fine dessert, but follow the dessert rules: put a serving at each plate when you set the table, let your child eat it before, during, or after the meal, but allow only one helping. As my granddaughters taught me, if you allow it, children will fill up on bread and jam and not eat anything else.

Variation: Baked Tuna Noodle Casserole Put the tuna noodle mixture in an ovenproof casserole dish, sprinkle on some packaged bread crumbs and some grated cheese, and heat at 350° F uncovered for 20 minutes. If you prefer to heat in the microwave, use a microwave-safe dish, sprinkle with the cheese of your choice (bread crumbs will just get soggy in the microwave), cover, and heat for 4 to 5 minutes on high. Uncover and sprinkle on crushed potato chips. Voilà! For another variation, used canned salmon instead of canned tuna.

FIGURE 8.1 COOKING PASTA
For pasta that's well cooked and doesn't stick together, use plenty of water and keep it boiling rapidly the whole time the noodles cook. Fill a 4 1/2-quart pan half to two-thirds full of water to give room for the noodles and for the water to boil. Add 1 teaspoon salt per quart of water to flavor the noodles. Bring to a hard, rolling boil. Add the noodles all at once and stir to keep them from sticking together. *Watch the pot* until it boils again and turn it down to keep it boiling but not boiling over. Otherwise, it will overflow all over the stove, as mine has done many times. Estimate the cooking time according to the package directions, but test for doneness 1 to 2 minutes before the package says to. Check by tasting. The noodles should be soft but give your teeth just a bit of resistance: That's what is meant by *al dente*.

FIGURE 8.2 OIL- OR WATER-PACKED TUNA
I chose water-packed tuna because that is about all I could find in my grocery stores. You may prefer oil-packed tuna, and that's fine if you can find it. Some people think it's more flavorful. Just drain the fat and throw it away.

FIGURE 8.3 MERCURY IN CANNED TUNA
Being a long-lived fish, tuna is potentially high in mercury. To limit your mercury exposure, use light tuna and eat tuna or other large fish no more than once a week. Avoid eating tuna at all if you are pregnant or planning to become pregnant. In general, canned light tuna is lower in mercury than white tuna, but sometimes it contains just as much, or more. For more information, go to www.consumerreports.org and search on "mercury in tuna."

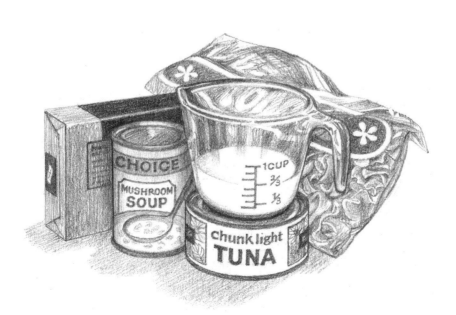

Macaroni-Tomato-Hamburger Casserole

In the cycle menu, which I introduce in chapter 11, "Planning to Get You Cooking," I call this a *dinner of last resort.* It is the Friday night, don't-feel-like-cooking meal. We all need these meals: They are the fast and easy throw-together meals that you can practically prepare in your sleep. **Tuna Noodle Casserole** is another good last-resort meal because everything can be kept on hand. Other good last-resort meals are **Spaghetti Carbonara** and **Spinach-Feta Frittata** (or any other kind of frittata). On page 138 in chapter 9, "How to Keep Cooking," I give you a list of additional grab-and-dump meal suggestions.

INGREDIENTS
1/2 lb dry macaroni
1 large onion, chopped
1 lb ground beef
28-oz can and *15-oz can diced tomatoes*

MENU
Macaroni-tomato-hamburger casserole
*Fruit, like apple wedges, banana chunks, canned
     mandarin oranges, or fruit in season*
Chewy bread
Butter
Milk
Ice cream and store-bought cookies

METHOD
Summary: Boil and drain noodles, brown ground beef and onion, and then gently mix it all up with tomatoes.

Fill a 4 1/2-quart pan about half to two-thirds full of water, add 1 teaspoon salt per quart of water, and bring to a rapid boil. Add *1/2 pound dry macaroni* and boil until al dente. Taste for doneness. Drain in a colander.

While the water for the macaroni heats, chop *1 large onion.* In a large skillet at medium heat, break up and brown *1 pound ground beef* (a potato masher works well) and cook the chopped onion. There will be enough fat in the meat to grease the pan and cook the onion. Cook until the meat loses all its red or pink color and the onion is clear.

Combine everything: Put the macaroni back in its pan (or the skillet, whichever is bigger) and add the cooked ground beef and onions.

Add a *28-ounce can and a 15-ounce can diced tomatoes* (can sizes vary, so come as close as you can to this amount).

Cook the mixture over medium heat, stirring occasionally. Don't stir too energetically or you will break up the macaroni.

RECIPE NOTES
Fast tip: Keep chopped onion refrigerated in a glass jar with a tight-fitting lid. The jar won't leak odor into your refrigerator. Chopped onion keeps for a week or two, and having it on hand speeds cooking time considerably. Some grocery stores carry frozen chopped onion, which tastes pretty good, although not as good as fresh. To speed cooking and to save wear and tear on the macaroni, heat the tomatoes before you combine them with the beef and noodles.

The night before: Find the canned tomatoes and the cooking pans. Place the frozen ground beef in the refrigerator to thaw. Line up the other ingredients for this recipe and for the other menu items.

Involving your children: Children can open tomato cans and macaroni packages, and they can wash and cut up apples and bananas. If you can live with a little mangling, even a toddler can use a plastic picnic knife to cut up bananas and peeled apple wedges.

Adapting this meal for children: This meal is another good one for children. The casserole is moist, soft, and easy to chew. It is also slippery, so remember that it qualifies as finger food. Beginning eaters may have this as long as they have been introduced separately to all of the ingredients.

Because macaroni-tomato-hamburger casserole has no added fat, it is a low-fat dish. Children need more fat. With this meal, you depend on butter on the bread and fat in the milk to give children the fat they need. Make these foods available to your children, and let them do the regulating. They will eat as much or as little fat as they need.

Variation: Use canned tomatoes with seasonings. Check out the tomato shelf in the grocery store. You will find Italian, Cajun, and Mexican tomatoes, tomatoes with onions and garlic, and others. Use a variety of macaroni and noodle shapes and sizes.

FIGURE 8.4 GROUND BEEF

Ground beef is out of favor these days. Well, it is and it isn't. Many people won't buy it in the grocery store because they think it isn't good for them. Then they end up at dinnertime with nothing to eat, so they scoot to the drive-through and get quarter-pounders with fries. It's crazy but understandable: If it is "bad" for you, you can eat it only when you don't think about it too much. So, forget about the "bad" label and *think* about it.

You don't have to be afraid of ground beef, but you do need to treat it respectfully. Ground beef is subject to contamination because harmful bacteria on the surface of the meat can be mixed throughout in the grinding process. Ground beef is rarely contaminated, but the *E. coli 0157* that is typical is particularly nasty. Illness from *E. coli 0157* can lead to kidney failure. Handle all ground beef as if it were contaminated. Don't let meat juices drip into raw produce, and wash your hands, utensils, and countertop with soap before and after you handle it. Cook it to an internal temperature of at least 160° F. For more about handling food safely, see figure 11.4, "Food Safety," on page 183.

You and your family can feel comfortable about eating ground beef. It is the key to many satisfying meals, and beef is highly nutritious (see "Enjoy Red Meat," pages 207 to 208). Ground beef is easy for kids to eat; it cooks quickly and is easy to freeze and keep on hand. For the recipes in this book I use ground chuck. Ground chuck is often labeled *lean ground beef.* It may also be labeled *80/20,* which means that 20 percent of the weight of the ground beef is in the form of fat. The level of fat is moderate but not so low that you lose flavor. So little fat cooks out that you may not even have to drain it. If you want leaner ground beef, check the total fat percentage declared by the Nutrition Facts label. However, don't forget that the idea is to use fat to make food taste good, not to avoid it altogether. Having said all that, the bottom line is experimenting until you find a ground beef with a fat content that gives you the results and flavor that you want.

To be tender, ground beef and other meats need to be cooked at moderate temperatures. Keeping the heat somewhere around medium also keeps fat from splattering all over your stove and wall and cuts down on cleanup. To me, "browning" ground beef means cooking until all the pink color is gone. To you, browning may mean cooking until it actually develops a brown color, which gives it more flavor but also dries it out more. If you like your ground beef really brown, you may want to cook your onions separately because they, too, will get brown and develop a pronounced caramelized flavor. On the other hand, you may like that. Who am I to say?

Keeping ground beef on hand is easy. When you get home from the grocery store, separate it into 1-pound packages in 1-quart zip top bags, flatten the bags, and freeze them. Flattened packages thaw quickly—but do be sure to thaw them in the refrigerator.

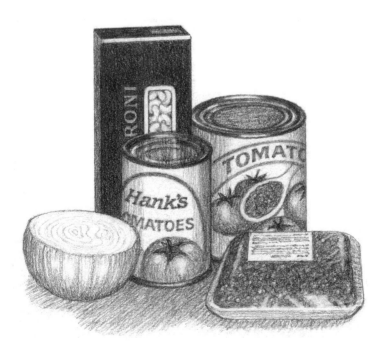

icken and Rice

If you are at home to put food in the oven and give it time to bake, there is no easier way to cook for a family than making oven meals. Your food can be assembled before the just-before-mealtime jitters hit. A well-constructed oven meal does most of the last-minute work for you; you just take it out of the oven and put it on the table. You can clean up the kitchen early and know dinner is taken care of. You can also use the hot oven to prepare other foods, like warming French bread or baking a dessert.

For all those reasons, and because it *tastes* good and is filling and satisfying, chicken and rice was one of my standbys when my children were growing up. They have all, in turn, made it in their own kitchens.

INGREDIENTS

1 1/2 cups uncooked enriched white rice
10-oz can cream of mushroom soup
1 packet dry onion soup mix
1 3/4 cups water
2 Tbsp fresh or 2 tsp dried parsley
6 boneless chicken breast halves or boneless thighs
*   or both, about 1 1/2 lb*
Sprinkle paprika
1/4 tsp black pepper

MENU

Chicken and rice
Glazed carrots (page 155) or vegetables in season
French bread warmed in the oven
Butter
Milk
Apple custard (page 163) or fruit in season

METHOD
Summary: Combine uncooked rice, canned soup, dry soup mix, and water. Top with chicken, cover, and bake.

Preheat oven (see the next column for temperature). Mix together in a 9 × 13-inch glass baking dish *1 1/2 cups uncooked enriched white rice*, a *10-ounce can of cream of mushroom soup*, *1 packet dry onion soup mix*, and *1 3/4 cups water*. Sprinkle dried or fresh parsley over the top.

Lay *1 chicken, cut in pieces*, or *6 chicken breast halves (about 1 1/2 pounds)*, over the top of the rice and soup mixture. Sprinkle on *paprika* and about *1/4 teaspoon black pepper* to give a little color and flavor.

Cover the dish with aluminum foil and bake until the chicken is tender and the rice is done. Baking time depends on the temperature: 2 hours at 300° F, 1 1/2 hour at 325° F, 1 hour at 350° F. To brown the chicken, remove the foil during the last 5 to 10 minutes of baking. Don't bake uncovered too long or the rice will dry out.

RECIPE NOTES
Fast tip: You can make use of the variation in cooking temperatures for your convenience in timing or to allow you to cook other foods at the same time. Cooking at 300° F will give you time to run an errand. The higher temperature will let you finish baking your apple custard while you cook dinner. The French bread can be warmed at any of the temperatures, but you have to watch it more closely at the higher temperature.

The night before: Find the cooking pan and the rice. Place the frozen chicken in the refrigerator to thaw. Be sure that you put even a seemingly impervious zip top bag in a dish or pan to thaw the chicken so that if the bag leaks it won't get *Salmonella* all over your refrigerator and produce. Check the recipe for the other menu items and get those ingredients lined up as well.

Presentation: This is a pretty dish. Plan to put it right in the middle of the table and serve it from there. Of course, plan to keep the hot dish out of reach of very small children. To make it easier for your child to serve herself, cut up some of the chicken breasts as you prepare this dish. She can scoop up just the right sized piece of chicken and the rice to go with it. If you have a large, flat, oval baking dish, use it to dress up the presentation and make this recipe look festive and sophisticated. Put on a few sprigs of parsley for garnish.

Involving your children: Children can measure the uncooked rice, open the canned soup and dry soup mix, and combine them. Once you are satisfied that your child has mastered sanitation procedures for raw chicken, she can assemble the whole thing. An adult also needs to put the dish into the oven and take it out again. That's hard for a child to do without getting burned.

A young child will be able to use a plastic picnic knife to chunk up cored apple pieces for the **Apple Custard**. In fact, the apple custard is a good recipe for an older child to make alone.

You may have to help her pour the mixture from the blender into the baking dish, and you will need to put the dish in the oven and remove it when it's done.

Adapting this meal for children: At the table, cut up the chicken finely and across the grain for young children, and mix it in with the rice. It should be quite moist, but if it is dry, add a little milk. Young children do better if some food is moist and soft. Dry, hard food seems to get stuck in their mouths.

Variations: This wonderfully convenient recipe is versatile, if you vary the liquid and spices. The trick is to keep the proportion of liquid to rice about 2 to 1. That is, it takes a cup of water to cook 1/2 cup of rice, so this recipe should have 3 cups of liquid for the 1 1/2 cups rice. Reader and family chef Suzanne Podurgiel experimented with substituting short-grain brown rice for the white rice and found that adding 2/3 cup more water was just enough to cook the rice without having the dish be watery. Other suggestions: Try golden mushroom soup instead of regular mushroom soup. Substitute dry vegetable soup mix for the onion soup mix. Substitute chicken broth, cream or sour cream, or tomatoes for the canned soup and get the total liquid to add up to 3 cups. Top each piece of chicken with a little pesto or stir it in. Add some Parmesan cheese. When you have the time and want to make something a little more challenging (to eat as well as to make), consider trying the **Jambalaya** recipe (page 134). While the principle of cooking the rice and chicken together is the same, the variety of vegetables and seasonings makes it an altogether different dish.

For ease of preparation, I have called for preboned chicken. It is certainly all right to use chicken pieces—roughly double the weight of preboned chicken to compensate for the weight of the bones. "Best of fryer" makes a good choice for chicken pieces—it has the boniest parts removed.

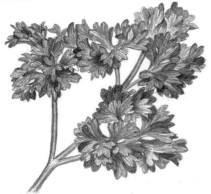

FIGURE 8.5 KEEPING CLEAN WHEN YOU COOK CHICKEN

Whenever I handle chicken, I have a flashback to learning sterile procedure during my dietetic-intern days. Before going into a room with patients who had contagious diseases, we had to carefully gown up and put on a face mask and rubber gloves. Then, even if we hadn't touched anything, we had to discard the whole works and wash up when we left. I think about it because you have to be about that careful when handling raw chicken.

Chicken won't hurt you if you handle and cook it right. However, do assume that chicken is contaminated with *Salmonella* bacteria. Unlike ground beef, which becomes contaminated only if something goes wrong in the meatpacking plant, most chicken is contaminated with *Salmonella*. Illness from *Salmonella* is unpleasant for anyone, but it's especially serious for children because the nausea, diarrhea, and fever can dehydrate them. Be careful not to let chicken touch or drip on other food or anything you can't wash in hot, soapy water. Rinse the chicken under cold water to start with, and consider everything that touches the raw chicken to be contaminated: your hands, the colander for rinsing the chicken, the knife and cutting board, the countertop, the sink, and the fork for turning it in the frying pan. As soon as you finish handling the raw chicken, wash all your utensils, the countertop, and the sink with hot, soapy water.

Do not touch *anything* before you wash your chickeny hands. *Your hands are contaminated, so keep your mind on what you are doing.* According to urban rumor, this point was made beautifully by a television news program. Raw chicken was coated with a substance that showed up only under ultraviolet light (Germ Glo), and a young mother was taped as she got it ready for cooking. See if you can detect her cross-contamination. She unwrapped the chicken and got out her knife and cutting board. Then she got the shortening out of the refrigerator and the pan out of the cabinet. She rinsed off the chicken, and then got out the colander to drain it. Then her son came in and wanted a drink of water, so she got out a glass and filled it for him. Then she finished cutting up the chicken and started frying it. When the area was flooded with ultraviolet light, the knife, cutting board, and sink glowed purple. And, to the mother's horror, so did the drawer, cabinet, cupboard, the outside and inside of the refrigerator, the cold-water tap, the glass, and *her son's hands and mouth*. For more about handling food safely, see figure 11.4, "Food Safety," on page 183.

Broccoli Chowder

Here is another canned soup recipe that is easy and very good. I suggest the frozen bread with it to remind you of its availability. The dessert is more elaborate than usual because the chowder is a little sparse, as main dishes go. The peach cobbler will help you and your diners to fill up and feel satisfied. You can bake the dessert at the same time as the bread.

INGREDIENTS

4 slices bacon
1/2 onion, minced
10-oz package frozen chopped broccoli
10-oz can condensed cream of potato soup
2 cups milk
1/4 tsp salt
1/2 cup shredded Swiss cheese or *cheese of your
  choice*

MENU

Broccoli chowder
"Homemade" bread from frozen bread dough
Butter
Peanut butter, jam
Fruit in season
Milk
Peach cobbler (page 162) or peach crisp (page 164)
Ice cream

METHOD

Summary: Brown the onion and cook the frozen broccoli; combine with milk and canned soup, and then purée in batches in a blender. Heat and stir in cheese.

Cut *4 slices bacon* into 1/4-inch pieces and cook until lightly browned. Remove the bacon and sauté *1/2 onion, minced* in the drippings until golden.

While you sauté the onion, cook a *10-ounce package frozen chopped broccoli* in 1/2 cup water until just crisp-tender. Don't drain.

In a large saucepan, combine the cooked bacon, sautéed onion, and cooked, undrained broccoli with a *10-ounce can condensed cream of potato soup,* *2 cups milk,* and *1/4 teaspoon salt.* While still cool, purée in a blender or food processor in batches. Return the puréed soup to the pan and heat thoroughly. Alternatively, use an immersion blender, otherwise known as an electric hand blender, to puree the chowder in the cooking pan.

Just before serving, stir in *1/2 cup shredded Swiss cheese* or *cheese of your choice.*

RECIPE NOTES

The night before: Find the canned soup and the cheese, and put the frozen broccoli in the refrigerator to thaw. Read the directions on the frozen bread dough and do what they say. Find the dessert ingredients; prepare the topping for the peach crisp if that's what you plan to have for dessert.

Involving your children: Children can open the broccoli; they can also open the cream of potato soup and pour it into the pan. Then they can measure the milk into the pan. Together you can do the blending. Your young child may want to push the buttons on the blender while you do the pouring.

The bread dough is a great find for children. They can put the dough in a greased loaf pan and bake it as is. Or you can let your child pinch off pieces, dip them in melted butter, and put them in muffin cups to rise and bake.

An older child can make the peach dessert.

Adapting this meal for children: This meal is surprisingly easy for children to eat if you let the soup cool a bit and put it in a cup or bowl with handles so they can pick it up and drink it.

Variations: Add one cup cooked rice after blending the soup. Substitute 2 tablespoons precooked real bacon bits (which come in a can) and 1 tablespoon butter, or for **Vegetarian Broccoli Chowder** skip the bacon and use 2 tablespoons butter.

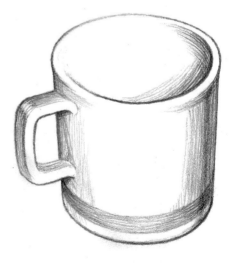

FIGURE 8.6 BACON

Most anyone who eats meat likes luscious bacon—and feels guilty about eating it. In fact, I have a friend who calls herself a baco-vegetarian. Bacon is one of those much-maligned foods that have been subjected to a variety of food alarms over the years. Allow me to dispel those alarms. First of all, the fat: Bacon does contain a lot of fat, and it certainly counts as your high-fat food when you have it on the menu. However, in this recipe, the bacon fat is thoroughly diluted by the soup, so the fat per serving is low. The highly flavorful bacon and bacon drippings add interest, which is the reason for using it.

Second, what about heart disease? The fat in bacon is the same as in (shudder, gasp) lard, a thoroughly defiled grease if there ever was one. But wait! Let us regard—*lard!* Lard is actually 15 percent polyunsaturated fat and 40 percent monounsaturated fat, so even the dietary enthusiasts must still their tongues about condemning lard. Not only that, but 30 percent of the remaining fat in lard is stearic acid, proven to neither raise nor lower blood cholesterol. For more on this arcane topic, see appendix N, "A Primer on Dietary Fat."

Third, what about nitrate and nitrite? There is lingering worry about bacon and other processed meats like hot dogs, luncheon meats, and sausage because they contain sodium nitrite. A couple of decades ago a nitrates-and-cancer scare erupted. Frying bacon at high temperatures can convert excess nitrites and nitrates in bacon to nitrosamine, which may contribute to cancer when you eat a lot of it. It is all different now. Nitrite is used instead of nitrate. It works better and is therefore used in smaller amounts. However, by way of being cautious without being self-sacrificing, it is better not to save bacon grease and use it for high-temperature frying. If you still worry about cured meats, keep in mind that danger relates to dosage and frequency. You control any food risk by using modest amounts as we do in the recipe, by eating it infrequently, or both.

Sodium nitrite used in processed foods retains color and prevents spoilage. Consumers nowadays are leery of such preservatives, feeling they don't want to eat either aging food or chemicals. Not to worry. Check the "sell-by" date. Sodium nitrite is a good chemical. It retards the growth of bacteria that produce the deadly *Clostridium botulinum* toxin, a guaranteed hazard.

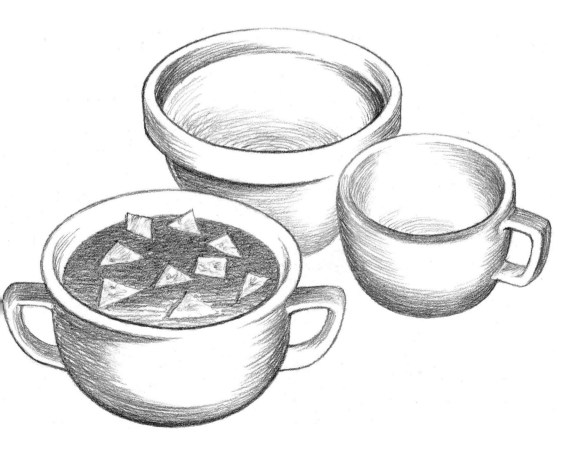

Spaghetti Carbonara (Yellow Spaghetti)

I asked each of my children, in turn, what food they remembered from their growing-up years. Each responded, "Yellow spaghetti." It was my dinner of last resort, so it showed up on the menu every couple of weeks. Carbonara means "in the manner of a charcoal maker." Despite my best efforts, I do not know what the charcoal maker does to stamp this as his dish, but there it is. I have served it to many people, most of them children, and have yet to be turned down. One young guest who disliked eggs was highly skeptical, but with reassurance from my children that it was good and from me that he didn't have to eat it if he didn't want to, he tasted it. He liked it.

INGREDIENTS
1 lb fettuccini or *other spaghetti*
1/2 lb bacon
6 eggs
1 cup grated Parmesan or *Asiago cheese (packaged or fresh)*

MENU
Spaghetti carbonara
Additional grated Parmesan or Asiago cheese
Mixed Vegetables (frozen or canned)
Green salad or fruit salad
Toasted bagels
Milk

METHOD
Summary: Start the spaghetti water heating, start the bacon frying, and put the eggs in a bowl of hot tap water to begin warming them up to room temperature. Mix the warmed, beaten eggs together with the cheese. Arrange to get them all ready at one time. Quickly toss hot, not thoroughly drained cooked pasta with hot, browned bacon and hot bacon fat. Add beaten eggs and cheese. The heat of the pasta/bacon mixture cooks the eggs.

Fill a 4 1/2-quart pan about half to two-thirds full of water, add 1 teaspoon salt per quart of water, and bring to a rapid boil. Boil *1 pound fettuccini* or *other spaghetti* until it's al dente. Drain, shake the colander to remove most but not all excess water, return the pasta immediately to the pan, and place it back on the burner set at the lowest heat.

While the water heats, peel off and drop *1/2 pound bacon* slices into a frying pan. Fry until lightly browned, stirring as you cook. Use a slotted spoon to lift onto a cutting board and chop into 1/4- to 1/2-inch wide pieces. Pour off all but about 2 tablespoons bacon grease. Put the bacon back in the pan with the reserved grease and hold over low heat.

While the bacon cooks, bring *6 eggs* to room temperature by letting them stand for 5 minutes in your hottest tap water. (Be sure the eggs are not cracked. If they are, throw them away.) Beat the eggs with *1 cup grated Parmesan* or *Asiago cheese (packaged or fresh)*. (Asiago is a hard, zesty, nutty-tasting cheese.)

Timing is important here. Try to get the bacon and spaghetti cooked at the same time so they are both hot enough to cook the eggs. Because you need to put the eggs in while the spaghetti and bacon are as hot as possible, have the egg mixture ready by the time you finish cooking the bacon and spaghetti.

Assemble the dish by pouring the hot bacon and bacon fat into the cooked spaghetti. Toss to distribute evenly. Add the egg and cheese mixture, stirring and tossing to combine it evenly with the spaghetti-bacon mixture.

In the finished product, the egg needs to be semisolid, as in a very soft scrambled egg. It should be thick enough to cling to the spaghetti and not pool in the bottom of the pan, but not so cooked that it turns into chunks of egg. To cook egg that is still runny, heat the pan gently to thicken the egg, stirring as you heat.

RECIPE NOTES
The night before: The cycle menu in chapter 11, "Planning to Get You Cooking," lists spaghetti carbonara as a Friday, clean-out-the-refrigerator meal. The main dish is fresh, but for the other menu items, I suggest potential discoveries from the archeological dig of the refrigerator. You may find bits of vegetables that can be combined to make a satisfactory hot vegetable dish, or you might be able to marinate leftover vegetables in salad dressing to include in the salad. Bits of cheese can go in the salad or on the vegetables. You may have enough odds and ends of fruit to make a fruit salad, or you might have enough for **Fruit with Brown Cream Sauce** (page 164). On the other hand, if what you find in your refrigerator is not appealing, throw it away. There is nothing to be gained by traumatizing

yourself and others in the name of economy. I know a grown man who still turns green when he remembers the leftover French fries that showed up in his mother's casseroles.

Presentation: Save a little crumbled bacon to sprinkle over the top of the dish.

Involving your children: Children love to crack eggs. It is especially fun to crack them by tapping them together. Surprisingly, cracking eggs together or on a flat surface makes it easier to avoid getting shell in the bowl. Australians, who reportedly bet on anything, bet on which egg will crack first. A child could have fun predicting which egg will be the first to go. Have children crack each egg separately into a small bowl so it is easier to fish eggshell back out again and so you can discard any egg that doesn't look just right. Use a clean spoon rather than the egg shell to scoop up stray bits of shell. The shell works better but introduces a slight risk of contamination.

Adapting this meal for children: Spaghetti is only hard to eat if you are concerned about social niceties. In a child's mind, spaghetti is a finger food, so get ready. Children love to suck up strands of spaghetti, and that's fine, if you can stand it. They also love to watch you twirl spaghetti around your fork and will try to imitate you. However, they will revert to using their hands. This spaghetti sticks together, so it is somewhat easier to eat than **Spaghetti and Meatballs** (page 114). It is tasty and can become a favorite with anyone who has been introduced to all the parts. To prevent allergies, it is best to wait until a baby is 7 to 9 months old before introducing her to egg whites and wheat.

Variations: Instead of the bacon, you can use 3 tablespoons of butter or olive oil. But before you reject the bacon, read figure 8.6 on page 103.

You can also make **Vegetarian Spaghetti Carbonara** by leaving out the bacon, sautéing a variety of vegetables in the butter or olive oil, and combining them with the egg/spaghetti mixture.

FIGURE 8.7 EGGS

Yellow spaghetti raises the issue of egg safety, both from the point of view of cholesterol content and *Salmonella* contamination. About cholesterol, as I say in "Enjoy Eggs," page 208, in chapter 13, "Choosing Food," because the cholesterol in food has a minimal impact on blood cholesterol, and because eggs are so convenient and nutritious when you are cooking for a family, I recommend that you eat eggs.

I carefully researched the safety of eggs for this recipe because *Salmonella* finds its way into the yolks of about 1 in 10,000 eggs before they are laid. I checked with the American Egg Board and with food scientists and satisfied myself that, if you follow the directions, the recipe will be safe. The goal is to get the temperature of the egg-spaghetti-bacon mixture up to about 160° F, the instant-kill temperature for *Salmonella*. To help achieve that safe temperature, bring the eggs to room temperature before you crack them by putting them in hot tap water for 5 minutes (but don't let them stand around for long at room temperature). Be careful to have the bacon and spaghetti as hot as can be when you mix in the eggs and cheese. The bacon and spaghetti will cook the eggs, but if the eggs are still runny, do a final heating until the egg mixture is at the very-soft-scramble stage, which is 160° F or more. In this recipe, the eggs are diluted with cheese, which lets them get to above 160° F and still be soft-scrambled. For your general information, eggs that are soft-scrambled or cooked until the white coagulates and the yolk begins to coagulate are cooked to a safe temperature.

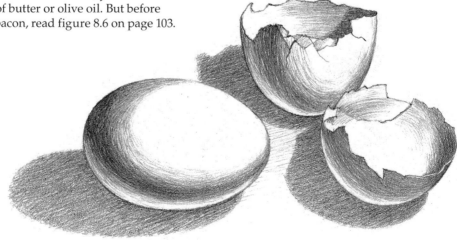

Swiss Steak

This is a good recipe for company. It looks pretty, it's easy to serve, and it can be prepared for baking ahead of time. I have also used it as a way of introducing you to clear oven cooking bags. These cooking bags are great for preparing pieces of meat and roasts. The food in the bags browns but stays moist. The recipes on the package say to set the oven temperature at 350° F. That works great for poultry and fish, which are tender and cook fast. However, for the tougher beef cuts, I find a lower temperature allows for the longer cooking time necessary to make the meat tender. You can also prepare this recipe in a covered casserole in a 300° F oven for 1 1/2 hours, or in a slow cooker on low for 4 to 6 hours.

INGREDIENTS

1 small clear oven cooking bag
2 lb round steak, cut into helping-sized pieces
28-oz can seasoned tomatoes
1 packet dry onion soup mix

MENU

Swiss steak
Mashed potatoes (page 157)
Steak cooking liquid for gravy
Gingered broccoli (page 156)
Oven-browned rolls
Butter
Milk
Apple custard or another baked dessert

METHOD

Summary: Combine round steak, canned tomatoes, and dry soup mix in an oven bag and bake.

Preheat the oven to 300° F.

Follow the cooking-bag directions about putting flour in the *clear oven cooking bag*. Put the bag in a cake or jelly roll pan (10 × 15 1/2 × 1-inch pan). Place *2 pounds round steak, cut into helping-sized pieces, a 28-ounce can seasoned tomatoes*, and *1 packet dry onion soup mix* in the bottom of the bag.

Close the cooking bag and cut steam vents according to the package directions. Bake for 1 hour. Remove the pan from the oven. For safety, let stand for 15 minutes before you open the bag.

RECIPE NOTES

Fast tip: This is a great way to cook and tenderize beef for other recipes. You can cut the leftover beef into cubes, refrigerate or freeze it, and use it later in your **Beefy Shortcut Stroganoff** (page 108) or in **Minestrone Soup** (pages 128). You can even freeze it as is and have it weeks later as the same meal all over again.

The night before: Place the frozen steak in the refrigerator to thaw. Find the cooking bag. Line up the other ingredients. Wash the broccoli and apples, and find the rest of the ingredients for the apple custard.

Added touch: Before baking, top the steak-tomato mound with sliced mushrooms or green pepper rings.

Presentation: This looks great served straight from the cooking bag. Transfer the cooking bag to a platter, peel back or cut away the edges, and serve from the platter. Because the food is very hot, you may have to help your child get her serving, or you may be able to scooch the platter around the table. Since the steak is cut into helping-sized pieces, she can then serve herself.

Involving your children: When your child has mastered sanitation procedures, she can make this whole recipe. Until then, your child can open the can of tomatoes and pour it over the beef, and sprinkle the onion soup on top. She can help wash the potatoes and even mash them. She can break the broccoli into florets if you cut the stems to the length you want.

Adapting this meal for children: This meal works well for children because the meat is so tender and moist that even beginning eaters can manage it. Just cut the meat pieces across the grain to shorten the fibers. Let your child eat the broccoli with her fingers. You may find yourself doing the same!

Variations: You can add potatoes and carrots to the cooking bag and have a one-dish meal. In fact, now that you have the braised, one-dish meal idea, you can stray even further from this recipe and make that traditional favorite, **Pot Roast**. A center-cut chuck roast tenderizes beautifully when baked at 325° F for 3 to 4 hours in a covered Dutch oven or in a clear cooking bag (reduce the temperature to 300° F), or in a slow cooker for about double that time. Half-cover the meat with a braising liquid of a 15-ounce can each of beef broth and diced tomatoes and a 10-ounce can of golden mushroom soup. For extra flavor, consider adding a half-cup of beer or wine. When the meat is almost done, add any vegetables you fancy: potatoes, carrots, onions, cabbage, turnips, rutabagas, or celery. Salt and pepper the vegetables as you add them. Continue cooking for 30 minutes to an hour. The broth, tomatoes, and soup give this dish an "automatic" gravy.

FIGURE 8.8 COOKING BEEF TO MAKE IT TENDER

Round steak is inexpensive, nutritious, convenient, and low in fat. It is also *tough*. Like other low-fat beef (see figure 12.1, "Fat in Meat, Poultry, and Fish," on page 194), round steak has to be specially prepared to make it tender and enjoyable to eat. For **Swiss Steak**, we braise it: We put it in a small amount of liquid and cook it for a long time at a low temperature. We could also stew it, like we do for **Beef Stew** (page 124): Put it in a large amount of liquid and cook it for a long time. (Are you beginning to get the principle?) It helps even more if the liquid has acid in it, like tomato juice and vinegar do, because the acid breaks down the connective tissue in the meat.

For the **Pot Roast** described in the variations, the method again is braising. Slow-cooker cooking is the ultimate in braising, featuring as it does very low temperatures and long cooking times. A pot roast in the slow cooker is a set-it-and-forget-it recipe that allows you to run lots of errands while dinner takes care of itself. Since the slow cooker fad has passed, you may not get one for a gift, but you can probably find one at a garage sale. Even new, they are inexpensive. My favorite slow cooker is the oblong one, with a separate base and roughly 5-inch-deep metal pan that fits on the base. Food cooks evenly, and the cooking pan is easy to clean and refrigerate. It doubles as a keep-warm server.

Another strategy for cooking low-fat beef is to tenderize the meat ahead of time. Presumably, you could marinate it: Soak it overnight (in the refrigerator) in a liquid that has acid and seasonings. While marinades taste good, I don't find them too helpful for tenderizing. If you want to grill or broil steak, you might have to buy a cut that has more fat in it, such as sirloin. You could also use a low-fat cut and treat it with prepared meat tenderizer. Meat tenderizers contain *papain*, an enzyme extracted from papayas, or *bromelin*, an enzyme extracted from pineapple or related plants; the enzymes break down the connective tissue. Also look for packets of preseasoned tenderizer-marinade, which adds flavor as well as tenderizes. Follow the package directions to treat the meat before grilling or broiling.

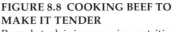

Beefy Shortcut Stroganoff

This is essentially a PPM (pre-prepared meal, otherwise known as leftovers) using the **Swiss Steak** from the previous recipe. In the cycle menu, the Swiss steak is on for Sunday and the beefy shortcut stroganoff is on for Tuesday. If you use the beef that quickly, you can refrigerate it. If you keep it longer, freeze it.

INGREDIENTS
2 cups leftover Swiss steak, chunked
Leftover tomatoes and sauce from Swiss steak
1/2 cup sour cream

MENU
Beefy shortcut stroganoff
Noodles or mashed potatoes (page 157)
Green salad
Fruit in season
Bread and butter
Milk
Ice cream and store-bought cookies

METHOD
Summary: Heat leftover cubed meat and tomatoes, add sour cream, and serve over boiled noodles or mashed potatoes.

Gently heat *2 cups leftover Swiss steak, chunked,* and the *leftover tomatoes and sauce from Swiss steak.* Stir in *1/2 cup sour cream.* Add more tomatoes or tomato juice to get the consistency you want.

Serve over hot cooked noodles or mashed potatoes.

RECIPE NOTES
The night before: Locate the beef cubes; if they are frozen, put them in the refrigerator to thaw. Locate the sour cream and the other ingredients. Wash the salad greens and put them in a tight container to crisp (see figure 10.2 "Prepackaged Salad Greens or Do-It-Yourself? on page 151). Check out your fresh fruit supply. If you can't find any, check your supply of canned fruit.

Added touch: Add fresh or canned mushrooms.

Involving your children: A child can mix the ingredients for the main dish. She can also spin the greens for the salad, tear them up, and put them in the bowl.

Adapting this meal for children: This meal has a number of dishes, so your child is likely to find something on the table that she finds appealing. Don't feel she has to eat the stroganoff—noodles or mashed potatoes with butter are just fine.

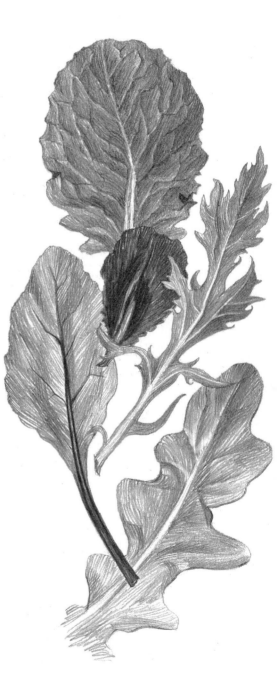

Mostaccioli with Spinach and Feta

This strange-sounding recipe is surprisingly appealing and popular with most people, even those who don't usually like feta cheese. Feta has a strong flavor and a distinctive, crumbly texture. Until your diners develop a taste for feta cheese, the secret seems to be in crumbling it finely—into pieces about half the size of peas. That way, the taste isn't too concentrated in any one bite. This recipe does wonderful things for spinach and lets you serve your vegetables, starch, and protein all at one time.

INGREDIENTS

8 oz mostaccioli, penne, ziti, or other tube-shaped pasta
10-oz package frozen chopped spinach, thawed
3 medium raw tomatoes or 6 Roma tomatoes
6–10 green onions: bulbs and most of the tops
2 Tbsp olive oil
8-oz package mild feta cheese, finely crumbled

MENU

Mostaccioli with spinach and feta
Scalloped corn (page 156)
Toasted English muffins
Milk
Plum cobbler (page 162) or peach crisp (page 164)
or fruit in season

METHOD

Summary: Drain thawed frozen spinach and combine with al dente pasta, raw tomatoes, and onion. Crumble in feta cheese and gently heat.

Fill a 4 1/2-quart pan about half to two-thirds full of water, add 1 teaspoon salt per quart of water, and bring to a rapid boil. Cook *8 ounces mostaccioli or other tube-shaped pasta* until al dente.

While the pasta cooks, pour a thawed *10-ounce package frozen chopped spinach* into a colander and squeeze out the excess liquid.

While the pasta cooks, chop *3 medium tomatoes or 6 Roma tomatoes*. Cut crosswise into 1/4 inch or less slices *6 to 10 green onions* (bulbs and most of the tops).

Drain the pasta and put it back in the pan, then add the spinach and *2 tablespoons of olive oil*.

Combine the tomatoes and onions with the pasta and spinach and add an *8-ounce package mild feta cheese, finely crumbled*.

Mix and warm gently in the original cooking pan or in a glass dish in the microwave.

RECIPE NOTES

Fast tip: Have tomatoes at room temperature to speed the final heating. To preserve flavor, unless they are getting too ripe, don't refrigerate fresh tomatoes. A critical flavor component of tomatoes disappears when they are chilled.

The night before: Take the spinach out of the freezer and refrigerate to thaw. Wash the green onions and other vegetables. Find the corn and crackers for the scalloped corn. Make the crisp mix or find your stored jar of it in the refrigerator.

Presentation: The mostaccioli is very pretty. It looks great in a clear or white bowl.

Involving your children: Children can open the package of spinach and put it in the colander. They can toast the muffins and cut up the plums and put them in the baking pan. If you have crisp topping on hand, they can sprinkle that over the top. They can open the corn, put it in the pan, and crunch in the soda crackers.

Adapting this meal for children: As with other one-dish meals, this is a sink-or-swim meal, so be sure to give additional options. My menu is rather odd because scalloped corn doesn't really "go" with the main dish, but it is delicious, easy to like, and filling. The English muffins should be pretty neutral, and the dessert is filling and nutritious while it gives a fruit serving.

Variation: Instead of spinach, add a variety of sautéed vegetables, like bits of carrot, broccoli, zucchini, mushrooms, or green or red peppers.

FIGURE 8.9 FETA, BRIE, AND PREGNANCY

If you are pregnant, be sure that the label on any soft cheese such as feta, brie, fresh mozzarella, and queso fresco clearly states that it is made from pasteurized milk. Unpasteurized (raw) milk and foods made from it can contain harmful bacteria. Most concerning during pregnancy is listeria, which can harm the fetus. For more information, go to www.cdc.gov and do a search on "listeria and pregnancy."

All cheese produced in the United States for the domestic market must be either aged for at least 60 days or made from pasteurized milk. Either process—aging or pasteurizing—destroys pathogenic bacteria. Imported cheese is not subject to these regulations.

Herb-Baked Fish

This basting sauce contains ginger, reportedly helpful in toning down or taking away the fishy taste of fish. Fish aficionados say if fish is fresh, it shouldn't have a strong fishy taste or odor. It should smell like a "fresh sea breeze," and, I suppose, taste as light and delicate as that breeze smells. But for some of us, even a fresh sea breeze tastes like fish, and ginger will offset that flavor. The menu for this meal specifies scalloped potatoes or corn pudding, both of which have fat in them. The fat in the high-carbohydrate side dish helps to balance out the relative dryness of the fish. However, even with that addition, this is a relatively low-fat, low-calorie meal, so the **Pineapple Upside-Down Cake** helps to make this a filling and satisfying meal.

INGREDIENTS
2 Tbsp butter, softened or *olive oil*
Fish Seasoning:
   1/2 tsp salt
   1/4 tsp pepper
   1/4 tsp dried thyme
   1/4 tsp dried oregano
   1/4 tsp ground ginger
   1/4 tsp onion powder
   1/4 tsp garlic powder
2 lb low-fat white fish: cod, halibut, whitefish, turbo, pollack, or your preference

MENU
Herb-baked fish
Boxed scalloped potatoes prepared in oven or microwave, or corn pudding (page 159)
Green salad
Whole wheat bread or toast
Butter
Milk
Fruit in season
Pineapple upside-down cake (page 162)

METHOD
Summary: Combine herbs and butter and brush the herbed butter on the fish before and during baking.
   Preheat oven to 325° F.
   Make an herb basting sauce by combining *2 tablespoons softened butter* or *olive oil* with Fish Seasoning prepared by mixing these ingredients: *1/2 teaspoon salt, and 1/4 teaspoon each pepper, thyme, oregano, ginger, onion powder,* and *garlic powder.*

   Wash *2 pounds fish* in cold water and pat excess off excess moisture with paper towels. Put the fish on a rack over a pan to catch the juices (a cooling rack over a jelly roll pan will do). Brush fish with herb sauce.
   Bake for 10 to 20 minutes, brushing with herb sauce once or twice during baking.
   The fish is done when it turns white and flakes easily with a fork. If you want more precise cooking times, begin with the "10-minute rule." Measure the fish at its thickest point and cook 10 minutes per inch. That is, cook a 1-inch thick piece of fish 5 minutes on each side. Double the cooking time for frozen fish that has not been defrosted. However, don't follow the 10-minute rule slavishly or the fish could get dried out. You'll learn with practice when to stop cooking. Fish is done when it is white and flakes and reaches an internal temperature of 130 to 140° F.

RECIPE NOTES
Fast tip: Quadruple (or more) the Fish Seasoning recipe and store it in a small labeled jar. The next time you make herb-baked fish, combine 2 teaspoons of Fish Seasoning with the butter or olive oil. Use Fish Seasoning to make the seasoned flour for **Fried Fish** (page 136).

The night before: Prepare the Fish Seasoning. Put the frozen fish in the refrigerator to thaw. Find the scalloped potatoes or corn pudding ingredients. Find the canned pineapple.

Added touch: To serve, lay a thin lemon slice on top of each piece of fish.

Presentation: If you would rather use a plainer carbohydrate side dish, like rice or boiled potatoes, you can make your fat source in this menu tartar sauce or a creamed vegetable dish, like creamed peas or spinach, or broccoli with cheese sauce. You can also make more of the herbed butter sauce and put it on the table for family members to use on their fish and vegetables.

Involving your children: Children can tear greens for the salad and grate the cheese for the corn pudding. They can also use a pastry brush to put the first layer of basting sauce on the fish. A child will enjoy laying out the rings of pineapple and decorating with maraschino cherries for the upside-down cake. The batter for the cake is so easy that an older child could mix it up.

Adapting this meal for children: If you buy boneless fish, this is a fine meal for children. Dress the salad lightly so your child can pick it up with his fingers.

Variations: Grilled Fish with Herbed Butter
This adds a great taste. Combine 2 tablespoons butter with 2 teaspoons fish seasoning and baste the fish with the herbed butter as it grills, the same as you would in the oven. To make heating up the grill worthwhile, grill corn on the cob or skewer tomatoes and peppers and grill them at the same time. Continue to follow the 10-minute rule for cooking time (10 minutes per inch of thickness), and cook to an internal temperature of 130 to 140° F.

Poached Fish Bring to a slow boil enough water, chicken or vegetable broth, and milk or cream to cover the fish. Add 2–3 teaspoons fish seasoning, plus a couple of teaspoons lemon juice. Add the fish and bring the liquid back to a simmer. Apply the 10-minute rule for cooking time (10 minutes per inch of thickness) and internal-temperature rule (130 to 140° F). The acid in the lemon juice keeps the flesh firmer and whiter.

Sautéed Fish Heat olive oil or melt butter in a medium-temperature frying pan, sprinkle in some fish seasoning, lay in the fish and cook for about 5 minutes on each side until it is gold-brown and reaches an internal temperature of 130 to 140° F.

Baked Fish You can use the same herbed butter, or experiment with **Mustard-Honey Butter**: Thickly brush the fish with equal parts melted butter and mustard. Drizzle on honey and top with buttered bread crumbs. Bake at 400° F for 10 minutes or until it passes your doneness tests. Wait to give your child honey until she is at least 1 year old.

FIGURE 8.10 FISH
When you prepare fish, use the same clean technique that you use with chicken or meat. Wash your hands and all utensils after you handle fish, and be careful not to cross-contaminate. Thaw frozen fish in the refrigerator to reduce moisture loss and prevent spoilage; then rinse with cold water and dry with paper towels before you prepare it. You can also purchase fish individually wrapped and frozen. This thaws fast in cold water.

When you purchase fish, know what you are getting. Frozen fish is perfectly acceptable if it has an appropriate freshness date, no freezer burn, and an undamaged package (for purchasing tips, see chapter 12, "Shopping to Get You Cooking," page 187). While the word *fresh* implies that fish has not been frozen, some seemingly fresh fish in some markets is defrosted frozen fish. If you cook the fish right away, it is simply a truth in marketing issue. But if you take it home and refreeze it, both the quality and the safety will be compromised. Ask whether your "fresh" fish has been frozen and thawed, or read the fine print on the package.

Fish that is truly fresh has never been frozen. Because fish so rapidly develops off flavors and odors, fresh fish must be kept clean and cold and moved rapidly from catch to market to table. To purchase fish that is really fresh, deal with a reputable fish market that is expert about moving fish quickly and cleanly, and cook it the day you buy it. The staff in a dedicated fish market will be able to give you advice on what to buy and how to cook it.

You can purchase fish whole, as fillets, or as steaks. Fish fillets are most common. They are sides of flesh cut from the backbone and ribs, with the skin on or off. Your supermarket frozen fish case probably has perch, cod, haddock, and pollack fillets, lean fish with a mild flavor and white or light color flesh. Salmon, swordfish, tuna, and other large fish may be sold as fillets or as steaks, cut 1/4 to 1 1/2 inches thick. The oil and muscle development in the flesh of these moderate-fat fish gives them a more pronounced flavor and a firm, meaty texture. As mentioned earlier, because of their mercury content, tuna and other large fish should be eaten no more than once a week.

Most challenging of all—to cook and to eat—is the whole fish. If you do any fishing yourself, you know all about it. You also need to know which fish taken from which waters are free from industrial contaminants and are therefore safe to eat. If you don't know, check your fishing license. The rest of us can have our whole fish by purchasing whole rainbow trout.

What about bones? All cuts of fish may or may not be boneless, depending on whether the pin-bones have been removed. Your fish market will be able to tell you and can teach you about boning fish. For supermarket fish you will have to look and feel. Take the bones out of your child's portion, and be careful when you eat your own.

Meat Loaf

Consumer research tells us we are looking for comfort food: meat loaf, chicken soup, dumplings, mashed potatoes. Your idea of comfort food may be lots different from mine, because comfort food is good-tasting, familiar food with positive memories associated with it. Your feel-good food might be hoppin' John (rice and black-eyed peas), wonton soup, refried beans, or Twinkies.

Here is my favorite meat loaf recipe, perfected over decades. You may have one in your family as well. If you want to start a conversation in a group of experienced cooks, ask for a meat loaf recipe!

INGREDIENTS
1⅓ cups dried stuffing mix
1/4 cup dried onion flakes or *1/2 cup finely chopped onion*
1 3/4 cups milk
2 lb ground beef
1 egg, beaten
4 tsp Worcestershire sauce
1 1/2 tsp salt
1/8 tsp dried sage
1/4 tsp dry mustard
1/4 tsp black pepper

MENU
Meat loaf
Scalloped potatoes
Carrot and celery sticks
Herbed peas (157)
Bread or toast
Butter
Milk
Old-fashioned bread pudding (page 164) with raisins, or fruit in season

METHOD
Summary: Soak dried stuffing mix in milk, add ground beef and seasonings, shape into a loaf, and bake.

Preheat oven to 325° F.

In a large mixing bowl, combine *1 1/3 cups dried stuffing mix, 1/4 cup dried onion flakes* or *1/2 cup finely chopped onion*, and *1 3/4 cups milk*. Soak 10 minutes.

Add all at once: *2 pounds ground beef, 1 beaten egg, 4 teaspoons Worcestershire sauce, 1 1/2 teaspoons*

salt, 1/8 teaspoon dried sage, 1/4 teaspoon dry mustard, and *1/4 teaspoon black pepper*. Mix with a spoon or with your carefully washed hands.

Reserve half the recipe for meatballs or Salisbury steaks (see variations). Pack the remaining mixture into an 8 1/2-inch bread pan or mold into an oblong shape and place it on a jelly roll pan. (The bread pan gives a moister, softer meat loaf. The free-form meat loaf is firmer and has a more browned crust.)

Bake for 30 minutes. Use a meat thermometer and remove the meat loaf from the oven when it reaches an internal temperature of 160° F (if you use ground poultry, cook it to 170° F). If you take it out promptly when it's done, it will be juicy. If you cook it too long, all the good juices will cook out and it will be swimming in juice. Let it stand for 15 minutes to set before you serve it.

RECIPE NOTES

The night before: Put frozen ground beef in the refrigerator to thaw. Find the meat loaf ingredients, the bread pan, and the ice cream scoop. Wash the celery and refrigerate it in a zip top bag to crisp. Chop the onions and refrigerate in a tightly sealed container (so they don't smell up your refrigerator). Make the **Herbed Butter** (page 111) or locate your stash. Find the stale bread and cube it up for bread pudding, or set out your hoarded bread cubes to thaw.

Added touch: Squirt a ribbon of ketchup down the middle of the meat loaf before you bake it. Grate a little cheese into the mixture, or lay fancy shapes of cheese on the top.

Presentation: Serve the whole meat loaf on a platter; slice it at the table.

Involving your children: Children can wash and peel the carrots and measure the bread crumbs, onions, and milk. Some children will love getting their hands into this goopy stuff. However, to be allowed to work with raw meat, a child has to be older and must have demonstrated that she knows proper procedures for handling raw meat. Children will also love scooping out the meatballs and putting them on the jelly roll pan (see the variation). An older child can make the bread pudding.

Adapting this meal for children: Children do well with this meal because everything is soft and easy to chew. Because children under age 2 might choke on carrot and celery sticks, give them soft, fresh fruit that has been cut into bite-sized pieces so they can eat it with their fingers.

Variations: Meatballs Make frozen, ready-to-eat meatballs for **Spaghetti and Meatballs** (page 114) or to warm up for the occasional fast meal. Using a size 30 ice cream scoop (see figure 8.12, "Ice Cream Scoops," on page 113), portion balls of the remaining meat loaf mixture onto a jelly roll pan. Refrigerate until the rest of the dinner is done. Then bake the meat balls at 325° F until they are done, about 20 minutes. Freeze the meatballs before you bag them up so they don't stick together. Spread them out on a second jelly roll pan lined with parchment or waxed paper and freeze them before you transfer them to a zip top bag. Store them in the freezer.

You can also use the meat loaf mixture to make **Salisbury Steaks**, which are simply hamburger steaks mixed with extra bread and seasonings, formed into patties, and cooked. Heat a tablespoon or two of butter in a frying pan at medium heat. Add the steaks when the oil is sizzling gently. Sauté steaks for 3 to 5 minutes on each side or until they reach an internal temperature of 155° F.

Gravy is a fine accompaniment to Salisbury steaks. Once you master gravy-making, you can make gravy with any meat or poultry that leaves you with pan drippings, which is the fat left in the pan after you fry or sauté. Move the Salisbury steaks to a plate and cover to keep them warm. Blend 4 tablespoons of flour into the pan drippings. Cook for about a minute. Remove from the heat. Stir in 2 cups water, broth, or milk. Bring to a boil, stirring constantly, and boil for 1 to 2 minutes to thicken. Add 1/2 teaspoon salt (unless the broth was salty) and 1/4 teaspoon pepper. If the gravy lacks flavor or color, add a little beef broth concentrate or commercial gravy seasoning. Serve with **Mashed Potatoes** (pages 157).

Note: It's important to cook the flour in drippings to destroy the amylase, an enzyme in the flour. Otherwise the amylase could break down the flour and take away its thickening power.

FIGURE 8.11 PURCHASING AND USING A MEAT THERMOMETER

Color is not a reliable indicator that food is thoroughly cooked. A food thermometer is the only way to tell if food has reached a high enough temperature to destroy bacteria. But purchasing a meat thermometer can be complex. Some types of thermometers can be left in foods while they cook or bake, and others can't. The ones that can be left in don't work well for thin foods like hamburgers. If you are willing to check foods at the end of cooking and *not* leave the thermometer in place while food cooks, a digital thermometer is a good, all-purpose tool. It registers the food's temperature in 1 to 20 seconds, and because it has to be inserted only 1/2 inch deep, it works well for thin foods like burgers. I *love* my Thermapen, but it is pricey—it costs almost $100. Thermometers that can be left in place, liquid-filled or bimetal thermometers, have to be inserted 2 to 3 inches deep and take 1 to 2 minutes to get a reading. If you roast a lot, you might want to investigate a programmable thermometer with or without a remote pager. The unit has an alarm to alert you when the food reaches the stated temperature. Any thermometer that can be left in place is best for roasts, turkeys and meat loaf.

Target internal temperatures:
- Ground beef: 160° F
- Beef, veal, or lamb roasts, steaks, and chops: 145° F for medium rare, 160° F for medium, 170° F for well-done
- Poultry or ground poultry: 165° F
- Pork or ground pork: 160° F for medium, 170° F for well done
- Eggs: 150° F (the point at which the white is set and the yolk is starting to set).
- Reheating food, heating bread dressing: 165° F

FIGURE 8.12 ICE CREAM SCOOPS

Ice cream scoops are great time-savers because you can quickly portion out with one hand dumplings, cookies, meatballs, or muffins. If yours is marked with a size, it will be on the narrow piece that sweeps out the bowl. Size 30 works well for large drop cookies, meatballs, and regular-sized muffins. Size 60 works well for dumplings, small drop cookies, and itty-bitty muffins. The size numbers refer to scoops per quart. The 30 holds 2 tablespoons, and the 60 holds 1 tablespoon.

Spaghetti and Meatballs

Here is the shortest recipe in the book. It is short because you use the frozen meatballs you made when you prepared the **Meat Loaf** meal. Here you get your reward for planning and cooking ahead.

INGREDIENTS
Dry packaged spaghetti
Olive oil
12–16 frozen meatballs, thawed
1 or 2 32-oz jars prepared spaghetti sauce

MENU
Spaghetti and meatballs
French bread
Butter
Tossed green salad
Apple and orange wedges or fruit in season
Grated Parmesan cheese, fresh or otherwise
Milk

METHOD
Summary: Heat prepared spaghetti sauce and frozen meatballs. Serve over spaghetti with grated cheese.

Fill a 4 1/2-quart pan about half to two-thirds full of water, add 1 teaspoon salt per quart of water, and bring to a rapid boil. Add *dry packaged spaghetti* (1 pound or however much your family needs), and boil until al dente. Drain and toss with a little *olive oil* to keep it from sticking together.

Heat up the thawed meatballs (the ones you made when you prepared the **Meat Loaf**) in the microwave. If you heat them on top of the stove, you will have to stir them, and that may break them apart.

Warm up *one* or *two 32-ounce jars prepared spaghetti sauce*, whichever brand you prefer. Dilute the sauce with water if you wish. Put the heated meatballs in the hot spaghetti sauce.

Serve sauce and meatballs in one dish, the cooked spaghetti in another.

RECIPE NOTES
Fast tip: Store the cheese grater in the refrigerator with the block of Parmesan cheese, and wash the grater only when you add a new block of cheese. Put the grater and cheese on the table on a plate, and let family members grate their own cheese.

The night before: Put the frozen meatballs in the refrigerator to thaw. Locate the spaghetti sauce. Wash and crisp the greens for the salad (see figure 10.2 "Prepackaged Salad Greens or Do-It-Yourself?" on page 151). Locate fruit and French bread and put them in a handy place. Locate the Parmesan cheese and the grater.

Added touch: Enrich the sauce with more vegetables by sautéing any or all of the vegetables in the **Marinated Chicken Stir-Fry** (pages 132); add them with the meatballs for the final warm-up. Keep in mind, however, that you are *adding* these vegetables, not *hiding* them.

Involving your children: Children can spin and toss the salad and peel the oranges.

Adapting this meal for children: Depending on your eaters, you may want to start by keeping the meatballs separate from the sauce. Children often don't want sauce on spaghetti, but spaghetti and a meatball makes a nice meal. For the youngest eaters, the ones who feed themselves with their fingers, consider using mostaccioli, penne, ziti, or another tube-shaped pasta instead of spaghetti. Those shapes are far easier to pick up and eat.

The vegetables add extra interest for those who have mastered each of them. However, do not try to sneak vegetables into your child by hiding them in the sauce. That is dirty pool—your child will be on to you in a flash, and his liking for vegetables will have a setback. With the tomatoes in the sauce, you are already offering lots of vegetables, so you do not have to resort to such a sneaky tactic.

Variations: Vegetarian Spaghetti Leave out the meat, add a drained can of chickpeas (garbanzo beans) or other cooked dried beans, and have vegetarian sauce.

Meat Sauce Instead of meatballs, brown ground beef with onions and put it into the spaghetti sauce.

Italian Sausage Spaghetti Sauce Cook Italian sausages, cut them up, and add them to the sauce instead of ground beef or meatballs.

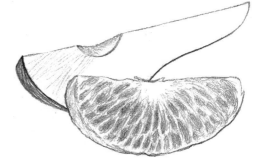

Spinach-Feta Frittata

A frittata is an unfolded omelet with vegetables, cheese, or meat or all three. This can be another last-resort dinner. It can also be breakfast or Sunday brunch. For more about eggs, see figure 8.7 on page 105.

INGREDIENTS
4 to 8 oz fresh spinach
1 to 2 tsp butter
6 to 8 eggs
1/3 cup cool water
4 oz feta cheese

MENU
Spinach-feta frittata
Fruit salad or vegetable salad
Bread or toast
Butter
Milk
Ice cream

METHOD
Summary: Beat eggs until frothy and pour them into a frying pan. Press in fresh spinach and add cheese; cover and cook until set.

Wash and spin dry *4 to 8 ounces fresh spinach*.

Melt *1 to 2 teaspoons butter* in a nonstick frying pan using almost-the-lowest temperature on your range.

Bring *6 to 8 eggs* to room temperature by letting them stand for 5 minutes in your hottest tap water. (Be sure the eggs are not cracked. If they are, throw them away.) Crack the eggs into a deep glass bowl. Add *1/3 cup cool water* (1 tablespoon per egg). Beat with an electric mixer until the eggs are frothy. Pour mixture immediately into the frying pan.

Gently press the fresh spinach into the eggs, putting in as much as can be coated with egg, and finely crumble *4 ounces feta cheese* over the eggs.

Cover and cook slowly for 10 to 20 minutes or until the eggs are set to your liking.

Slip the frittata onto a plate, slice, and serve.

RECIPE NOTES
Fast tip: Frittata *is* a fast tip. It is a busy person's version of an omelet. With frittata, you don't have to hover and check and fold and check again. Write down the setting and burner you use and how long you cook the frittata. Next time you make it, you can set the timer and forget it.

The night before: This can be a clean-out-the-refrigerator meal. Investigate your resources for vegetables, cheese, and meat for the frittata or for fruit or vegetables for a salad.

Involving your children: Let children crack the eggs, wash and spin the spinach.

Adapting this meal for children: Be sure to have plenty of toast, milk, and a popular fruit. Even if she doesn't like frittata, your child will survive.

Variations: Potato Frittata Brown pre-prepared hash browns, add chopped onions and cook them until they are clear, and substitute grated cheddar cheese for the feta cheese. **Bacon or Ham Frittata** Add crumbled bacon or small pieces of ham to the potato frittata, sprinkle with cheddar cheese.

Ratatouille Frittata Substitute leftover **Ratatouille** (page 158) and use Swiss cheese instead of feta.

Almost any vegetable works well in a frittata, and almost any cheese. Warm up leftover vegetables from the refrigerator, add them to the beaten egg, and top with any kind of grated cheese you choose. Use your imagination!

For a crowd, double this recipe and bake it in a 9 × 13-inch pan at 325° F for 20 minutes.

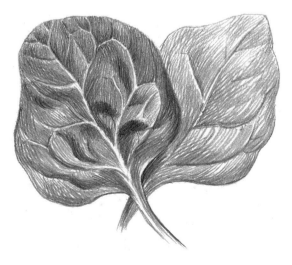

Lemon Chicken

This is a fast, easy, and wonderfully tasty chicken recipe that features prebrowning in store-bought mixed seasoning and olive oil or butter, then braising to get the chicken done inside.

I like butter for sautéing because it tastes good and browns well—the food develops a lovely golden color with relatively little heat and cooking time. But butter does burn easily, so you have to watch carefully when food is browning. A handy compromise is to combine butter with a high-monounsaturated oil such as peanut or canola oil or, if you want the flavor, olive oil. Whichever method you use, heat up your pan before you put in the fat. If your pan is the correct temperature, butter will melt quickly but not immediately burn, and oils will shimmer.

Lemon chicken makes a handy PPM. Put it on a bun for a hot or cold sandwich, or cut it across the grain into thin slices and toss the slices with a green salad for a quick lunch. Simply super.

INGREDIENTS
6 boned chicken breast halves (3 to 4 oz each),
*   boned skinless thighs, or a combination of the two*
2 Tbsp butter or *olive oil*
2 tsp lemon pepper
2 Tbsp water

MENU
Lemon chicken
Oven-roasted potatoes (page 161)
Creamed spinach (page 156) or vegetables in season
Peach cobbler (page 162) or peach crisp (page 164)
Fruit in season
Bread or toast
Butter
Milk

METHOD
Summary: Brown chicken in seasoned oil, add water to the pan, reduce heat, and cover. The steam finishes the cooking.

Wash, drain, and blot with paper towels the 3 to 4 ounce pieces *chicken breast or thighs.*

Heat *2 tablespoons butter* or *olive oil* at medium temperature in a nonstick frying pan. Add about *2 teaspoons lemon pepper*. Immediately add the chicken and brown on both sides. When the browning is finished, add about 2 tablespoons water to the pan and cover.

Reduce the heat to low, cover, and let the steam finish cooking the chicken—probably another 10 minutes. It's done when the chicken is white in the middle and cooked to an internal temperature of 165° F. Don't overcook it or it will get tough and stringy.

RECIPE NOTES

The night before: In separate pans, place the frozen chicken and spinach in the refrigerator to thaw. Locate the potatoes, and maybe wash them. Locate the pan and the parmesan cheese for the oven-roasted potatoes, and mix up the spices. Find the peaches and locate the dry ingredients for the cobbler (mix them up and put a plate over the top of the bowl), or locate your cache of crisp topping.

Presentation: Garnish with thin lemon slices.

Involving your children: Children can scrub the potatoes, mix up the potato topping, unwrap the thawed frozen spinach, put it in the colander, squeeze out the water, and put it in the cooking dish.

Adapting this meal for children: To serve so your child can help herself, cut some of the chicken breasts up into child-sized helpings as you put them on the platter. Let your child eat the potatoes with her fingers. Put the spinach in little bowls so she can eat it easily with a spoon.

Variations: Baked Lemon Chicken Brush the chicken with butter, sprinkle with lemon pepper, and bake at 400° F for 20 minutes or 325° F for 30 minutes to an internal temperature of 165 ° F.

Parmesan Chicken Smear the chicken breast with mustard, sprinkle with parmesan cheese, and bake at 400° F for 20 minutes or 325° F for 30 minutes to an internal temperature of 165° F. If you don't like the mustard, try mayonnaise, Italian dressing, or butter.

Mock Fried Chicken Flour chicken pieces with a mixture of 1/3 cup flour and 2 teaspoons **Meat and Poultry Seasoning**: 1 teaspoon salt, 1/4 teaspoon pepper, 1/2 teaspoon poultry seasoning, and 1/2 teaspoon paprika. Brown the pieces at medium heat in butter, reduce the heat to low, and cover them to finish cooking for 5 or 10 minutes. To get a crisper coating, finish cooking by putting the pieces on a rack in a baking pan and sliding them into an oven preheated to 325° F. Bake for 5 to 10 minutes.

Braised Pork Chops with Sweet Potatoes

Consider putting pork chops on your menus. Fresh pork is delicious, reasonably priced, high in protein, and particularly high in thiamine. Because grocery stores have difficulty convincing consumers to buy pork, prices are often relatively low. Today's pork is low in fat and is trichina-free. (Trichina seems to show up most often in bear meat, so be careful when you cook your bear!) Pork is tender and cooks quickly. You don't have to overcook it and dry it out to make it safe. Cook to an internal temperature of 160° F will make your pork chops juicy, tender, and appealing.

Adding sweet potatoes to this dish makes it tasty and expeditious. Not only are the potatoes an excellent source of vitamin A and carotene, but they are also filling and complement the taste of pork.

INGREDIENTS

4 sweet potatoes
1 to 2 Tbsp butter
1 to 2 tsp dried sage
6 3- to 4-oz boneless or *bone-in loin pork chops*
1/2 cup chicken broth or *apple juice*
Salt and pepper to taste

MENU

Braised pork chops with sweet potatoes
Microwave chunky applesauce (page 163)
Bread or toast
Butter
Milk
Ice cream

METHOD

Summary: Brown pork chops in butter and sage. Parboil sweet potatoes. Combine everything, cover, and braise until done.

Peel the *4 sweet potatoes* (which are sometimes called *yams*), wash them, and cut them into 1-inch slices. Parboil (partially boil) the sweet potatoes by cooking them for 5 minutes in boiling water salted with 1 teaspoon salt per quart. When you can just get a fork into the potatoes, remove them from the heat and drain.

While the potatoes cook, melt *1 to 2 tablespoons butter* at medium heat in a large frying pan that has a tight-fitting lid. Sprinkle *1 to 2 teaspoons dried sage* into the melted butter or rub on the pork chops. With the lid off, brown

6 3- to 4-ounce pork chops on both sides and remove them from the pan.

Pour off excess grease from the frying pan and add *1/2 cup chicken broth or apple juice*. Lay the parboiled sweet potatoes in the frying pan, lay the browned pork chops over the sweet potatoes, and add *salt and pepper to taste*. Cover, reduce the heat to low, and cook for an additional 10 to 20 minutes, or until the sweet potatoes are fork-tender and the pork chops are cooked to an internal temperature of 160° F.

RECIPE NOTES

Fast tip: Once you master cooking pork chops, they can be your fast tip. Pork chops are ready to cook, and they cook quickly.

The night before: Place frozen pork chops in the refrigerator to thaw. Find the potatoes, peel them, and cover them with water to keep them from darkening. For the microwaved applesauce, find and wash the apples and locate the dish for cooking them. The applesauce gets better with standing, so go ahead and cook the applesauce if you have the time and energy.

Involving your children: Children can peel the potatoes. A preschooler can cut up the apple wedges for the applesauce with a plastic picnic knife. An older child can make the applesauce, except for getting it in and out of the microwave.

Adapting this meal for children: This meal works great for children because the meat is so tender and the vegetables are appealing.

Variations: Make braised pork chops to combine with other menus by using the same technique given in the **Lemon Chicken** recipe. Brown the chops at medium heat in seasoned butter or oil (you can experiment with a variety of seasonings—or use none at all), and finish cooking by braising: Add a small amount of liquid, reduce the heat to low, and cook with the lid on the pan to an internal temperature of 160° F.

Make **Sautéed Pork Chops** by dredging them in a mixture of 1 Tablespoon **Meat and Poultry Seasoning** (recipe on page 116) and 1/2 cup flour. Brown them on both sides in butter. To finish cooking and preserve the crisp coating, slip the pork chops into a 325° F oven for 5 to 10 minutes to an internal temperature of 160° F.

Wisconsin Fish Boil

This is a variation on poached fish. Fish boil is a traditional meal in Door County, a lovely vacation spot that makes up the "thumb" of Wisconsin. For the full treatment, fish boil needs to be prepared in a huge cooker over an open fire. Since cherries are a major crop in Door County, the meal is only complete with a cherry dessert.

INGREDIENTS
1 1/2 lb cod or *haddock*
6 medium boiling potatoes
6 small whole onions
1 1/2 lb carrots

MENU
Wisconsin fish boil
Potatoes
Carrots
Onions
Melted butter
Bread and butter
Cherry cobbler (page 162)
Ice cream

METHOD
Summary: The idea is to cook all the vegetables and the fish in the same pot in the same water. Start the vegetables cooking first, and about 10 minutes before they are done, add the fish and finish cooking. Put the fish in a steamer insert before you lower it into the water to keep it from breaking up and to make it easier to remove from the pot.

Fill an 8-quart pan about two-thirds full. To leave room to cook both the vegetables and the fish, make the water level 2 to 3 inches above the top of the vegetables.

Heavily salt the water with 1 tablespoon salt per quart of water. (This is not a mistake. The extra salt helps the fish keep its shape. Don't worry—the food won't taste too salty.) Bring to a rapid boil.

Prepare the following: *1 1/2 pounds cod or haddock*, cut into helping-sized pieces, *6 medium boiling potatoes, 6 small whole onions,* and *1 1/2 pounds carrots*, peeled and cut into chunks, or baby carrots left whole.

Begin cooking the vegetables first by putting them in the salted, boiling water. When the vegetables have been boiling for 10 minutes, or when you can just get your fork into them, lower the fish-filled steamer insert into the boiling water, lower the temperature to a fast simmer, and cook

for 5 to 10 more minutes, until the fish reaches an internal temperature of 130° F to 140° F. Remove all the food from the water, arrange on a platter, and pass with melted butter.

RECIPE NOTES
Fast tip: To remove the fish, lift out the insert. Drain the vegetables in a colander, and you are ready to arrange the food on a platter and serve!

The night before: Place frozen fish in the refrigerator to thaw, find the cooking pot, and determine what you will use as a steamer insert for the fish. Locate the vegetables. For the cherry cobbler, put frozen cherries in the refrigerator to thaw. Locate the dry ingredients and mix them up.

Added touch: Melt butter and put it in a pitcher or gravy boat to serve. This is not really "added." It is essential!

Presentation: As artfully as you can, arrange the fish and vegetables on the platter and add a few slices of lemon and a few sprigs of parsley to dress it up. This meal is hard to arrange to make it look pretty, but if you don't forget the melted butter, it won't matter.

Involving your children: Children can help clean the vegetables and make the cherry cobbler.

Adapting this meal for children: As long as the fish is boneless, this is a great meal for children. The menu has a number of items, and they are all moist, soft, and easy to chew.

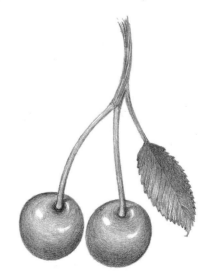

Hamburgers

Once you master your method, your table can be the place to get the best burgers in town. The key to juicy, flavorful hamburgers is cooking them until they are done—but no more.

INGREDIENTS
1 Tbsp butter
1 Tbsp Worcestershire sauce
1 1/2 lb ground beef

MENU
Hamburgers on buns
Dill pickle slices
Lettuce
Tomato slices
Chopped onion or thin onion slices
Mayonnaise
Ketchup and mustard
Potato chips
Carrot and celery sticks, pickle spears
Fruit in season
Milk

METHOD
Summary: Shape hamburger patties and fry them until they are done to your liking.

In a nonstick frying pan, heat *1 tablespoon butter* at medium temperature. Add *1 tablespoon Worcestershire sauce.*

Form *1 1/2 pounds ground beef* into 6 4-ounce patties (they will cook down to 3 ounces).

Harold McGee, author of *On Food and Cooking,* found in his laboratory that turning meat often cooks it more evenly. Flip your burgers every minute or so, and check the temperature after three or four flips. For done but not dried-out burgers, cook to an internal temperature of 160° F.

RECIPE NOTES
Fast tip: To keep hamburger patties on hand in the freezer, make them when you get home from the grocery store, lay them out on a jelly roll pan lined with waxed paper or parchment paper, freeze them, then store them in a zip top bag. Also consider purchasing pre-portioned, frozen beef patties. If the price and quality are agreeable, why not let someone else do your work for you?

The night before: Put frozen ground beef in the refrigerator to thaw. If they have been refrigerated (refrigerating tomatoes destroys an important flavor component), put the tomatoes on the counter to bring them to room temperature. Find the ketchup, mustard, mayonnaise, potato chips, and pickles. Clean and crisp the celery and carrots. Chop the onions and refrigerate them in a tightly closed jar.

Added touch: Sprinkle a little dill weed on the burgers as you begin to cook them. Search for some great buns. Buns make all the difference between a hamburger and a great hamburger. If you don't have buns in the house, consider making **Gravy** (page 113) with the pan drippings.

Presentation: Put out toppings and let family members doctor their burgers to taste.

Involving your children: Once your child is reliable about cleanliness when working with raw meat—when she can remember to wash her hands before and after she handles it and doesn't put her meat-juicy hands in her mouth—let her help shape hamburger patties. Making a fancy shape can be a fun treat occasionally, but don't get caught up in making food cute to capture your child's interest. If you do, you are probably trying to get your child to eat, and even though your attempts are creative and playful, they will backfire.

Adapting this meal for children: These hamburgers are big, so you might want to cut them in half for children. If you can find little buns, make the hamburger patties smaller. Kids enjoy food that is "their size."

Chapter
9
How to Keep Cooking

Let's take a look at your progress. Are you having some successes by now with your cooking, and—even better—are you starting to get some pleasure from cooking and from food you make yourself? Rather than finding cooking a mysterious and alarming business, are you developing rhythms and intuitions with food? When someone asks you for a recipe, do you have to stop to think about what you really *did* do? That means you are turning into a cook. Congratulations!

I do hope the process of food preparation holds some satisfaction for you, at least some of the time. If not, why not? Are your standards too high? Does your attitude need adjustment? Would you benefit from setting aside time occasionally to enjoy cooking? Like eating, cooking can be a creative act that gives you a change of pace and restores your energy. Why not let it be that for you? Take a clue from your meditating friends, and let your cooking be mindful. Tune in on it, enjoy it, and let it be restorative.

Can you make a few things well? Give yourself a pat on the back. Things didn't turn out the way you had hoped? Keep it to yourself. Your apologies just make your diners uncomfortable. You're not forcing anybody to eat, so they can take care of themselves. Make notes in your cookbook on how to make it better the next time, and forget about it. After experiencing more cooking failures than I care to think about, I finally concluded that if something turned out well the first time I made it, I was lucky. If it turned out well the second or third time, it was because I had adapted the recipe to my stove, my pans, and my methods, and it had therefore

become *mine*. No matter how good a recipe is, the nature of working with food is variation. As you develop your cooking skill and confidence, you will take those variations in stride.

More Recipes and Cooking Possibilities

The recipes in this chapter are a bit more complex than the ones in chapter 8, "How to Get Cooking," and they give you opportunities to learn about cooking dry beans, making soup (with its all-important broth), choosing and cooking rice, and frying. Although they have a few more steps, the recipes are still simple and accessible. Because we are cooking ahead to make PPMs (pre-prepared meals, otherwise known as leftovers), and because they keep well and taste even better the second day than the first, some of the recipes also make bigger batches. The recipes for **Beef Stew, Chicken Soup**, and **Savory Black Beans and Rice** make about 12 helpings, roughly twice the amount made by the recipes we worked with before.

In this chapter, you will also find short cuts, such as "last resort" ideas like grab-and-dump meals and prepackaged "convenience" meals, along with ideas for cooking for one person. In the discussion about the generic casserole we'll eke out some general principles of food composition and recipe construction that you can use when you want to improvise and create your very own signature one-dish meal. Finally, to help you continue to develop as a cook, we'll talk about cookbooks, television cooking shows, and cooking classes.

Chicken Soup

This recipe makes a big enough batch so you can eat it for lunch or freeze it for another dinner. Surveys tell us that chicken soup, like meat loaf, is one of our comfort foods. Chicken soup is also invested with curative powers. Does it really matter whether those powers are real or imagined? Whatever its appeal, there is no doubt that knowing how to make a pot of chicken soup comes in handy. Winter or summer, soup makes a convenient and satisfying meal.

INGREDIENTS

12 oz skinless, boneless chicken breasts and/
or thighs
Large (46-oz) can chicken broth
1 1/2 cups shredded carrots
1 large onion, chopped
1/2 cup chopped celery
6 oz wide egg noodles
Fresh or dried parsley

MENU

Chicken soup
Chewy bread
Butter
Fruit in season
Milk
Ice cream and cookies

METHOD

Summary: First poach the chicken in the broth, lift it out, and set it aside. Boil the vegetables and noodles in the broth. Cut up the chicken and add back to the broth.

Poach the chicken: Bring *12 ounces chicken* and *1 large (46-ounce) can chicken broth* to a boil in a large Dutch oven or soup pot. Turn off the heat, cover, and let stand for 20 to 30 minutes.

Using a long-handled slotted spoon, remove the poached chicken from the broth. Bring the broth back to a rolling boil and add *1 1/2 cups shredded carrots* and any other vegetables that can cook in about 5 to 10 minutes, such as *1 large chopped onion* and *1/2 cup chopped celery*. Along with the vegetables, add *six ounces wide egg noodles* (estimate the weight by dividing the 12- or 16-ounce package).

Reduce the heat to a medium boil and cook until the noodles are al dente. Meanwhile, cut the cooked chicken into bite-sized pieces using a sharp knife and a cutting board. When the noodles and vegetables are done, reduce the heat and add the cut-up chicken. Put in some fresh or dried parsley to give it a little color. Depending on how hot you like your soup, turn off the heat and let the room-temperature chicken cool it down a bit, or reheat it until it is again simmering. Be careful not to boil—boiling it at this point will overcook the chicken and break apart the noodles and vegetables.

RECIPE NOTES

Fast tip: To make this recipe even easier, buy canned, deboned chicken. Also consider purchasing shredded carrots. The shreds are long, so cut them crosswise to shorten them up a bit.

The night before: In the refrigerator, thaw frozen chicken in a pan to catch the drips. Unearth the soup pot. (In my house, it is in the basement. I use it infrequently, so I store it in an out-of-the-way place.) Wash and chop the onion and celery. Peel and shred the carrots, or locate your shredded carrots.

Presentation: Keep your eyes open at garage sales for an interesting soup tureen for serving this and other soups.

Involving your children: Children can help wash celery and peel onions. Chopping onions is tricky because of their shape, so keep that job for yourself. An older child can make the dumplings (for the variation).

Adapting this meal for children: For the child who eats with his fingers, separate the solids from the liquid so he can eat the solids with his fingers and drink the broth from a cup. Consider cutting the vegetables in pieces big enough to pick up easily. You can also give your child less broth, or add crackers to thicken the broth enough to make it easier to eat with a spoon or fingers.

Variation: Leave out the noodles and add **Ricotta Dumplings** (see next recipe) or make dumplings using the recipe and directions on the Bisquick box.

FIGURE 9.1 POACHING AND SIMMERING
Chicken cooks fast in water. The instructions say to *poach* the chicken in simmering water separately from the noodles because noodles need to be boiled, and boiling can make chicken tough and stringy. Poaching the chicken in the broth gives both the chicken and the broth a little more flavor. Liquid simmers when bubbles rise slowly to the surface and just barely seem to break.

FIGURE 9.2 BROTH
The stock is the essential ingredient of good soup, so don't skimp on it. This recipe calls for canned broth, which is tasty. The "real cook's" way of making a soup base is to cook bones and vegetables for a long time, simmer the cooking liquid down to concentrate it, then strain it. I won't teach you that because, after years of trying, I have given up on it. Instead, I discovered broth-concentrate paste. Some stores carry it in bulk; I generally can only find it in jars. It is concentrated in flavor and salty, so you have to be careful about how much broth base and added salt you use. Your grocery store might have a broth sold in a carton or a frozen soup base. You might like bouillon cubes or crystals (to me, they taste artificial). Explore until you find a soup base that you like. It will open up a whole world of soup-making possibilities for you.

Regular canned chicken broth has 1,000 milligrams of sodium per cup, which is high. (See the section, "Salt" in the "How to Cook" prologue, page 92.) Even low-salt broth varieties have 700 milligrams of sodium per cup. That's a reasonable amount unless you are on a salt-free diet. If you follow the package directions to substitute broth concentrate or bouillon cubes, you will get about 500 to 600 milligrams of sodium per cup of reconstituted broth.

FIGURE 9.3 SIFTING FLOUR
Because flour packs down in the bag or canister, many baking recipes call for sifted flour. To be measured properly, flour has to be sifted or fluffed up again. I find that stirring fluffs it enough and is a whole lot faster and easier than sifting.

Ricotta Dumplings for Chicken Soup

Since the dumplings cook somewhat into the soup, the dumplings give a thicker and more gravy-like broth.

After cooking for 30 years, I discovered that the secret of keeping dumplings from falling apart in the broth is to let the mixed-up dough sit for a few minutes before spooning it into the boiling broth. On the other hand, dumplings that break down in broth give it a delicious gravy-like consistency. Don't peek once you put the lid on the pan, or the dumplings will get hard. Hard is the way I like them, so when I was a little girl I regularly sneaked into the kitchen to lift the lid off the pot. However, that is not a prescribed dumpling-making technique.

INGREDIENTS
2 cups all-purpose flour, stirred before you measure
1 Tbsp baking powder
1 tsp salt
1/2 tsp dried thyme
1 Tbsp dried parsley flakes
1/2 cup ricotta cheese
1 egg
1/4 cup milk

METHOD
Summary: Combine the dry ingredients in one bowl and the wet ingredients in another. Mix the two together to form a dough. Let stand for 15 minutes, then drop spoonfuls into boiling broth and simmer.

In a medium-sized bowl mix together *2 cups all-purpose flour*, stirred before you measure, *1 tablespoon baking powder, 1 teaspoon salt, 1/2 teaspoon dried thyme*, and *1 tablespoon dried parsley flakes*.

In a small bowl, stir together *1/2 cup ricotta cheese, 1 egg,* and *1/4 cup milk* until well mixed.

Add the wet ingredients to the dry ingredients. Stir just until the dough holds together; if you stir the batter too much, the dumplings will be tough.

Let the dough rest for 15 minutes.

Using a tablespoon or a #60 ice cream scoop (see figure 8.12, "Small Ice Cream Scoops," on page 113), form dumplings and drop them into the gently boiling broth. Dipping the spoon or scoop in the boiling broth between scoops helps the dumplings drop out more easily. Cook uncovered 10 minutes and covered 10 minutes.

Beef Stew

This classic American recipe makes about 12 servings and is even better warmed over. This stew is much like a boiled dinner. It has a lot of broth that you eat with a spoon, and the vegetables are in big pieces that you eat with a knife and fork. It tastes great over purchased baking powder biscuits or the **Yorkshire Pudding** (page 126).

Braised beef cubes (beef cooked a long time in liquid in a covered pan, at a low temperature) can solo as beef cubes over noodles and substitute for Swiss Steak in **Beefy Shortcut Stroganoff** (page 108). Be sure to check the Variations: With a few changes in seasonings and vegetables, this stew can turn into a wonderful array of recipes that may become your standbys.

INGREDIENTS

2 Tbsp butter, margarine, or cooking oil
2 lbs stew beef, cut into 1-inch cubes
4 cloves garlic, minced
2 15-oz cans beef broth or 4 cups water with 4 tsp to 2 Tbsp beef broth concentrate
15-oz can diced tomatoes
10-oz can golden mushroom soup
1/4 cup red wine (optional)
1 Tbsp sugar
1 tsp salt
1 tsp ground black pepper
4 medium potatoes, washed, peeled, and cut in chunks
8 small onions, peeled and cut in halves or fourths
8 whole medium carrots, peeled and chunked or 15–20 peeled baby carrots
1/2 head celery, washed and cut crosswise in 1-inch pieces
Other slow-cooking vegetables as available: cauliflower, rutabaga, turnips, etc.

MENU

Beef stew
Baking powder biscuits or Yorkshire pudding (page 126)
Butter
Canned peaches or fruit in season
Cucumber slices
Milk
Pumpkin custard (page 148)

METHOD

Summary: Brown cubed stew beef in butter. Add minced garlic for the last 30 seconds, stir, and cook lightly. Add beef broth, tomatoes, golden mushroom soup, wine (optional), sugar, salt, and pepper. Simmer for 1 1/2 hours. Add the vegetables and continue to simmer for another hour or until the vegetables are tender when tested with a fork. Add enough salt and pepper to make it taste the way you like it.

In a Dutch oven, heat *2 tablespoons butter* or *cooking oil* at medium temperature until sizzling. Add *2 pounds stew beef cut into 1-inch cubes* and cook at medium temperature until beef cubes are light brown. At the very end of browning, add *4 cloves minced garlic*. Cook garlic briefly until it is golden but not brown. Add and bring up to simmering: *2 15-ounce cans beef broth* or *4 cups water with 4 teaspoons to 2 tablespoons beef broth concentrate* (read the package directions; use less concentrate than recommended, and taste to see if you need to add more). Also add the *15-ounce can diced tomatoes*, the *10-ounce can golden mushroom soup*, *1/4 cup red wine* (optional), *1 tablespoon sugar*, *1 teaspoon salt*, and *1 teaspoon ground black pepper*. The heating liquids will deglaze the pan for you—get the good stuff off the pan and into the cooking liquid. Simmer for 1 1/2 hours before adding vegetables.

Add the washed and peeled vegetables: *4 medium potatoes* cut in chunks, *8 small onions* cut in halves or fourths, *8 medium carrots, chunked* or 15 to 20 *peeled baby carrots*, and *1/2 head celery*, cut crosswise in 1-inch pieces. You may also add other slow-cooking vegetables, such as cauliflower, rutabaga, or turnips. Simmer for 1 hour or until the vegetables are done to your liking.

Instead of simmering on top of the stove, you can combine all the ingredients at one time and simmer in a slow cooker 3 to 4 hours on medium or 5 to 6 hours on low, or in a 250-degree oven for 4 to 6 hours. Make a note of how long it takes to get the stew done to your liking for next time.

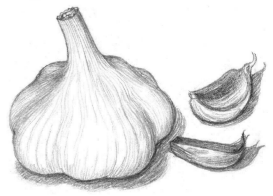

RECIPE NOTES

Fast tip: You can purchase stew beef in the meat case. For lower-cost and more consistently sized pieces of stew beef, cut up your own from chuck steak or sirloin tip steak. Sirloin tip is quicker-cooking and higher in fat, and therefore more flavorful and more tender. See figure 9.4 on this page for instructions on preparing your stew beef ahead of time.

Instead of cutting up onions, use canned or frozen tiny onions. It makes a nice touch and saves crying over onions. Add precooked onions toward the end of cooking so they don't get overcooked.

The night before: Put frozen beef cubes in the refrigerator to thaw. Locate all the ingredients. Consider preparing the vegetables and covering them with cold water. Get out the Dutch oven or slow cooker. Taste the wine to be sure it is okay. (Just kidding.)

Presentation: Set the table with flat bowls and eat with forks, knives, and spoons.

Involving your children: Your children can count out the baby carrots, wash the potatoes, and pound the garlic. Pulverized garlic still tastes like garlic, but you have to scrape it up to put it in the pot.

Adapting this meal for children: Most of the alcohol in wine boils off during cooking. It is up to you whether the trace that remains is concerning. Everything in this meal is soft, moist, and easy to chew. To give even more help to beginning eaters, cut the cooked meat *across* the grain. Cutting with the grain gives long fibers that are more difficult to munch or chew. Cut the vegetables in pieces big enough for finger-eaters to pick up and bite off. Older children like eating plain cucumber slices and consider them finger food. Because this is a one-dish meal and therefore sink-or-swim, I gave inexperienced eaters more options by putting canned peaches on the menu as well as pumpkin custard for dessert.

FIGURE 9.4 PREPARING BEEF CUBES
Prepare ahead by purchasing and cutting up several pounds of beef cubes from chuck steak or sirloin tip steak and freezing them in 1-pound zip top bags.

Precooked beef cubes: Prepare ahead even more by using your oven and a large roasting pan to make a great vat of precooked beef cubes that you can freeze in 12-ounce bags (a pound cooks down to 12 ounces). It takes time, but the oven-browning method works well and you clean up only once. Preheat oven to 350° F. In a roasting pan that can be covered, melt 1 tablespoon butter for each pound of stew beef. Add the beef, stir, leave the lid off the pan, and return to the oven. Roast for about 20 minutes, stir, roast again, stir again. Two or three 20-minute roastings should brown the beef cubes nicely. Put the lid on the pan, turn the oven down to 325° F, and braise until the beef cubes are tender. Sirloin tip steak takes about an additional 1/2 hour after browning. Chuck steak takes about 1 1/2 hours after browning. When the meat is done to your liking, divide it up in as many bags as you had pounds of meat to start with, and divide any broth among the bags. Freeze the beef cubes and broth. You can use these precooked beef cubes in any recipe that calls for stew beef: Each bag gives the equivalent of 1 pound raw beef cubes. Use the precooked beef cubes and broth as is over noodles or mashed potatoes, or add some sautéed onion and garlic to give additional flavor.

FIGURE 9.5 BROWNING MEAT
You brown meat, fish, and poultry to develop the flavor. Prescribed meat cooking technique is to brown at high temperatures to sear the meat and seal in the juices. According to Harold McGee (*On Food and Cooking: The Science and Lore of the Kitchen*), it doesn't work. Seared meat is no juicier than meat that has not been seared. Instead, brown meat at a high enough temperature to get the sizzle, but not so high that you get the smoking, mess, and splatter. Browning does not necessarily fully cook the food—the cooking has to be finished another way. When you brown, notice that at first water and juices cook out. The water and juices bubble up, making a soft, gurgling, water-in-a-brook sound. As the water cooks off, the sound changes to a more high-pitched, fat-splattering sound. That's when browning occurs. At that point, watch the food carefully, because it browns quickly. Brown to your taste. I find if I get beef cubes too browned, it dries them out too much, so I settle for only lightly browned. Butter browns foods more easily than other fats and adds a lovely flavor. However, it also burns more easily, so watch it more carefully during browning.

Variations: Start by browning 2 pounds stew beef. Add 4 cloves minced garlic for the last few seconds. Then add the liquid and spices called for by the variation and braise the meat for a total of 2 1/2 hours. Add the vegetables called for by the variation partway through cooking as directed. Add the quick-cooking ingredients at the end.

Beef Ragout What could be more sophisticated than a French dish? The word *ragout* comes from a French word meaning "to revive the taste." Might this recipe have originated as a way to use up leftovers? Serve it with cooked noodles.

Liquid: 4 cups beef broth and 1/2 cup dry red wine (optional)
Spices: 2 teaspoons dried thyme and 1/4 teaspoon black pepper
Vegetables: 15–20 peeled baby carrots and 2 medium onions, cut in wedges. Add 1 hour before the end of cooking
Quick-cooking: 8 ounces fresh mushrooms, sliced, or 16-ounce can mushroom stems and pieces, drained

Moroccan Stew This wonderfully tasty variation may strain your spice cabinet, but it is worth it. Moroccan cooking is highly spiced, although predominantly Islam Moroccans wouldn't include the beer. I include it because it adds flavor. Serve with couscous.

Liquid: 1 28-ounce plus 1 15-ounce cans diced tomatoes and 1 cup beer
Spices: 1/2 teaspoon pepper; 1 teaspoon each salt, paprika, turmeric, and coriander; 1 1/2 teaspoons ground cumin; 3 tablespoons orange zest (grated orange peel); and 3 cinnamon sticks, pounded into splinters
Vegetables: 1 pound carrots, cut into sticks. Add 30 minutes before the end of cooking
Quick-cooking: 2 15-ounce cans chick peas, drained

Balsamic Stew For added flavor in this and any other stew, use olive oil for browning the beef cubes. Serve with rice, couscous, potatoes, or noodles.

Liquid: 1 15-ounce can beef broth and 3 tablespoons balsamic vinegar
Spices: Salt and pepper to taste
Vegetables: 1 pound carrots, cut lengthwise into fourths, or 1 pound baby carrots; 3 celery stalks, sliced into strips; and 1 large onion, sliced
Quick-cooking: 1/2 cup chopped parsley

FIGURE 9.6 GARLIC
With your fingers, you can easily separate a head of garlic into cloves, each of which has a thin, dry skin. To prepare the garlic clove, get rid of the skin, cut off the stem end and mince it. To easily get the skin off and begin mincing at the same time, put the garlic clove on a cutting board and pound it lightly with a meat mallet, the bottom of a jar, or the flat side of a big knife. That breaks the skin away so you can remove it easily with your fingers. Then you can pulverize it by pounding it some more, mince it with a garlic press, or cut it very finely with a knife. *Or* forget the whole thing and buy garlic in jars or garlic powder. The container will tell you how much to substitute for cloves of garlic.

Fresh garlic tastes better if it is lightly browned before you put it in a recipe, but if you brown it too long, it gets bitter. Cook it for 30 seconds or so. Stop the browning by removing it from the pan or by adding liquid ingredients.

Yorkshire Pudding

A traditional British accompaniment to beef, Yorkshire pudding is an easy-to-make bread that is essentially a popover. When making it to accompany the **Beef Stew** dinner, bake it at the same time you bake the pumpkin custard.

INGREDIENTS
3 Tbsp cooking oil, lard, or *butter*
1 1/2 cups all-purpose flour
1/2 tsp salt
2 eggs
1 cup milk

METHOD
Summary: Put cooking fat in a dish and heat in the oven. Beat flour, salt, eggs, and milk into a batter and pour into hot baking dish with the melted fat. Bake.

Preheat oven to 350° F.

Put *3 tablespoons fat (cooking oil, lard,* or *butter)* in an 8 × 8 × 2-inch Pyrex dish and heat it in the oven for 5 minutes. To prepare the batter, beat together until very smooth *1 1/2 cups flour, 1/2 teaspoon salt, 2 eggs,* and *1 cup milk*. Pour batter into the hot baking dish with the melted fat and bake for 20 to 30 minutes. It will be a puffy and irregular golden mass with a crispy, delicate outside crust and a center that is soft and somewhat custard-like. Cut into serving-sized pieces and eat with a fork or your fingers.

Pesto-Parmesan Chicken

Clio (of "Clio's Excellent Adventure" in Chapter 5) has been making this dish ever since I have known her, and it is unfailingly delicious. It is company-pretty and enticing but family-friendly and easy-to-make.

INGREDIENTS

6 boneless, skinless chicken breast halves, about 1 1/2 lbs
1 1/2 cups grated Parmesan, Romano, or Asiago cheese, about 6 ounces
6 Tbsp pesto

MENU

Pesto Parmesan Chicken
Roasted Broccoli
Rice
Ciabatta bread
Butter
Fruit in season
Milk

METHOD

Summary: Rub chicken with pesto-cheese mixture. Press chicken breasts into grated cheese. Bake.

Preheat oven to 425° F.

Mix *2 tablespoons grated Parmesan, Romano, or Asiago* cheese with *6 tablespoons pesto*. Rub or pat pesto mixture onto *6 boneless, skinless chicken breast halves (about 1 1/2 pounds)*, until you have a light, even coating. Sprinkle the remaining cheese onto a plate. Press both sides of the chicken into the cheese to form a coating. You will probably need to refresh your plate of grated cheese several times. Be careful that you do not contaminate your container of cheese by handling it after you have handled the raw chicken.

Place the chicken into a 10 x 6-inch baking dish. Bake for 25 minutes to an internal temperature of 165° F.

RECIPE NOTES

Fast tip: You can, of course, make your own pesto from basil that you grow in your own garden. What an achievement! You can also purchase pesto at the framer's market or in the frozen-foods case at the grocery store. Look for a pesto where the first listed ingredient is basil, *not* oil or cheese or some other ingredient.

Use the chicken breasts as they come from the package—don't unroll them or flatten them out. Leaving the chicken in thicker pieces makes it easier to produce cooked chicken that is still moist. Keep a close eye on the internal temperature and take it out immediately when it reaches 165° F. Tent it with aluminum foil to keep it warm until you are ready to serve.

Consider making more chicken to have it for another dinner or to use in the variations suggested below.

The night before: In the refrigerator, thaw frozen chicken in a pan to catch the drips. Unearth the baking dish. Shred or grate cheese if necessary. Thaw the pesto.

Presentation: This dish is very pretty. Serve in the dish you bake it in. Tip the dish to dip up enough pan juices to flavor the rice or for dipping your bread.

Involving your children: This dish is easy enough that a child old enough to be aware of contamination issues can put it together with minimal supervision. Younger children can grate the cheese. Very young children can wash the broccoli.

Adapting this meal for children: At first, children may find the flavor of pesto and parmesan challenging—or not. You can't predict! Most children can eat rice, and the Ciabatta bread is appealing—especially with plenty of butter—so they can fall back on those. Roasted broccoli may be popular at your house—or not—you might want to substitute corn, and save the broccoli for a night when you have a more-popular entrée. And of course, there is always the fruit. If all else fails, children can eat fruit and bread and drink their milk.

Variations: Slice the leftover chicken pieces thinly across the grain and use them in sandwiches or in salads. You can even put leftovers in a quesadilla along with grated mozzarella cheese.

Minestrone Soup

This recipe makes enough for about 12 servings. I generally double it to make about 24 servings, but here I keep it to 12 so you can see if you like it before you produce it in quantity. Minestrone soup freezes and warms up well, so having some in reserve is both a treat and a help.

Cooking dry beans is quite easily done with a little planning and preparation. The main strategy in this recipe is to cook the beans and beef at the same time and let them flavor each other. Using canned beans, however, is perfectly okay, so don't feel obligated to start with dry beans if you don't want to.

INGREDIENTS

1/2 lb dried kidney beans
1 lb beef for stew, cut into 1/2-inch cubes
2 Tbsp butter
5 to 6 oz uncooked spaghetti, broken into 1-inch
   segments
2 to 3 Tbsp olive oil
1 large onion, chopped
2 cloves garlic, minced
2 medium carrots, shredded (about 4 oz)
2 medium potatoes, diced
4 oz cabbage, shredded (about 1/4 head)
15-oz can tomatoes with Italian seasonings
1 tsp salt
1/4 tsp pepper
2 tsp dried Italian seasoning

MENU

Minestrone soup
Oyster crackers or variety of snack crackers
Chewy bread
Butter
Milk
Apple wedges, orange slices

METHOD

Summary: Presoak beans and simmer slowly with browned beef 3 to 4 hours. Add spaghetti and continue to simmer for 10 to 15 minutes until the spaghetti is al dente. At the very end, add the sautéed vegetables, seasonings, and spaghetti.

Wash and soak overnight *1/2 pound dried kidney beans.* Brown *1 pound stew beef* in *2 tablespoons butter.* Drain the beans and put them in a large Dutch oven or soup pot with the browned beef. Cover the beans and beef with water (fill to about 3 inches above the ingredients) and add 1 teaspoon salt per quart of water. Put a little water in the frying pan you used for the beef and simmer it to get up the brown drippings from the meat. Add this to the soup, too.

Cook the soaked beans and beef slowly for 3 to 4 hours until the beans and meat are tender. The beans will soak up water and the water will cook off. Add water to keep the level at 2 or 3 inches above the ingredients. Toward the end of cooking, add *5 to 6 ounces uncooked spaghetti, broken into 1-inch segments and simmer for 10 to 15 minutes until the spaghetti is al dente.*

Sauté the vegetables in 2 to 3 tablespoons olive oil until they are as done as you like: *1 large onion,* chopped; *2 cloves garlic,* minced; *2 medium carrots,* shredded (about 4 ounces); *2 medium potatoes,* diced; and *4 ounces shredded cabbage.* When the spaghetti is done, add to the soup the sautéed vegetables and the *15-ounce can tomatoes with Italian seasoning.*

Also at the end of cooking, add about *1 teaspoon salt* (adjust this depending on your taste), *1/4 teaspoon pepper,* and *2 teaspoons dried Italian seasoning.*

RECIPE NOTES

Fast tip: Purchase preshredded carrots and cabbage.

Substitute canned beans for dry beans. Double the weight. That is, instead of the 1/2 pound dry beans called for by the recipe, use one 15-ounce can. Drain the beans before adding to the pot. You can substitute one kind of canned beans for another, depending on what you like. Get creative by using beans in any combination: kidney beans, garbanzo beans (chickpeas), white beans, or pinto beans.

The night before: Put frozen beef cubes in the refrigerator to thaw, sort and soak the beans, locate the other ingredients, and find the stew pot. Chop the onions and put them in a tightly covered jar in the refrigerator. Peel and shred the carrots and shred the cabbage; refrigerate together in a sealed container. Peel and dice the potatoes, cover with water to keep them from turning brown, and refrigerate.

Added touch: Grate fresh Parmesan or Asiago cheese over the soup.

Presentation: Serve this in a tureen or stew pot so you can dish it up at the table. Your children can tell you how much to put in the bowl for them. Be sure to listen—when you are doing the serving, they lose control and won't eat as well if you don't pay attention to their directions.

Involving your children: Your child can sort the beans. Since you definitely don't want to bite into a rock or a clump of dirt, make a routine of picking the beans over twice. You can take turns being the first one to do the picking. Your child can also cut up the potato, clean the garlic, and break up the spaghetti before you cook it.

Adapting this meal for children: This is generally an easy meal for children to eat, as long as you don't serve it too hot. All the tips for **Chicken Soup** (page 122) apply to minestrone, as well.

Variation: Vegetarian Minestrone Soup Skip the stew beef, use a vegetable soup base, and increase the beans to a total of 1 pound dry beans or 2 16-ounce cans. To compensate for losing the fat in the meat, increase the olive oil and/or butter to 1/2 cup. That 1/2 cup oil or butter seems like a lot, but it comes out to only 2 teaspoons fat per serving, which is moderate.

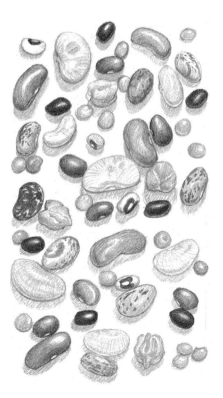

FIGURE 9.7 COOKING DRY BEANS
Dry beans need to be sorted, washed, soaked, and then cooked, generally for at least a couple of hours.

To sort: Spread the beans out by the handful on a plate and look them over carefully to weed out rocks, sticks, and beans that don't look healthy. Dump the plateful into a cooking pot full of water, and sort through another handful until you are done.

To wash: Let the beans sit in the water for a couple of minutes to loosen any dirt. Stir or swish briskly, then pour through a colander, rinse again by running water through the colander, rinse the pot, and then put the beans back in the pot. Cover with water to a couple of inches above the top of the beans.

To soak: Use the hurry-up or overnight method.
Hurry-up: Bring washed beans to a boil. Boil 1 minute, turn off power, cover and let soak for 1 hour. Drain and replace the water.
Overnight: Let the beans sit in water overnight. The next morning, drain and replace the water.

Supposedly, changing the water after you soak beans makes them less gassy. That is, you have less intestinal gas after you eat the beans. Even for your children, intestinal gas is a social issue, not a physical or medical one. If you eat beans a lot, gas is less of a problem. I am not sure whether this is because your intestine adjusts or your nose does.

FIGURE 9.8 SAUTÉING VEGETABLES
In contrast to the chicken soup recipe, here we sauté the vegetables to the crisp-tender stage to give extra flavor. Then we add them to the soup without cooking them any more. That gives the soup a fresh flavor and more texture than if you simply cooked the vegetables in the soup in the first place. It also adds a step, so you might not think it is worth it. In that case, put the raw vegetables directly into the soup as we did for the chicken soup. On the other hand, you may like this method enough to use it for your chicken soup. On the other *other* hand, tomatoes interfere with the softening of vegetables, so cooking the vegetables in this tomato-based soup will preserve their texture.

⌐ Black Beans

..ke this recipe because it is delicious and because it reminds me of my friend June, who taught me that children eat what I think of as challenging food. June came back from several years in Brazil with a craving for black beans and rice and a conviction that this to-me-exotic dish was to Brazilian children simply a familiar and well-liked food. Comfort food, you might say. It has since occurred to me that *gourmet* cooking is, in many cases, our attempt to duplicate some other country's everyday cuisine.

When first presented with black food, my children varied in their responses. Curtis, always the adventurous one, tried it willingly, immediately loved it, and ate it in great quantities. Lucas, the skeptical one, took a look and said he didn't like it. One of June's boys said, "Try it; it's really good." Lucas tried it and he, too, loved it and ate it in great quantities. Kjerstin said, "No, thank you." On black-bean nights, Kjerstin ate rice.

"The darker the beans, the greater the flavor," says June. If June says it, it must be so. However, these beans and the liquid they cook in are really black, so they might be challenging for your eaters at first, especially in the variations I suggest. Black bean tacos *are* a little strange. To make this recipe more accessible, try it with red beans or pinto beans instead.

INGREDIENTS

1 lb dry black beans or *2 15-oz cans black beans, drained*
1/4 lb bacon, cut into 1/2-inch pieces
1 large onion, chopped
2 cloves garlic, minced
3/4 tsp dried leaf oregano
1/2 tsp dried rosemary, crushed
1/4 tsp dried thyme
1/4 tsp black pepper
2 dried chilies (whole red peppers)
1 tsp salt

MENU

Savory black beans
Rice
Corn pudding (page 159)
Bread and butter
Orange rounds with parsley sprigs
A side dish of cooked sausages (your choice) if you have a dedicated meat eater at the table
Milk
Ice cream

METHOD

Summary: Combine cooked bacon and sautéed onion and garlic with presoaked or canned black beans. Season, simmer a couple of hours, and serve.

Wash, soak, and drain *1 pound dry black beans* (see figure 9.7 on the previous page for soaking methods), or use *2 15-ounce cans black beans, drained.*

Cook *1/4 pound bacon cut into 1/2-inch pieces* until golden brown. Put the bacon into the beans. Use the bacon fat to cook *1 large onion, chopped* until clear. Add *2 cloves garlic, minced* for the last 30 seconds of cooking.

Measure into the beans *3/4 teaspoon dried leaf oregano; 1/2 teaspoon dried rosemary, crushed; 1/4 teaspoon dried thyme; 1/4 teaspoon black pepper; 2 dried chilies (whole red peppers);* and *1 teaspoon salt.*

Put enough water into the pot to cover the beans with an inch or two to spare.

Reduce the heat and simmer about 2 hours until the beans are tender. If you started out with canned beans, simmer about 1/2 hour to blend the flavors.

Serve over rice.

RECIPE NOTES

The night before: Wash and soak the beans. Locate the bacon, onion, and garlic. Locate and line up or mix up the spices. Line up the ingredients for the corn pudding.

Presentation: Spruce up the presentation with chopped green onions and a dollop of sour cream. What, you may ask, is a dollop? Well, it is a glob. Always attentive to your image, I can tell you that you will seem to be a far more sophisticated cook if you use a *dollop* rather than a *glob.*

The traditional Brazilian accompaniment is a dish of orange rounds (peel the oranges and cut crosswise) with snips of fresh parsley. The sweet, slightly tart flavor complements the beans, and the color and shape dress up the plate.

Involving your children: Your child can pick over the beans. He can also crush the rosemary and measure the spices and herbs into a little dish so they are all ready to put into the beans. He can peel the oranges and tear the parsley into sprigs. An older child can mix up the corn pudding.

Adapting this meal for children: With the menu I have suggested, there are plenty of choices, so your child will be able to pick and choose and have a meal even if he doesn't feel ready to tackle the beans. The food in this meal is all soft and easy to chew, so even your least experienced eater will be able to manage it, provided he has been previously introduced to all the parts separately. Mash a younger child's beans with a fork to make them easier to mouth and swallow. A child who has mastered eating table food with his fingers can pick up the beans and rice and make a lovely meal of it—and a lovely mess as well. Wait to clean up until after the rice dries; it will sweep or vacuum up easily in no time at all. The beans are a little spicy, but most children are not put off by that, nor does it hurt them. In fact, they like it. Southwestern and Mexican children develop a preference for spicy foods at quite a young age.

Variations: If you don't want to use bacon, substitute 3 tablespoons butter or cooking oil.

This makes a big recipe, so you will have enough for a second meal. On the cycle menu I suggest **Black Bean Soup**, which you make by simply adding more water or broth and perhaps including some of the leftover rice. Other possibilities are refried black beans (mash them and add a little more fat), black bean tacos, black bean burritos, and a baked potato with black beans, cheese, and sour cream. You get the idea.

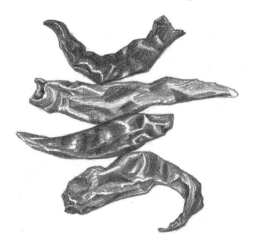

FIGURE 9.9 RICE
You have lots of choices with rice, all of them good. *White rice* is polished: It has the hull and bran layers removed in the milling process. *Polished enriched rice* is fortified by being sprayed with a solution of B vitamins. To conserve nutrients on the surface, don't rinse the rice, and cook it in as little water as possible. *Converted* rice is parboiled before milling, which forces the B vitamins in the outer coatings into the grain itself. *Short-grain or long-grain brown rice* is unpolished: It has only the hull removed in the milling process, so the B vitamin- and fiber-containing bran and rice germ remain. You will find interesting varieties of rice, such as basmati, an unpolished rice, and wehani, a polished rice. And of course there is quick-cooking, minute, or instant rice, which is available in either the white or brown variety.

The cooking method and the finished product depend on the rice you start with. Quick-cooking rice takes about 10 minutes, and directions are specific to the product; read the box. For converted white rice, cook rice in double the amount of water—that is, one part rice to two parts water. With brown rice or other varieties, read the directions on the box or on the bin of the bulk foods case. Bring the salted water to a boil (1 teaspoon of salt per quart of water), add the rice, stir, cover, and turn the heat to low. Converted rice takes 20 to 25 minutes to cook, and whole-grain (brown) rice takes about 40 to 45 minutes. If you like whole-grain rice and don't have time to cook it, consider cooking a large batch and freezing it in meal-sized quantities.

Quick-cooking, converted, and whole-grain rice tends to be dry, flaky, and easily separated when cooked. Polished rice may be dry or sticky, depending on the size of the kernel. *Indian* rice is long-grained and easily separated, whereas *Japanese* rice is short-grained and sticky.

FIGURE 9.10 FLAVORING BEANS
Black beans taste good on their own, but making them savory requires added fat, salt, herbs, and spices. The fat from 1/4 pound of bacon may seem like a lot, but it is not—it figures out to about two teaspoons of fat per cup of beans. This amount of fat conforms to the magic number of 35 percent or less calories from fat. Do not be tempted to delete the fat; it is important for flavoring the beans, and it gives them their stick-to-the-ribs quality. If beans are fat-free, they are only carbohydrate and protein, which don't stay with you. Herbs provide depth and complexity of flavor, and chilies add a gentle bite. They bite hard, however, if you happen to get one in your mouth! Use them for cooking, then remove them before you serve.

Marinated Chicken Stir-Fry

To keep stir-fry from turning out like Chinese stew, use a medium-high temperature and cook vegetables quickly and lightly to the crisp side of crisp-tender. You don't need a wok; a large skillet with a tight-fitting lid will do.

INGREDIENTS

1/3 cup rice vinegar
3 Tbsp chopped garlic
3 Tbsp soy sauce
2 Tbsp dark-brown sesame oil
1/4 tsp black pepper
1 1/2 lb chicken breast strips
1 Tbsp peanut or canola oil
3 cups raw vegetables, including any combination of
  the following:
  carrot sticks
  broccoli florets
  cauliflower pieces
  green or red pepper strips
  whole fresh or frozen snow peas
  zucchini rounds
  mushroom slices
  green onion, crosscut
  bean sprouts

MENU

Marinated chicken stir-fry
Rice
Fruit in season
Bread or toast
Butter
Milk
Old-fashioned bread pudding (page 164)

METHOD

Summary: Make the marinade and combine it with chicken breast strips. Refrigerate for 24 hours. Stir-fry chicken and vegetables, boil remaining marinade and serve it on the side.

Make a marinade by mixing together *1/3 cup rice vinegar, 3 tablespoons chopped garlic, 3 tablespoons soy sauce, 2 tablespoons dark-brown sesame oil, and 1/4 teaspoon black pepper.*

Combine *1 1/2 pounds chicken breast strips* with marinade in a zip top bag. Refrigerate for 24 hours, turning occasionally.

In a large nonstick skillet or wok, heat *1 tablespoon peanut or canola oil* on medium high. Using a slotted spoon, lift the chicken out of the marinade and place the chicken in the skillet. Brown it, add a little marinade, cover, and steam for 2 to 3 minutes to finish cooking. Remove.

Pour the rest of the marinade from the bag into a saucepan, heat to boiling, and boil gently for 3 minutes (this is to kill any *Salmonella*). Put in a separate dish to serve on the side.

In the same skillet you used for cooking the chicken, begin cooking *3 cups vegetables* chosen from the ingredients list in 1 to 2 tablespoons boiled marinade. The vegetables that need to cook longest are at the top of the list. Put those in first.

Add the cooked chicken to the cooked vegetables, heat, and serve.

RECIPE NOTES

Fast tip: The rice vinegar is a fast tip. It has a sweet flavor and provides the sweetness for this sweet-and-sour marinade. Drain the marinade from the chicken strips by snipping the corner off the zip top bag and letting the marinade drip into a small saucepan.

Along with the other marvelous helps you can find in the meat section of your grocery store, you can probably find chicken cut up into strips ready to go into stir-fry. It might be fresh or frozen. Either is a worthwhile investment because it saves you time, energy, and mess.

Frozen stir-fry vegetables may substitute passably for fresh vegetables.

Two nights before: Refrigerate frozen chicken (in a pan) to thaw.

The night before: Get the chicken started marinating. Locate the vegetables you will use. Clean the vegetables, and perhaps even cut some of them up.

Presentation: Serve the rice and stir-fry in separate dishes so your diners can pick and choose. Until your children become accustomed to this dish, you might even serve the chicken and vegetables separately.

Involving your children: A child can wash vegetables and help break the pieces apart. He can also mix up the marinade.

Adapting this meal for children: Everything in this meal is soft and easy enough to chew for children over age 2. For the toddler, you may want to leave out the harder, chewier bits. The first few times you have this, your children will probably just eat the rice, and that's fine. Then, they may have a small helping and eat just the foods that look familiar. Still fine. Serving food that they may not immediately like gives them an opportunity to learn to quietly push what they don't eat to one side and leave it. Then, they may want to paw through the serving bowl and find what they like. Not fine. That can spoil the dish for others at the table. Children need to learn to respect others' wishes and needs at mealtime as well as their own.

Variation: The marinade also tastes good with pork, which you can buy finely sliced and ready to cook. Follow the same procedure as for marinating chicken. To give your butcher the opportunity to make your life easier, call the day before you shop and ask to have stir-fry meat ready for you. Develop a relationship with your butcher people. You will find they use much ingenuity to prepare foods ahead of time and get them ready for you to cook.

FIGURE 9.11 SESAME OIL
The oil in this recipe is often called "toasted" sesame oil, although it may not say that on the bottle. It is dark brown, comes in a small bottle, and has a pronounced flavor. Experiment. If you think this marinade is too strongly flavored, cut the sesame oil to 1 tablespoon and use peanut oil for the other tablespoon. You can also buy clear sesame oil for general usage. It is nearly flavorless and behaves about the same as other seed oils.

Jambalaya

Jambalaya is a famous Creole-Cajun dish. The word *jambalaya* is probably derived from *jambon*, both Spanish and French for the ham typically used as an ingredient. The "a-la-ya" is probably an African exclamation.

INGREDIENTS
4 slices bacon
1 1/2 lb boneless chicken breasts or combination of boneless breasts and thighs
1 tsp salt
1/4 tsp black pepper
4 tsp Creole seasoning
1 green or red pepper, chopped
1 cup chopped celery
1 large onion, chopped
1/4 cup chopped fresh parsley or 1 Tbsp dried parsley
1 tsp dried thyme
4 cloves garlic, minced
15-oz can chicken broth
15-oz can diced tomatoes
1 1/2 cups uncooked enriched white rice
1 bay leaf

MENU
Jambalaya
Glazed carrots (page 155) or sweet-sour cucumber salad (page 155)
Cornbread and butter
Apple custard or fruit in season

METHOD
Summary: Fry and remove the bacon and use the fat to sauté the chicken and vegetables. Combine with the seasoning, hot liquids, and rice; bake covered in the oven.

Preheat oven to 325° F. Lightly brown *4 slices bacon* in a large Dutch oven and crumble. Lift out the bacon to drain and leave the drippings in the pan for browning the chicken and sautéing the vegetables.

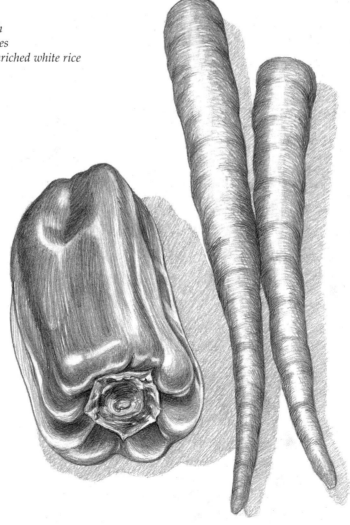

Wash the chicken pieces, dry with paper towels, and cut into roughly 1-ounce chunks. Add *4 tsp Creole seasoning* to the drippings (be careful not to breath any vapors from the hot spice) and heat to medium temperature. Brown the chicken pieces in the seasoned bacon fat. Remove the chicken.

In the remaining fat in the Dutch oven, sauté all together until the onion is clear: *1 green or red pepper, chopped*; *1 cup chopped celery*; and *1 large onion, chopped*. Toward the end of cooking, add *1/4 cup chopped fresh parsley* or *1 tablespoon dried parsley* and *1 teaspoon dried thyme*. At the very end, add 4 cloves minced garlic and cook about 30 seconds.

While you sauté the chicken and vegetables, heat one *15-ounce can chicken broth* and a *15-ounce can diced tomatoes* to nearly boiling. Pour into the sautéed vegetables. Add *1 1/2 cups uncooked rice*, browned chicken, bacon, and *1 bay leaf*.

Cover and bake for 30 minutes; check once during baking to add more hot broth or water if the jambalaya begins to dry out. Remove the bay leaf, add salt and pepper if needed, and serve. Put hot sauce or crushed red peppers on the table for any family members who don't think it's hot unless they cry.

RECIPE NOTES

The night before: Find the cooking pan and the rice. Locate the spices and put them where you can find them easily. Clean the vegetables, and perhaps even chop them. Put frozen chicken in the refrigerator to thaw. Find the bacon. Check the recipes for the other menu items and get those ingredients lined up as well.

Presentation: This is a beautiful, hearty, colorful dish. Bring it to the table in a good-looking pan, like your Dutch oven.

Involving your children: Children can wash and dice the vegetables, measure the rice, and open the cans of broth and tomatoes.

Adapting this meal for children: While this dish is mildly seasoned, it *is* seasoned. Given the seasoning and the mixture of a number of foods, this may be a challenging dish for your child. However, Cajun children eat it enthusiastically. Your child may, too, or he may need time to get accustomed to the mixtures and the seasonings. Eating bread or drinking milk with spicy dishes helps cool the burning sensation in the mouth. Fruit with the meal gives a cooling side dish.

Make the meal more accessible by cooking the rice plain, then combining all the other ingredients as a sauce and serving separately. Children can generally manage the rice if the jambalaya is too challenging. Consider replacing the cornbread on the menu with a popular bread.

Variations: Ham and Chicken Jambalaya
Reduce the amount of chicken to 1 pound, and add 1 cup diced ham just before you put it in the oven. You can also use shrimp in jambalaya, either alone, as a substitute for chicken, or with the chicken and/or the ham.

Chicken and Sausage Jambalaya Again, reduce the amount of chicken to 1 pound, and add 1/2 pound sausage. Polish sausage is good, or for adventurous eaters try 1/4 pound each Polish sausage and Andouille sausage (Andouille is usually quite spicy.)

I put glazed carrots on the menu because they are easy to like and give a sweet contrast to the spicy flavor of the main dish. The traditional but more challenging vegetable with this meal is greens. For experienced eaters, try substituting **Greens and Bacon** (page 156) for the carrots, then add back the sweet flavor by using **Sweet-Sour Cucumber Salad** (pages 155), or simply have some sweet pickles.

Fried Fish

Fried fish is last on the list of recipes because it is the most difficult. While restaurants make it seem so simple, it is tricky to fry food well and safely. I debated about whether to include this recipe and finally decided to leave it in for its teaching value. Fried food, like other food that is relatively high in fat, is perfectly acceptable some of the time. Anything can be good for you—or not so good. It all depends on the dose and frequency. You can overdose on *water*, if you drink too much of it.

My developmental editor, Paulette Sharkey, says she would never fry fish. When it's time for fried fish, says Paulette, it is time to eat out or stop at the seafood market for take-out. Well, I can understand that. It makes a mess and it stinks up the house. In Wisconsin, restaurants and churches have wonderful fish fries on Friday nights, a heritage of our German-Catholic forebears. However, like a lot of foods, I like fried fish better if I make it at home, so I think it is worth the mess and the smell.

Even if you fry only once in a while, you need to know what you are doing. Frying involves using relatively large amounts of fat, heated to a relatively high temperature—350° F. That can be dangerous. Use a fresh liquid oil that has a relatively high smoke point, such as peanut, soybean, cottonseed, or safflower oil. These oils have smoke points that are 60 to 100 degrees higher than the cooking temperature.

The smoke point is very close to the point at which oil bursts into flames. If you use fresh oil and keep the cooking temperature around 350° F, you shouldn't have trouble with fire. However, to put out an oil fire, slap the lid on the pan, use a fire extinguisher, or sprinkle salt or baking soda on the fire. *Don't* use water—it will float the fire and make it spread. You can prevent grease fires by not reusing fats. Even one use of fat at a high temperature can decrease by 100 degrees the point at which it will burst into flames.

To have the coating adhere well to the fish, make sure the eggs are cold and the fish is dry. The fat should be about 1/2-inch deep in the pan so that the fish will float in the hot oil rather than being immersed in it.

INGREDIENTS
2 lb boneless fish fillets: cod, halibut, whitefish,
*   turbo, pollack, or your choice*
Seasoned flour:
*   1/2 cup flour*
*   3 tsp Fish Seasoning (page 110)*
2 eggs
2 Tbsp cold water
1/2 lb saltines
Oil for frying

MENU
Fried fish
Tartar sauce
Baked potatoes with sour cream
Green salad
Fruit in season
Bread or toast
Cherry cobbler (page 162)

METHOD
Summary: Dip the fish fillets three times: first into seasoned flour, then into egg, and finally into cracker crumbs. Fry in hot oil.

Thaw *2 pounds boneless fish: cod, halibut, whitefish, turbo, pollack, or your choice*. Wash in cold water, cut into helping-sized pieces, drain, and pat dry.

Make seasoned flour by combining *1/2 cup flour* with 2 teaspoons Fish Seasoning. Get out three shallow bowls for dipping the fish. Put the seasoned flour in the first. In the second, thoroughly blend *2 cold eggs* with *2 tablespoons cold water*. In the third bowl, spread cracker crumbs that you have purchased or made. (In the blender, blend *1/2 pound saltines* on high until they become fine crumbs. It's best to use regular salted saltines with salted tops.)

Begin heating the oil so it is hot by the time the fish is coated. Frying temperature for fish is 350° F. To gauge the temperature, use an electric frying pan set to 350° F, use a frying or candy thermometer, or test the temperature with part of the egg-cracker coating. The oil will be hot enough when the coating floats, sizzles, and slowly browns. If it browns immediately, it is too hot.

To coat the fish, dip each piece in the seasoned flour, then in the egg, then in the cracker crumbs. As each piece is coated, immediately place it in the hot oil. Use a pancake turner or serving tongs to keep your fingers safe. Fry until bubbles start to appear on the upper surface of the fish, then gently turn one time only. The fish will be done when it is white and flakes easily, about 10 minutes per inch of thickness or to an internal temperature of 130 to 140° F. If the fish is thinner than one inch, fry it only briefly on the second side, just to cook the egg coating. Drain the fried fish on paper towels.

RECIPE NOTES

The night before: Find the potatoes and wash them. Wash the greens, spin them, and return them to the refrigerator, in the spinner, to crisp. (See figure 10.2 "Prepackaged Salad Greens or Do-It-Yourself?" on page 151.)

You can purchase already-prepared **Tartar Sauce.** I prefer the flavor and texture of one I make quickly myself, with 1/2 cup Miracle Whip, 2 to 3 tablespoons sweet pickle relish, 2 to 3 tablespoons dried onion flakes, and 2 to 3 tablespoons dried parsley flakes. Mix it together (I use a jar) and add extra milk to make it soupy. It thickens as the dried onion and parsley hydrate. Let it stand in the refrigerator for a half-hour and add more milk if it needs it. You can keep this tartar sauce for a month or two. It can be mixed with tuna to make great tuna salad sandwiches.

Presentation: Serve the fish on a pretty platter and garnish with lemon wedges.

Involving your children: Children can break and beat the eggs, wash and pierce the potatoes with a fork, spin the salad greens, and tear them into bite-sized pieces.

Adapting this meal for children: Children generally do well with this meal because they like fried food. Choose boneless fish. Dress the salad lightly or not at all so children can eat it with their fingers. Show your child how to mash some butter or sour cream or both into the potato.

Variations: This fish warms up great in the toaster oven or microwave. Have it again for lunch the next day or make it into a sandwich with lettuce and tartar sauce.

Try making **Sautéed Fish** for a tasty variation on fried fish that takes less fat and less heat and makes less of a mess. Dip washed, drained, and blotted fillets in the seasoned flour mixture. Sauté in 1 to 2 tablespoons butter in a nonstick frying pan at low-medium to medium temperature until the fish is nicely browned on both sides, it flakes easily and it reaches an internal temperature of 130 to 140° F. Serve immediately.

FIGURE 9.12 FAT FOR FRYING
Peanut oil, canola and sunflower oil are the best oils for frying. They brown well, and they are high in monounsaturated fat, which is more heat resistant than polyunsaturated fat. (See appendix N, "A Primer on Dietary Fat.") Olive oil also works well, but it does add its own distinctive flavor. Saturated fat is also more heat resistant, which makes corn oil, cottonseed oil and soybean oil, with their relatively higher percentages of saturated and monounsaturated fat, good choices for frying. An oil labeled "vegetable oil" is likely to be either cottonseed or soybean oil: Read the ingredients list. Butter works well for the lower heat of sautéing, but it is likely to burn at the higher temperatures used in frying. Margarine breaks down. Low-trans-fat hydrogenated shortenings work well. Lard browns well, but not everyone likes its smell.

I hesitated to recommend peanut oil because some children are allergic to peanuts. However, the Food Allergy & Anaphylaxis Network (www.foodallergy.org; 800/929-4040) says that peanut oil doesn't carry the peanut allergen unless it is cold-pressed.

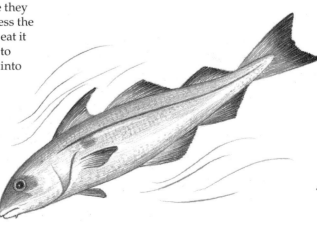

Grab-and-Dump Meals

The early menus in chapter 8, "How to Get Cooking," are so simple that it may be hard to imagine scaling them down, but it can be done. Every cook needs to keep a few meals on hand that they can throw together quickly. Here are my ideas; you undoubtedly have your own. These are real meals; you can serve them and know you have done your job of getting a meal on the table.

Consider these possibilities, all of which are nutritious:

- Hot dogs, canned baked beans, and potato chips, with ice cream for dessert.
- Macaroni and cheese (packaged dinner) and canned or frozen green beans, peas, or Mixed Vegetables. You can add tuna to increase the protein.
- Bologna or any deli-meat sandwiches with lettuce and mayonnaise, canned grapefruit slices, and store-bought cookies for dessert.
- Tuna salad sandwiches or hot tuna sandwiches on buns (foil-wrap tuna salad and cheese on a bun and bake 15 minutes at 325° F), with canned peaches for dessert.
- Canned "hearty" soups with oyster crackers (read the label to find ones that have at least 5 to 7 grams of protein per serving), and ice cream for dessert.
- Canned beef stew with Bisquick dumplings or canned biscuits, and canned fruit.
- Canned spaghetti dinners like SpaghettiOs or mini-raviolis (aggressively orange and slippery, these are more popular with children than with adults), pineapple–cottage cheese salad, and instant pudding for dessert.
- Canned corned beef hash, poached eggs, and canned apricots.
- Rice meal from the recipe on the box of herb-seasoned rice or minute rice (they tell you the protein to add), and canned fruit or vegetable.
- Boxed bean dishes like red beans and rice. Add butter or sausage for fat and flavor, and put together a dish of grapefruit sections and orange rounds.
- Pancakes with syrup or applesauce-yogurt topping and sausages on the side.
- Pancakes with chicken or hamburger gravy.
- Toaster waffles, scrambled eggs and orange juice.

Prepackaged "Convenience" Meals

Prepackaged meals jump-start your cooking by giving you ideas and gathering up the ingredients for you, and they may require reduced cooking times. For instance, if you have a package of Tuna Helper on your shelf, you can lean on the cupboard door and get an idea for dinner. All the ingredients (except the tuna, of course) are pulled together in one place so all you have to do is find the pan, the colander, the tuna, and the water. If you were to prepare the **Tuna Noodle Casserole** from chapter 8, "How to Get Cooking," you would also have to find the noodles and the cream of mushroom soup. Tuna Helper costs only about 10 percent more than the tuna noodle casserole you make yourself, and it has about 10 percent more salt, still a reasonable amount. You still might want to add more noodles as well as more vegetables. Is it worth it to buy the mix? You decide. Only you know how you feel when you are leaning against the cupboard door seeking dinner. If you have gone into survival mode, rounding up noodles and mushroom soup may be more than you can bear.

Of course, the preassembled idea can be taken to a ridiculous extreme, such as in the prepackaged bowl, spoon, cereal, and milk I saw in the dairy case. I suppose that could be helpful when you are out camping or on the road and looking for a quick breakfast at a picnic bench, particularly since the milk is processed at ultrahigh temperatures so you don't have to refrigerate it until after it's opened. However, the advertising implies that you can just hand these to your kids in the morning and expect them to eat while you do something else. That's like feeding a dog. It takes the nurturing out of feeding.

The same is true of the special kids' meals that the food industry promotes. The idea with kids' meals is that you feed your child a separate, special dinner. With these products, the food industry is pandering to consumer research that says family meals are going the way of the covered wagon. Ironically, with all the advertising, parents get the idea that it is okay to feed kids this way, whereupon advertisers promote the concept all the more. Not a good idea. Handing kids food takes the loving out of feeding, and I don't recommend it.

However, you have my blessing to buy any prepackaged meals *for the whole family* that take your fancy. What's important is having family meals and doing what you have to in order to make those family meals happen. Using pre-packaged meals will cost you extra, but, surprisingly, not always that much extra. Buying mixes is *certainly* less expensive than eating out. "Helper" mixes, as I said earlier, cost about 10 percent more than preparing your own comparable dish. Freeze-dried soup starters cost about 20 percent more than making a comparable soup from scratch, and they save time and trouble—they take just a few minutes to mix up and 90 minutes to simmer until done. Frozen vegetable and vegetable-and-pasta mixes cost about 20 percent more than such dishes you assemble yourself; they give you menu ideas and save some time and trouble. There are also the frozen dinners where everything is included: You just bake or microwave. Of course, anything labeled "gourmet" is likely to cost more, so be sure you are willing to pay for the value-added expense.

Fast Meals for One

Any of the meals offered so far are good choices for one person. However, they raise the obvious problem of what to do with so much food. Of course, you can eat chicken and rice or meat loaf 5 days in a row, as my son Lucas did when he was in college. If you have freezer space, you can purchase a supply of "disposable" storage containers and freeze meal-sized, homemade PPMs (pre-prepared meals, if you recall) to heat up in the microwave when you want them. If you have a good memory or a way of keeping track, you can accumulate a variety of these homemade PPMs.

Here are a few quick and easy but nourishing meals for one. Highlight the ones that seem appealing and accessible; ignore the others. All the meals provide protein, fat, and carbohydrate. Many include vegetables. To round out the meal, toast yourself some great bagels with cream cheese or have French bread with butter, open a can of fruit, and pour yourself a glass of milk.

- Baked potato with toppings. Thoroughly scrub a big, lovely potato and bake it in the toaster oven. (Ask the produce manager which are the baking potatoes.) For a soft skin, wrap the potato in aluminum foil. For a crisp skin, don't wrap the potato. For a tasty skin, butter it. Bake at 425° F for about an hour. The potato is done when you can easily pierce it with a fork. For a faster meal, bake the potato in the microwave. Pierce the potato 10 or 15 times with a fork to keep it from exploding, and read your microwave manual for time. Five minutes or so should do it. Split it open and load it with toppings: cheese, bean salsa, sour cream, canned bacon bits, chopped green onion.

- Fresh tortellini in broth. Purchase fresh tortellini in the refrigerator case. Take out as many as you think you can eat. Seal the package tightly for another meal; freeze it if you won't want them for a while. Cook according to the package directions, except substitute chicken or vegetable broth (canned or from a paste concentrate) for the water. At the end of cooking, sprinkle in a little dried parsley for color, or drop in some fresh spinach. The spinach will cook in a minute or less. Grate Parmesan cheese over the top.

- Ramen noodles. These aren't just for college students, although sooner or later, nearly every young adult resorts to Ramen noodles due to their wide availability, very low cost (often less than 25 cents per package), and ease and speed of preparation. According to a Japanese poll, instant noodles were the most important Japanese invention of the twentieth century! The noodles are manufactured by being boiled with flavoring; deep-fried with canola, palm, or cottonseed oil to remove moisture; then dried into a noodle cake. A package of Ramen noodles gives the nutritional equivalent of two slices of bread with 2 teaspoons butter. To consider the fat-saturation issue, see appendix N, "A Primer on Dietary Fat." Because the noodles are made with enriched hard wheat flour, they provide B vitamins and iron as well as 10 grams of incomplete protein per package, which is the equivalent of 1 1/2 ounces of meat. Any of the suggestions that follow will balance out the incomplete protein. Ramen noodles are high in salt, but is it more important to you to avoid salt or to have dinner? For more about salt, see appendix O, "Sodium in Your Diet."

Here are some variations that will give you the total protein equivalent of 3 ounces of meat: *Drink a glass of milk.* Adding high-quality protein to a Ramen noodle meal can be that simple! *Make egg-drop soup.* Stir a beaten egg into the hot cooked noodles and broth along with the packet of seasoning mix. *Make peanut butter noodles.* Stir 1 1/2 to 2 tablespoons peanut butter and enough hot noodle water into cooked, drained noodles to make the mixture as liquid as you like. Add Asian hot sauce to your taste. Eat as is or serve over fresh or frozen cooked vegetables. *Go back to the source.* Ramen is a Japanese dish of noodles served in a meat-, poultry-, or fish-based broth with toppings such as thinly sliced pork, beef, chicken, fish, or tofu.

- Stock your freezer with quick-cooking meats or poultry. Freeze individual, meal-sized pieces of chicken breasts or thighs, sirloin tip steaks (tender and tasty but not too expensive), or ground beef patties to thaw and cook a portion at time. To prepare portions that are easy to pull out, separate the pieces on a jelly roll pan lined with waxed paper or parchment paper and freeze. Package the frozen pieces in a zip top bag and label. You *can* purchase packages of portion-sized cuts of all these foods, but generally the packages are pretty big and they are expensive. Do you have the freezer space? Is it worth the expense? Only you can decide.
- Use shortcuts for cooking meats, fish, or poultry. Use the method for **Lemon Chicken** on page 116 to sauté yourself a single chicken breast. Use the same method to make yourself a sirloin tip steak, except use Montreal Steak Seasoning instead of lemon pepper. Make **Parmesan Chicken** (page 116) in your toaster oven. Make extra to thinly slice and eat in a sandwich, on a main-dish salad, or over ramen noodles. Purchase individually wrapped fish pieces and make **Herb-Baked Fish** (page 110) in your toaster oven. Mix your own **Fish Seasoning** (page 110) or use lemon pepper or a premixed fish seasoning from the spice aisle. Cook yourself a **Hamburger** (page 119).
- For a side dish, mix up some dried mashed potatoes, microwave part of a package of frozen vegetables, or open a small can of vegetables. Prepare instant brown or white rice, couscous or pasta. Get your vegetables and carbohydrate by microwaving part of a package of frozen vegetables with potatoes or vegetables with pasta. Voila! Dinner!
- Make a great main-dish salad with thinly sliced leftover chicken or steak, warm or cold. Use prewashed salad greens and add some very thin red onion slices, cherry tomatoes cut in half, cucumber slices, garbanzo beans, bacon bits, hard-cooked egg—the list goes on. (See figure 9.13 on the next page for egg-cooking instructions.) Add a cheese or two of your choice: cheddar, American, feta, Parmesan. Add croutons or cubed French bread to provide carbohydrate, or depend on your bread and milk for carbohydrate. Toss with your favorite dressing, or use the **Best-Yet Oil and Vinegar Dressing** recipe on page 152. For other main-dish salads, also consider the **Tomato and Fresh Mozzarella Salad** on page 153 or just pile some cottage cheese on a tomato.
- Consider a frittata. Make yourself an individual **Spinach-Feta Frittata** (page 115). Use a small pan and start with as many beaten eggs as you want, pat in as much spinach as the eggs will coat, and pile on as much feta as fits on top. Cook according to the directions. Frittata refrigerates well—you can make the whole recipe, take it out a portion at a time, heat it in the microwave, and eat it for several days. Make the frittata variations on page 115, or make up your own.
- Continue the egg theme. Consider fried egg sandwiches, egg salad sandwiches (use some of the **Tartar Sauce** I talked about on page 137, hard-cooked eggs on a spinach salad, deviled eggs (stir Miracle Whip, a little mustard, and salt and pepper into the hard-cooked yolks), and scrambled eggs, alone or with a topping of chopped tomatoes (fresh salsa if you like it), green onions, and cheese.
- Precook ground beef. Crumble and cook a pound of ground beef, then use it for making a variety of dishes: chili (dried onions, canned chili beans, and canned diced tomatoes), hamburger soup (broth, onions, and frozen or canned Mixed Vegetables), taco salad (season the meat with packaged taco seasoning), tacos (the same meat, just a different presentation), burritos (include canned refried beans), sloppy joes (add ketchup, dried onions, and a little steak sauce or Tabasco).

- Get creative with cooked dried beans. Prepare a vegetarian meal by cooking frozen beans or draining a can of beans: lima, butter, black, pinto, white, kidney, or black-eyed peas. Flavor the beans with sautéed onions (or dried onions), garlic, and other vegetables if you want, such as tomatoes or greens. Add other flavorings to your taste: cilantro, parsley flakes, chili powder, or Tabasco. Prepare a portion of instant rice, spoon on the beans, and melt cheese over the top. Yum!

- Consider hummus. Spread hummus on a slice of bread, whole grain if you like. Or spread it on a flour tortilla and top with greens, tomato, cucumber, and red or green pepper and roll it up. Add vinegar, oil, salt, and pepper if you feel it needs more oomph. Or use pita bread, and fill the pocket with hummus and vegetables. You can also use hummus as a dip for raw vegetables.

- Don't forget peanut butter to make your favorite sandwich—with jelly, honey, bananas, sugar, dill pickles, or sweet pickles. Peanut butter is high in protein. Peanut and wheat protein together give high-quality protein. If you are in doubt, drink a glass of milk with your peanut butter sandwich.

FIGURE 9.13 MAKING PERFECT BOILED EGGS

Choose clean eggs that are free from cracks. Bring eggs to room temperature by letting them stand 5 minutes in hot tap water. Prewarmed eggs are less likely to crack during cooking than eggs straight from the refrigerator. In a saucepan, cover the eggs with cold water and heat on high, without the lid, until the water reaches a hard boil. Put the lid on the pan and set it off the burner to finish cooking the eggs: 5 minutes for soft, 10 minutes for medium, and 15 minutes for hard. At the end of cooking, to keep the yolks from turning dark around the outside, drain off the hot water and immerse the eggs in ice water.

Hard-cooked eggs are easier to peel if they aren't too fresh. Fresh eggs are a pain to peel—the shells won't let go of the egg and the resulting product is pockmarked, albeit tasty.

You can also cook eggs in the microwave, but to do it safely, you must crack them into a dish, pierce the yolk and white a number of times with a fork or toothpick, and cover loosely. Start by cooking on medium for 40 seconds. Write down how long your microwave takes to make eggs the way you like them. You can add butter or cream if you like before covering.

The Generic Casserole

Nutritionally, a casserole is like an ordinary sandwich, which gives you two slices of bread, 2 to 3 ounces of protein (poultry, fish, peanut butter, cheese, etc.), about 2 teaspoons of fat (butter, mayonnaise, or margarine), and maybe some vegetables (lettuce, tomato, pickles, etc.). From a serving of casserole you hope for the same: two servings from the bread group, 2 to 3 ounces of meat, 2 teaspoons of fat, and some vegetables. Prepackaged casseroles, soups, and mixes are good meal substitutes if they give you the nutritional equivalent of a sandwich.

Like the child who learns to run the day after he learns to walk, you are now ready to turn cooking skills into *improvising*! Turn that bit of sandwich-equivalent information into a **Generic Casserole** formula that you can use to throw together your own casseroles from whatever you happen to have on hand. You can also use it to evaluate other recipes to determine whether they are likely to work.

Generic Casserole is *not* the alarming dish that shows up on the table after someone cleans out the refrigerator. It is a potentially new and delightful creation. It may become the dish your children fondly remember when someone asks them, "What food do you think of when you remember eating meals at home?"

THE GENERIC CASSEROLE FORMULA

Each helping of casserole gives the following:

> 2 ounces meat, poultry, fish, dry beans, eggs, or nuts
> 2 servings bread, cereal, rice, or pasta
> A liquid of some sort: canned soup, canned tomatoes, broth, or white sauce
> About 1/4 teaspoon salt
> About 2 fat equivalents

To make **Generic Casserole**, you first have to figure out how much raw food to cook to make a helping. Let's start with the starch for **Generic Casserole**. Figure that your two servings of bread, cereal, rice, or pasta, after cooking, is—tah-dah!—1 cup!

Coming now to the crux of the matter, *how much is that before it is cooked?*

Starchy Ingredients:
What Cooks to Make a Cup?

1/3 cup uncooked rice
1/2 cup uncooked macaroni
1 cup uncooked noodles
3 to 4 ounces uncooked spaghetti (1/2 cup, but it's hard to measure)
8 ounces potato
1/2 cup dry beans

The alert reader will note that *potatoes and beans are not cereals!* Well, who cares? They are starchy, and that is what we are after for our **Generic Casserole**: a source of complex carbohydrate to mix in with the protein. In scalloped potatoes and ham, you use potatoes for the starch. In baked beans and ham, you use beans for the starch. You'll get a higher-protein casserole if you use cooked dried beans for the starch, but it won't hurt you.

The Protein for Generic Casserole
Coming to another crux of the matter, if you will allow me the liberty of two cruxes, what about the protein? To answer that question, it is easier to talk about ounces than servings. For six servings of **Generic Casserole** you need about 12 ounces of cooked meat equivalent, or about 1 pound raw. Ounce-sized portions of high-protein foods are given in the following list. Each contains about 7 grams of protein. Notice that the ever-versatile beans show up yet again, this time as a source of protein.

Protein Ingredients:
What Counts as an Ounce?

1 ounce cooked meat, poultry, or fish
1 egg
1 ounce hard cheese (like cheddar)
1/2 cup cooked dried beans, peas, or lentils (1/4 cup dry)
2 to 3 tablespoons nuts or seeds
1/4 cup cottage cheese
2 tablespoons peanut butter
1/3 cup tofu

The Fat for Generic Casserole
To substitute one fat for another, it is easiest to think in terms of equivalents for a teaspoon of butter or margarine.

A teaspoon of butter or margarine gives about 5 grams of fat, a modest amount. So do 3 tablespoons of half-and-half, a tablespoon of sour cream, and 1/3 cup of cream of mushroom soup. You can estimate fat by reading the nutrition label. It will tell you how much *total fat* there is in a serving and give it to you in grams. Amounts of fatty foods that give 5 grams of fat per serving are summarized below. No, I am not turning on you and becoming a fat-gram cop, but knowing the numbers and what they mean will set you free. Just look at how much half-and-half or sour cream you can substitute for a teaspoon of butter!

Equivalents for 1 Teaspoon of Butter or Margarine

1 teaspoon cooking oil or solid shortening
1 teaspoon mayonnaise
1 tablespoon Miracle Whip
1 tablespoon cream cheese
2 tablespoons Neufchâtel (looks and tastes like cream cheese)
3 tablespoons half-and-half
1 tablespoon whipping cream
1 tablespoon sour cream
3 tablespoons low-fat sour cream
1/2 cup whole milk
3 tablespoons medium white sauce or gravy (made with 2 tablespoons butter, 2 tablespoons flour and 1 cup liquid)
1 tablespoon hollandaise sauce

Isn't this fun? It's a little odd to put whole milk on this list, because it has more protein than other fatty foods. However, 1/2 cup whole milk has the same amount of fat as a teaspoon of butter and gives you another way of adding fat to your mashed potatoes and cream soups.

At the risk of repeating myself, allow me to again reassure you about fat. In light of all the hysteria about fat and the conviction that *less is better,* you may be tempted to forgo fat altogether or to substitute the fat-free versions of, say, margarine, sour cream, or mayonnaise. *Don't do it!* You will ruin the taste and texture of the recipe and discourage yourself from being a cook. Fat makes food taste good and contributes to browning and smoothness. If you don't get fat at home, you will have to sneak off to get a grease fix at the local fast-food place. Most of us need those fixes from time to time, but if yours get too frequent, something is the matter with your strategies for making meals at home.

Using the knowledge that we have so carefully accumulated, figure 9.14 lists the possibilities for your very own **Generic Casserole**. Combining these foods in the amounts suggested will give you about six helpings.

The Generic Soup

You can adapt the **Generic Casserole** formula to improvise **Generic Soup**. To make six servings of soup, start with the same amount of protein ingredient: 1 pound raw weight. Increase the liquid to 6 cups, then add three to four cups starch and vegetables, combined. How much you add depends on whether you want a thick or a thin soup. A 1 1/2 cup serving of a main-dish soup gives you roughly two servings of starch, 2 ounces of protein, about 2 teaspoons of fat, and some vegetables.

Cookbooks

Where does this leave you? Do you want to learn more about cooking, or have you had enough? With what you have learned in these two chapters, and with what you *will* learn in chapter 10, "Enjoy Vegetables and Fruits," you will have an adequate and flexible tool kit to manage family dinners. Keep working with these tools until you feel comfortable with them and can feed your family with a minimum of stress and strain.

If you want to learn more, the choices are vast, but we can narrow them down a bit. For books that deal with cooking at about the same level as these chapters, you might consider *Cheap, Fast, Good*, written by food column authors Beverly Mills and Alicia Ross, which "cuts through both the budget dilemma and the time dilemma." You might also consider *Desperation Dinners*, an older but still popular book by the same authors. If you can still find it, *Cooking with 5 Ingredients* by Barbara C. Jones is a fine book packed with easy, fast, and accessible recipes. Consider the popular *Fix-It and Forget-It* cookbooks by Phyllis Pellman Good. Branded "unfashionable American cooking," *New York Times* writer Ginia Bellafante went on to observe, "Her books dispute the perceived notion that cooking is a pastime and food a powerful expression of status and style." It seems to me that the last thing you need when you are getting dinner on the table is to be worrying about status and style!

FIGURE 9.14 GENERIC CASSEROLE
Select one item from each column. Combine in a 2-quart casserole dish and bake at 350° F for 30 to 45 minutes. Makes six helpings.

Protein ingredients	Liquid ingredients	Starchy ingredients
1 lb raw weight, 12 oz cooked weight, or 1 1/2 to 2 cups cubed or chunked:	1 1/2 to 2 cups:	6 cups:
Tuna fish	Broth or bouillon	Bread, cubed
Canned meat or chicken	Milk	Cooked rice
Cooked meat or poultry: chicken,	White or cheese sauce	Cooked macaroni
ground beef, sausage or sausages,	Canned tomatoes	Cooked spaghetti
beef, pork, turkey, ham	Cream soups: mushroom, potato,	Cooked noodles
Hard-cooked eggs	broccoli, celery, chicken, cheese	Cooked barley
Dried beans or peas (6 cups	Tomato soup	Cooked bulgur
cooked or 3 cups dry)	Tomato sauce	Cooked potatoes
Cheese	Shredded cheese plus milk	
	Evaporated milk	

Some of the liquid ingredients, like cheese sauce and mushroom soup, add fat. Others, like tomato sauce and broth, do not. If the liquid ingredient does not contain fat, your casserole will taste better and have a more stick-to-the-ribs quality if you add fat—up to 12 fat equivalents. This is particularly important if dried beans or beans are your main ingredient. This startling amount works out to only 1 teaspoon of fat per 1/2 cup of beans.

How-to-cook books for older children make great primers for adults as well as a good introduction to cooking for youngsters. The Bayless's *Rick and Lanie's Excellent Kitchen Adventures* features a father and daughter preparing foolproof, easy, well-written recipes full of the love of good eating. Micah Pulleyn and Sarah Bracken's *Kids in the Kitchen* and Marion Cunningham's *Cooking with Children* are both good choices in this category, as are the Williams Sonoma cookbooks for kids.

A step up from the beginner books are the standard, all-purpose cookbooks, like *Better Homes and Gardens, Betty Crocker,* and *The Fannie Farmer Cookbook.* The *Joy of Cooking* is a dense version of the other three, more of a cooking encyclopedia than a cookbook. It helps to have at least one all-purpose cookbook on hand for looking up obscure questions like "How do you make muffins so they don't have tunnels?" or "How do you poach an egg?"

For still another step up, into books that emphasize fine cuisine rather than straightforward good cooking, consider *The New York Times Cookbook*, another oldie but goodie. As editor Craig Claiborne comments in his preface, "Cooking is one of the simplest and most gratifying of the arts, but to cook well, one must love and respect food." Also consider *Vegetarian Cooking for Everyone* by Deborah Madison, who observes that in her cooking classes, "many students regard cooking as a quirky process that's hard to grasp. Unnerved, they fail to notice that ... cooking is guided by common sense and even logic."

Poke around to find a book that addresses your regional foods. My favorite is Suzanne Breckenridge and Marjorie Snyder's *Wisconsin Herb Cookbook*, which includes "recipes to challenge and recipes to start you on your way to confident (herb) cooking." The authors tell how to grow herbs as well as how to cook with them. They comment enticingly, "Herbs have a sneaky way of becoming an obsession when given half a chance."

I feel the same way about cooking. If you have been bitten by the food and cooking bug, you might want to challenge yourself in another direction, with a couple of books that are for the scientifically curious. Shirley Corriher, author of *CookWise: the Secrets of Cooking Revealed,* bills herself, justifiably, as a "culinary food sleuth." A research biochemist, food scientist, and accomplished chef, Corriher gives

recipes that "not only please the palate but demonstrate the roles of ingredients and techniques." Corriher accessibly teaches the science of food and cooking.

If you like your science straight, with no recipes, also check out Harold McGee's classic, *On Food and Cooking: The Science and Lore of the Kitchen.* McGee's book blends culinary lore, scientific explanation, and historical and literary anecdotes to examine the history and makeup of food, as well as what happens when it's cooked. McGee's huge, fact-packed book makes a great reference for anyone who wonders about food.

Even though we have been talking about other authors, our own lessons on food and cooking aren't done yet. In chapter 10, "Enjoy Vegetables and Fruits," you'll find still more easy and nutritious ways of making your meals satisfying and delicious.

Television Cooking Shows

I am a fan of PBS's *America's Test Kitchen.* I enjoy the orderly scientific approach and the logic about the principles of cookery. Presented by the same folks who publish *Cooks Illustrated* magazine, the program reviews equipment as well as cooking methods. The show spins off a number of cookbooks that you can find by going to their website.

My daughter-in-law Laurie Gonzagowski Satter enjoys another cooking program featured on PBS, *Everyday Food.* The program features young cooks who offer "quick, easy, and practical solutions to the challenges of everyday cooking, and includes easy-to-make recipes along with smart tips and kitchen techniques." There is also an *Everyday Food* magazine, which Laurie likes a lot.

I haven't gotten in the habit of watching the Food Network, but others wouldn't be without it. My librarian friend Ann Michalski compiled a list of popular programs. Ann points out that each program host has a distinctive personality that attracts a specific audience. Some personalities may please you; others may not.

• Rachel Ray's *Thirty Minute Meals.* Ray is bubbly and casual—both about her audience and her cooking. She doesn't measure, but instead uses a handful of this and a pinch of that. She emphasizes quick, healthy food for one, two, or a crowd.

- Giada de Laurentiis's *Everyday Italian*. De Laurentiis is a sophisticated cook who trained at Cordon Bleu in Paris. She cooks for one or two or large gatherings and emphasizes easy, healthy food and talks often of the importance of family.
- Paula Deen's *Paula's Home Cooking*. Deen emphasizes southern home cooking, uses butter liberally, and is not ashamed to use shortcuts such as cake mixes and rice mixes. She has no formal cooking training—she started catering out of her home to support herself and her family. Deen now owns a huge restaurant in Savannah, Georgia.
- Sandra Lee's *Semi-Homemade Cooking*. Lee offers interesting recipes and emphasizes easy ways to prepare foods, often combining prepared mixes and sauces with fresh ingredients.
- Ina Garten's *Barefoot Contessa*. I refer to Garten a couple of times in the recipe sections. Many of Garten's recipes are simple and easy to make, and she's good at explaining cooking techniques. Her upscale lifestyle is featured in the show, which may intrigue—or bother—you.

All of the programs have spun off cookbooks, DVDs, and Web sites. This is obviously not an exhaustive list, but it gives you a place to start.

Cooking Classes

Cooking classes can inspire you, give support for your commitment to cooking, dignify your art, teach you shortcuts, and introduce you to like-minded people. What could be better? Look for cooking classes at vocational schools, cookware stores, and cookware departments in department stores. Sometimes grocery stores give cooking classes as part of a promotion for certain foods. Cooking classes for kids are fun and helpful, too, if you remember that the point is not to teach your child how to cook dinner *for* you, but rather to interest him in cooking dinner *with* you.

University extensions, technical schools, and community colleges offer cooking classes as well. Look them up in your city or county telephone directory. "We promote MyPyramid," say my friends in these programs. "How can you recommend our programs when you disagree with what we teach?" I recommend them because I know they have far more to offer than teaching the rules—they teach cooking, planning, budgeting, and shopping. Some programs even go into homes to teach food skills.

I hope by now you have caught the cooking bug and are feeling successful with getting meals on the table. It wouldn't hurt my feelings one bit to find out you have grown beyond what you have learned here and are well into creating your own path with providing family meals. On the other hand, I wouldn't be at all disappointed to find you are cooking because it is a chore that you simply must do. The commitment involved with respect to reliably providing yourself and others with meals is the same either way.

Chapter

10

Enjoy Vegetables and Fruits

In our culture, vegetables and fruits are considered challenging. Most of us are the product of feeding lore teaching parents that children must be coerced if they are to eat their vegetables. Though the nutrients in fruits and vegetables are no more or less important than those in any of the other food groups, nutrition policy makers consider vegetables to be "marker foods" that give a snapshot of the overall quality of the diet. Thus, we get exhorted and reminded to eat our vegetables, which makes them seem ominous. Like children, we wonder, "If they are so good, why do I have to be persuaded to eat them?" As a result, generations of grown-ups feel obligated to eat their broccoli before they can have dessert, or they have been so traumatized by broccoli that they won't allow it at the table.

To get the vegetables and fruits you need, eat them because you enjoy them, not because you feel obligated. Vegetables and even fruits can be challenging: They have a variety of textures and flavors, some of them strong, sharp, or biting. You may be a *supertaster*, which means you are sensitive to the bitter compound 6-*n*-propylthiouracil (PROP) found in cabbage-family vegetables such as broccoli and greens such as kale, and chard. If you are a supertaster, you may also be more sensitive to sharp and salty foods and to the capsaicin in hot peppers. An estimated 25 percent of us are nontasters,

50 percent are medium tasters, and 25 percent are supertasters. However, being a supertaster doesn't mean you can't learn to enjoy strong-flavored vegetables and fruits. It will just take you longer, and you may enjoy them more if the strong flavors are toned down with salt, fat, sauces, herbs, and spices.

The recipes in this chapter help you sneak up on fruits and vegetables and learn to like them. To interest you in fruits and vegetables, in this chapter I am putting the cart before the horse. To expose you to the possibilities, I begin with delicious recipes and wind up with basic principles. My recipes start out by diluting and disguising vegetables. Then I progress to flavored butters and sauces for dressing up vegetables. After that, I give you recipes that use a lighter hand in enhancing the flavor of vegetables with salt, fat, and other seasonings. After a basic lesson on salads, we turn to fruits. After *that*, we turn to the generics: the basic principles of purchasing and preparing vegetables and fruits.

Vegetables in Disguise

This little section of recipes is for people who don't much care for vegetables but would like to learn. The vegetables are well diluted with other ingredients, including the fat and salt that are so necessary for toning down the flavor of vegetables.

PUMPKIN CUSTARD

Pumpkin is a wonderful vegetable that's high in vitamin A. Pumpkin custard contains eggs, vegetables, and milk, and is so nutritious that it doesn't have to be relegated to dessert. Double this recipe and put it on the table for breakfast. Have it for a snack.

Preheat the oven to 400° F.

Beat the following together in a large bowl:
15-oz can pumpkin
15-oz can milk (use the pumpkin can to measure the milk)
3 eggs

Mix the following together in a separate bowl:
1 cup sugar
1 tsp cinnamon
1 tsp nutmeg
1 tsp ginger
1/4 tsp cloves
Pinch (about 1/8 tsp) salt

Combine the two mixtures and pour them into a 2 1/2-quart glass casserole dish. Bake uncovered for 1 hour. Serve plain or with whipped cream.

Fast tip: Leaving the crust off the pumpkin pie is the fast tip. If you are a whiz at making pastry (or you've found a good store-bought pastry) and your pumpkin pie isn't the same without it, go for it.

SPINACH LOAF

Seasoned bread stuffing shows up in a number of my recipes. I like it for its ease of use and for its seasonings. In this recipe, the bready texture gives the spinach more body and the seasonings take away that tooth-scrubbing sensation you get from eating it.

Preheat oven to 350° F.

Combine:
1 10-oz package frozen chopped spinach, thawed and drained but not squeezed
1 egg, well-beaten
1/2 cup grated sharp cheddar cheese
1/2 cup seasoned bread stuffing, crumbled
1 Tbsp vinegar
1/2 tsp salt
Dash pepper
1/4 tsp paprika

Pour into a 1-quart casserole dish. Let stand for a few minutes for the bread stuffing to hydrate.

Bake for 30 minutes or until a knife inserted near the middle comes out clean. If all goes well, this will be while the spinach is still a nice, bright green.

BROCCOLI PUFF

The salt and fat tone down the broccoli taste and may make it more appealing to the confirmed broccoli skeptic.

Preheat oven to 350° F.

Shake together in a jar:
3/4 cup milk
1 Tbsp flour
1 egg
1/4 cup mayonnaise
1/2 tsp salt

Combine with:
1 10-oz package frozen broccoli, thawed
2 oz cheddar cheese, shredded

Topping:
1/4 cup bread crumbs
1 Tbsp melted butter

Bake for 45 minutes.

ZUCCHINI AND CARROT PATTIES

I hope you like these. I think they are absolutely smashing, and everyone I have served them to asks for more. Sebastian, Clio's son, eats them by the handfuls. I have tried grating the vegetables in the food processor, but it doesn't work as well. It seems that the patties depend on the long strands of the grated vegetables to make a lattice to hold them together while they fry.

Mix together and let stand to hydrate:
2 cups seasoned bread stuffing mix
4 eggs
1/4 cup milk
1 tsp salt
1/4 tsp pepper

Coarsely grate *2 cups zucchini* and *2 cups carrots* onto a piece of waxed paper using the large grating side of a box grater. Mix with the hydrated stuffing mix. The mixture will be very loose, but it will become firmer with cooking. Heat a large frying pan over medium heat and melt *2 teaspoons butter* and *2 teaspoons oil* together in the pan. When the fat is hot but not smoking, lower the heat to medium-low and drop size 30 ice-cream scoops of batter into the pan. Gently flatten into patties and fry in oil for 2–3 minutes per side. To choose your oil, see figure 9.12 "Fat for Frying."

ZUCCHINI PANCAKES

I seem to be on a zucchini kick, but these pancakes are just *so* good! My associate Clio says she likes them even better than the zucchini and carrot patties. I haven't tried them yet on Sebastian.

Preheat the oven to 300° F.

Combine:
2 medium zucchini, about 2 1/2 cups coarsely grated
2 Tbsp finely grated red onion
3 large eggs, beaten
6–8 Tbsp all-purpose flour
1 tsp baking powder
1/2 tsp salt
1/4 tsp freshly ground black pepper
Unsalted butter and vegetable oil

Grate the 2 medium zucchini and immediately stir in the 2 tablespoons grated red onion and 3 large eggs, beaten. Stir in 6 tablespoons flour, 1 teaspoon baking powder, 1/2 teaspoon salt, and 1/4 teaspoon pepper. If the batter is too thin from the liquid in the zucchini, add another 2 tablespoons flour. Alternatively, salt the grated zucchini in a colander, let it stand for a few minutes and squeeze out some of the water.

Cook on a lightly greased 350° F griddle or frying pan. A drop of water will dance and sizzle when the pan is ready. Cook the pancakes about 2 minutes on each side, until browned. Place the pancakes on a sheet pan in a 325° F oven to keep warm and to cook a little more. Continue to grill the pancakes until all the batter is used up. Serve hot.

BROCCOLI CASHEW SALAD

My daughter-in-law Angela Emmons Satter did a bit of web research and duplicated this deli salad. She substituted Miracle Whip for the mayonnaise and sugar called for in most recipes. This relatively high-fat salad pairs nicely with a low-fat entrée such as broiled fish.

Thoroughly wash *1 large head broccoli (about a pound)*, drain, and cut into bite-sized pieces.

Combine with broccoli and chill several hours:
1/4 cup bacon bits (real if you can get them, otherwise use the imitation ones made from soy)
1/2 cup raisins or Craisins
1 small red onion, chopped
1 1/2 cup Miracle Whip

Chill for several hours. Stir in *1 cup cashew halves or pieces* just before serving.

Enticements for Vegetables

If you are a novice eater of vegetables and fruits, the enticements of toppings and sauces may help you. You can also turn to the other vegetable and fruit recipe sections for more ideas to help you and your children be successful with vegetables and fruits. Glazed carrots are still carrots. The sweet flavor makes them more appealing to people just beginning to establish a relationship with carrots. Fruits can be baked into desserts. The plum cobbler (page 162) has all the nutrients of fresh plums, with some embellishment.

HERBED BUTTER

Mix the following ingredients together:
1/4 cup butter, softened
4 Tbsp fresh herbs of your choice: chopped dill, chives, mint, basil, parsley

Store the mixture in a labeled, covered jar in the refrigerator and use as needed for flavoring vegetables.

FIGURE 10.1 HERBS IN COOKING
You can purchase fresh herbs at the grocery store or grow them in your garden or on your window sill. All the herbs listed in the herbed butter recipe are also easy to grow fresh and keep on hand. Be careful of mint—it spreads and will invade your whole garden patch.

To keep fresh herbs on hand, wash them and then freeze them in water in an ice cube tray. When you are ready to use them, thaw as many cubes as you need and blot the herbs with a paper towel. To easily sliver basil, roll several leaves into a long cylinder and slice them across the grain or cut them with kitchen shears.

To substitute dried herbs for fresh herbs, cut the measurement in 1/3. Be careful not to use too much of the dried herbs—they are strong-tasting, and their flavor can easily overwhelm the mixture.

CHEESE SAUCE

This is a white sauce with cheese mixed into it that you can use for broccoli or cauliflower. The method for making white sauce is the same as the one for making **Gravy** on page 113.

Melt over low heat:
2 Tbsp butter

Mix together and blend into the melted butter:
2 Tbsp flour
1/4 tsp salt
1/8 tsp black pepper

Cook for about a minute, then remove from heat. Stir in *1 cup milk*. Bring to a boil, stirring constantly.

Remove from heat. Stir in *1/4 cup shredded sharp cheddar cheese* and *1/4 teaspoon dry mustard*. Stir until the cheese melts and blends into the white sauce.

To make **White Sauce** in the microwave, melt the 2 tablespoons butter in a 2-cup glass measuring cup for about a minute on medium-low. Stir in the 2 tablespoons flour and microwave on medium-low for 1 minute. Add milk to just over the 1-cup line, stir, and microwave in 45-second installments, stirring after each installment. (The frequent stirring prevents the flour from cooking in a mass in the bottom of the measuring cup. Those lumps don't stir out.) When the white sauce begins to boil, reduce the power to low and cook for 1 minute. Add the seasonings and grated cheese.

MUSTARD BUTTER
This is good with peas, brussels sprouts, cauliflower, broccoli, and green and wax beans.

Mix the following together well:
1/2 stick softened butter
1 tsp herb mustard or Dijon mustard
1/2 tsp lemon juice

Add the following to the mixture and mix well:
1 tsp fresh dill weed or 1/4 tsp dried
1 tsp chives, minced
Dash pepper
Dash salt

Store in a labeled covered jar in the refrigerator.

OLIVE OIL WITH GARLIC
Try this on peas, green and wax beans, brussels sprouts, cauliflower, and broccoli.

Combine the following ingredients in a blender:
8 cloves garlic, minced
1/4 cup olive oil

Heat gently in a frying pan or in the microwave until the garlic bits are light brown. Store in a labeled, covered jar in the refrigerator.

Variation: Toss vegetables with the mixture, then add 1/2 cup prepackaged Italian-seasoned bread crumbs, and toss again.

OLIVE-CREAM CHEESE SPREAD
This works well as a dip for pretzels or raw vegetables. It also melts nicely on hot vegetables. It is surprisingly tasty with brussels sprouts. The strong flavor of the topping competes nicely with the strong flavor of the vegetable.

Finely chop:
1 Tbsp stuffed green olives

Mix with:
1/4 cup cream cheese or Neufchâtel
A couple teaspoons olive juice

Store in a labeled, covered jar in the refrigerator.

Salads

The two criteria I used in choosing these salad recipes and all the other vegetable recipes are that they taste *good* and they are *fast and easy*.

GO-EVERYWHERE GREEN SALAD
You will develop your family favorites and standbys for green salads. Many families have the same salad over and over again and don't seem to get tired of it. You can vary it by changing the salad greens or by dressing it up with herbs or a variety of cheeses.

You can serve this salad with **Best-Yet Oil and Vinegar Dressing** (p. 152), but the dressing is up to you. For many children, a very light dressing or none at all works well because it makes it easier to pick the food up with their fingers. However, you and your child may like bottled salad dressing and plenty of it, and that's fine. You can also buy packets of pre-mixed salad dressing seasonings that you mix yourself with vinegar and oil.

Combine with salad tongs, 2 big spoons, or your carefully washed hands:
About 1 to 1 1/2 handfuls washed salad greens per
*   adult*
Additional ingredients from the variations list
Salad dressing of your choice

Use a small amount of dressing—less than you think you will need. Toss well until all the leaves have some dressing on them. Taste and add salt or more dressing as needed. Dressing makes the lettuce wilt, so don't add it until the last minute.

Variations: Add croutons, grated carrots, thinly sliced green onions, thinly sliced red onions (very pretty), parsley, chives, black or green olives, cucumbers, tomatoes, or leftover cooked vegetables marinated in salad dressing. You can also make a **Main-Dish Salad** by adding chopped hard-cooked eggs, thin slices of cold leftover meat or poultry, and chunks or shreds of cheese.

Cauliflower Blue Cheese Salad Some combinations benefit from more salt, as does this wonderful salad made up of romaine, thinly sliced cauliflower, thinly sliced red onions, thinly sliced black olives, and crumbled blue cheese. Make the dressing with 2 tablespoons vinegar, 2 tablespoons oil, a crushed garlic clove, and 1 1/2 teaspoons salt.

Adapting this salad for children: A child will generally eat less of this salad than an adult.

Put a half- or quarter-handful in the bowl for each child, depending on how old the child is and how much they generally eat. Salad can be challenging and even out of the question for young children. While children don't need teeth to eat soft, cooked food, they do seem to need their molars—which come in around age two years—in order to eat raw vegetables and green salad. After that, the problem is logistical. Since even adults have difficulty spearing salad greens with a fork, why not turn a child's green salad into a finger food? Serve it without dressing so your child can easily pick it up with her fingers. Give her a little side dish of salad for dipping. A sweeter dressing rather than a more savory one might be more appealing for the inexperienced eater. Or not. Children continually surprise me with their eating capabilities.

FIGURE 10.2 PREPACKAGED SALAD GREENS OR DO-IT-YOURSELF?

It is up to you whether you buy bagged, prepackaged salad fixings or the type you have to core, sort, and wash. Prepackaged salad is a value-added product that costs more per portion than the do-it-yourself variety. The salad greens that offer the dressing and other condiments are the most costly. With the plain prepackaged salad greens the cost difference is smaller, especially when you consider your time, water, and what you have to throw away when you buy in bulk. Whether or not you have to *wash* these prepackaged products depends on what it says on the package. The words to look for are *washed*, *prewashed*, and *ready to eat*.

Harmful bacteria have been removed from the varieties that are "washed" and "ready to eat." Large manufacturers use a state-of-the-art cleansing process that kills bacteria better than you could at home. However, the process isn't foolproof, as evidenced by serious *E. coli 0157* and *Salmonella* outbreaks caused by prepackaged, prewashed spinach. Other "scares" are media-generated rather than real. Uninformed reporters sounded the alarm on prepackaged fruits and vegetables when their laboratories found high bacterial levels in many packages of precut vegetables. "You're probably better off eating raw ground beef than you are eating this produce," warned one newscaster. What the reporters didn't bother to find out is that the bacteria in their lab tests were completely harmless. Anything grown in the ground has germs on

it. Only a few of those germs will make you sick, and those illness-producing germs were *not* present in the prepackaged produce.

How can you benefit from using these prewashed greens and still protect your family? Let's start with easy and work up to difficult. If you don't see specific words that indicate that products are washed and ready for consumption, wash the greens yourself before you eat them. Always wash salad greens from a bulk display or from the farmers market, even if it says—and looks—ready to eat. Customers can touch them or sneeze on them, so they are subject to contamination.

Whether you wash prewashed salad greens depends on how much risk you are willing to tolerate in order to have the convenience of using those greens directly out of the bag. Even if you wash them, you are just rinsing, which is lots easier than washing produce to get rid of dirt and grit. If you choose to wash them, Yvonne Bushland, reviewer and food scientist, says to rinse three times in "a large excess" of water. Use a big salad spinner to make the job easier. Pile the greens loosely in the basket and cover them with water. Using the basket, lift the greens out of the water, dump out the water and do it again—and again. If you don't have a spinner, use a big bowl and a colander. Lift the greens out of the water to get them away from the contamination rather than pouring the water through the colander.

I hope before this book is revised that the controls will be good enough that we won't even have to consider washing prewashed greens.

BEST-YET OIL AND VINEGAR DRESSING

I like homemade salad dressing best—it tastes fresh. An oil and vinegar dressing is always a work in progress, but this one has been around for a while. This dressing is simple and keeps as long as you want it. The recipe makes 1 1/2 cups of dressing, enough to keep on hand and use as you need it. Refrigerate it: The garlic and onion powders could introduce clostridium botulinum, which could grow at room temperature and produce toxin in the airless medium of the dressing. Combining vegetable oil with olive oil makes the dressing liquid and pourable at refrigerator temperature. Olive oil alone gets semisolid at refrigerator temperature.

Combine:
1/2 cup olive oil
1/2 cup salad oil
1/2 cup wine vinegar
1/2 tsp garlic powder
1/2 tsp onion powder
1/2 tsp salt
1/2 tsp black pepper
1/2 tsp dry mustard

Refrigerate when not in use.

Variations: Sweet Dressing Add 3 tablespoons sugar. Sweetening the dressing makes a salad that is more appealing to inexperienced eaters.

Herb Dressing If you will use this dressing immediately, add finely chopped herbs, such as parsley, chives, or basil. Herbs in dressing get strong-tasting when they are held for longer periods.

SPINACH, RED ONION, AND ORANGE SALAD WITH POPPY SEED DRESSING

You can find very small red onions in early summer. They taste good and add a beautiful, festive appearance.

10–12 oz fresh spinach
1 small red onion or 2–3 very small red onions
2 oranges
1 cup blue cheese
Poppy seed dressing (page 153)

Trim, wash, and spin dry *10 to 12 ounces fresh spinach*, and tear it into bite-sized pieces. (Salad needs less dressing if the greens are dry.) Slice *1 small red onion or 2 to 3 very small red onions* thinly, and break the slices apart into rings. Peel *2 oranges*, halve them end-to-end, and slice. Crumble *1 cup blue cheese.*

FIGURE 10.3 SALAD OIL
Choose your salad oil based on taste, price and the fatty-acid content. Olive oil, of course, lends its own distinctive flavor, which you may or may not enjoy. The major vegetable, seed and nut oils—peanut, canola, sunflower, corn, cottonseed, soybean, and sesame—are supposed to be tasteless, but some people swear they can taste the difference. There is a difference between plain sesame oil, which has little or no flavor, and *toasted* sesame oil, which has a distinctive flavor and a dark-brown color. Toasted sesame oil is a distinctive flavor ingredient to be used in small quantities. Single-ingredient oils vary in price, but corn, soybean and cottonseed oil tend to be the least expensive. Oil labeled "vegetable oil" is likely to be soybean or cottonseed oil or a combination of the two—read the ingredients list. To inform your oil decision based on the fatty acid content, see appendix N, "A Primer on Dietary Fat."

Just before serving, combine all ingredients and dress lightly until all the ingredients are coated with poppy seed dressing. You can also try the sweetened version of the best-yet oil-and-vinegar dressing.

Fast tip: Prepare the dressing and put the amount needed in the bottom of the salad bowl. Cross a long-handled serving fork and spoon on top of the dressing, then pile the prepared greens on top of the crossed utensils. The fork and spoon keep the greens from touching the dressing. Cover the salad bowl with plastic wrap and refrigerate until serving time. Toss just before serving.

It is particularly worth purchasing prewashed spinach. Spinach has so many little wrinkles that can hold on to sand and dirt, and it takes so many changes of water to get it all out that it can be quite discouraging to cook with fresh spinach. Even if you decide to wash it before you use it, it will be lots easier than starting with unwashed.

Adapting this dish for children: About the blue cheese: It's always a mistake to assume children won't be able to handle something and start adapting the dish before children have been given an opportunity to learn to like the food. However, the blue cheese in this salad might be challenging for many children. Unlike the red onions, which will also be challenging, they can't eat around it. It permeates everything. To start with, put the crumbled blue cheese in a separate bowl and pass it.

Variations: Vary this salad by using different fruits, greens, and cheeses. For instance, try a spinach-grape-feta salad with poppy seed dressing. Or substitute mixed salad greens.

Make this into a main-dish salad by adding cold, thinly sliced cooked chicken. The **Lemon Chicken** (page 116) works great with this recipe.

POPPY SEED DRESSING

Not only does this dressing taste great on the **Spinach, Red Onion, and Orange Salad,** it is also wonderful in the **Poppy Seed Coleslaw** (page 155). It is also good with fruit salad. You'll have your own ideas.

In a blender or food processor, combine the following ingredients and blend until pulverized:
1/3 cup sugar
3/4 tsp dry mustard
1/4 cup red wine vinegar
1 Tbsp grated onion or juice
3/4 tsp salt
  Add:
1/8 medium onion, coarsely chopped

Drizzle into the blender, mixing constantly at medium speed until the dressing is smooth and thick:
2/3 cup salad oil

At the end, stir in:
1 Tbsp poppy seeds

Fast tip: Coarsely chop the onion and let the blender do the grating. Double or triple this recipe and keep it in a glass jar in the refrigerator. It will be all ready to use for a sweet vegetable salad or fruit salad.

TOMATO SLICES WITH VINAIGRETTE

When tomatoes are farm fresh and vine-ripened, they don't need any help to make them taste wonderful. Just slice them and serve with salt and pepper or with sugar. However, toward the end of the season, if you or your neighbor have a tomato plant that just won't stop, you might appreciate pepping up those tomato slices with this vinaigrette.

You can keep this vinaigrette in the refrigerator, and just before you serve it, take out a

portion and add fresh herbs. The fresh herbs become strong and unpleasant if they are left in the oil for any length of time.

In a jar with a tight-fitting lid, shake together the following ingredients:
2 Tbsp wine vinegar or lemon juice
1/4 tsp salt
dash freshly ground black pepper
1/4 tsp prepared mustard
1/4 tsp dry mustard
6 Tbsp salad oil

Just before you use the dressing, shake it and take out 1/4 cup. To that 1/4 cup, add *1 tablespoon chopped fresh herbs.* Experiment with herbs to find out what you like and write it down. I have used dill, basil, parsley, and chives. Occasionally I use thyme, but only in a very small amount because it has a strong flavor.

TOMATO AND FRESH MOZZARELLA SALAD

Fresh mozzarella is different from the mozzarella on pizza. It is white and has a rubbery consistency and a delicate flavor. You will find it in the cheese case. This salad dressing has a lot of salt, but it has a purpose. The salt wilts the red onions and makes them less challenging. It draws some of the juice out of the tomatoes and adds flavor to the dressing. And it adds flavor to the fresh mozzarella cheese. This salad is also great with feta cheese, but if you use feta, leave out the salt. To make it with firm tofu, experiment with the amount of salt that tastes good.

Mix together ingredients for the dressing:
1/4 cup good white wine vinegar
6 Tbsp good olive oil
1 Tbsp salt
1 tsp freshly ground black pepper

Pour over:
2 medium red onions, thinly sliced

Let stand at room temperature for an hour or so to allow the onions to wilt.

Just before serving, gently stir in the rest of the ingredients:
2 pints grape or *cherry tomatoes, cut in half*
1 Tbsp chopped fresh basil leaves or *1 tsp dried*
1/4 cup chopped fresh parsley leaves
8 oz fresh mozzarella cheese, cut in small cubes

POTATO SALAD

I was never happy with my potato salad until I discovered Ina Garten's cooking method for potatoes. See figure 10.4 for more of my discoveries about cooking potatoes.

3 lbs small red or white boiling potatoes
6 hard-cooked eggs, sliced (optional)
1/2 cup chopped celery
1/2 cup chopped red or white onion

Mix together ingredients for the dressing:
1 cup mayonnaise
1/4 cup buttermilk, milk, or white wine
4 Tbsp Dijon or whole-grain mustard
1/4 cup chopped fresh dill or 1 Tablespoon dry dill
1 tsp freshly ground black pepper
1 tsp salt

Cook *3 pounds small red or white boiling potatoes* according to Ina Garten's method, described in figure 10.4. When the potatoes are cool enough to handle, cut them into bite-sized pieces. Place the cut potatoes in a large bowl. Add *6 hard-cooked eggs, sliced (optional), 1/2 cup chopped celery, and 1/2 cup chopped red or white onion.* Using a rubber scraper, gently stir in enough dressing to moisten. (As the salad sits, you may need to add more dressing.) Toss well, cover, and refrigerate for a few hours to allow the flavors to blend. Serve cold or at room temperature.

ALL-AMERICAN POTATO SALAD

Prepare *3 pounds small red or white boiling potatoes* according to figure 10.4.

Using a rubber spatula, toss potatoes with:
3 Tbsp white vinegar

Let stand. In the meantime, combine:
3/4 cup mayonnaise
3 Tbsp sweet or dill pickle relish
1 tsp powdered mustard
1 tsp celery seed
1 tsp salt
1/2 tsp black pepper
3 Tbsp minced fresh parsley leaves

Toss gently with cooked potatoes.

Add the following ingredients and toss gently:
3 Tbsp minced red onion
1 medium celery rib, chopped fine (about 1/2 cup)
3 hard-boiled eggs, sliced (optional)

HERBED POTATO SALAD

Prepare *3 pounds small red or white boiling potatoes* according to figure 10.4.

Using a rubber spatula, toss potatoes with:
3 Tbsp white vinegar

Let stand. In the meantime, combine:
2 Tbsp good dry white wine
2 Tbsp chicken broth
2 Tbsp lemon juice
2 garlic cloves, minced
1/2 tsp Dijon mustard
1 tsp freshly ground black pepper
2/3 cup olive oil

Toss gently with cooked potatoes and any combination of the optional ingredients:
1/4 cup minced scallions (white and green parts)
2 Tbsp chopped fresh flat-leaf parsley or 2 tsp dried parsley
2 Tbsp minced fresh dill or 2 tsp dried dill weed
2 Tbsp sliced fresh basil or 2 tsp dried basil

FIGURE 10.4 COOKING POTATOES FOR SALAD

The key to good potato salad is perfectly cooked potatoes. The Food Network's *Barefoot Contessa*, Ina Garten, recommends this surefire method—and it works.

Scrub and rinse small boiling potatoes. Cut larger potatoes in pieces to approximate the size of the smaller potatoes. Cover the potatoes with cold water and add salt. Bring to a boil and lower to a simmer. Cook for 10–15 minutes, until the potatoes are barely tender when pierced with a fork. Drain the potatoes in a colander, then place the colander with the potatoes in it over the empty cooking pot off the heat. Cover the potato-filled colander with a clean, dry kitchen towel and leave to steam for 15 to 20 minutes, until the potatoes are tender but firm.

Culinary authority Harold McGee, author of *On Food and Cooking*, explains that low-temperature cooking allows potatoes and other vegetables such as carrots, cauliflower, tomatoes, and beets to develop a "persistent firmness." McGee's low-temperature method is to bake vegetables at 130 to 140° F 20 to 30 minutes. McGee points out that vegetables cooked in this way keep their firmness when they are cooked more, even for prolonged times.

Last but not least, Shirley Corriher, food scientist and author of *CookWise*, points out that cooking potatoes makes their starch granules swell. Cooling after cooking lets the starch granules in the potatoes recrystallize so they aren't soluble in water. That allows potatoes to keep their shape when you slice them for potato salad or American fries.

SWEET-SOUR CUCUMBER SALAD

This is a variation on a traditional Scandinavian dish. You can keep the sweet-sour sauce for up to a week, adding more sliced cucumbers as you eat them.

Bigger, thicker cucumbers have coarser seeds and don't taste as good. If you can find dill-pickle-sized cucumbers, they are the best. The skins are often tender, and the seeds are small.

Scrub or peel (see fast tip) and slice as thinly as you can (paper thin, if you can manage):
2 large European-style cucumbers (often called burp-less) or 4–5 slim cucumbers, 7 or 8 inches long

Make a sweet-sour sauce by mixing together the following ingredients until the sugar is dissolved:
1/2 cup white wine vinegar
1/4 cup sugar
1/2 tsp salt
Dash pepper
4 tsp chopped fresh dill or 1 tsp dried dill weed

Pour the sauce over the cucumbers and refrigerate for 3 hours to allow the flavors to blend. Drain the cucumbers and serve. After you eat these cucumbers, you may add more to the sauce and have cucumber salad for another meal.

Fast tip: You don't have to peel cucumbers if the skins are tender and good tasting. Taste them to find out. If you object at all to the skin flavor, peel them.

Stemmed, cleaned, spun-dry fresh dill can be kept fresh and tasty in a zip top bag in the refrigerator for a week or more. To keep it longer, chop it up, freeze it in water in an ice-cube tray, and store the frozen dill cubes in a zip top bag.

Variations: Serve your cucumbers plain and more thickly sliced, or cut them into wedges. Your children might enjoy them more that way. Also, add thinly sliced sweet or red onion.

POPPY SEED COLESLAW

If you can, make this about 30 minutes to an hour before mealtime to give the flavors a chance to blend.

Chop the vegetables until they are as fine as you like them:
6 oz shredded cabbage
4 oz shredded carrots

Mix in a large bowl and, if you like, add 1/2 cup raisins. Mix in **Poppy Seed Dressing**, page 155, to taste.

Fast tip: Purchase your cabbage and carrots already shredded.

Stove-Top Vegetables

I hope at least one recipe among this group will become a family standby. My main contenders are **Creamed Spinach** and **Gingered Broccoli**. We will begin with three recipes—**Glazed Carrots**, **Stewed Tomatoes**, and **Scalloped Corn**—that are so surefire and easy that it is embarrassing to even call them recipes.

GLAZED CARROTS

Even without added sugar, cooked carrots taste sweeter than raw carrots. The brown sugar makes them even sweeter. Because almost everybody likes sweets, this recipe is a great way to introduce kids—and grown-ups—to carrots.

I like fresh carrots best for this recipe. You may peel carrots and make carrot rounds or sticks, or use the little prepeeled baby carrots and cook them whole or cut them up.

Boil *2 cups carrots, fresh* or *frozen* in a medium sauce pan in enough water to cover until almost tender, or about 5 minutes. Drain thoroughly and put back in sauce pan. If you are using canned carrots, skip the boiling and put the carrots straight into a medium saucepan.

Add the following ingredients to carrots in the saucepan and heat on the stove on medium heat until the brown sugar dissolves:
2 Tbsp brown sugar
1 Tbsp butter
Salt to taste (about 1/2 tsp)

STEWED TOMATOES

This is a homey, easy vegetable recipe that tastes surprisingly good. My daughter, Kjerstin, remembers it fondly.
15-oz can stewed tomatoes
1 cup tough or dried out bread cubes

In the microwave or on the stove, heat a *15-ounce can stewed tomatoes*. The can will say "stewed"—the tomatoes are cooked-looking and they have added sugar. When the tomatoes are hot, add *1 cup tough or dried-out bread cubes*. Let stand a minute or two for the bread to soak up the tomato juice. If the tomatoes taste too sharp, add sugar. That's all there is to it.

Serve in sauce dishes or custard cups.

:D CORN
wing ingredients together:

m-style corn
*1/2 cup slightly crushed soda crackers
   (approximately 10)*
1/4 cup milk or half-and-half
*Pinch pepper; salt to taste (you can also put in dried
   parsley and onions, if you like)*

Heat the mixture gently on low.

CREAMED SPINACH
This is my nomination for a recipe you will make again and again. I discovered it in a fine eating establishment in Birmingham, Alabama. I don't remember what I had for the entrée, but I do remember the spinach!

2 10-oz packages frozen chopped spinach
1/4 cup half-and-half or whipping cream
1/4 cup grated Parmesan or Asiago cheese

Thaw *2 10-ounce packages frozen chopped spinach.* Squeeze the thawed spinach until it is as dry as you can get it. Empty it into a microwave-safe glass dish. Heat in the microwave until the spinach is hot—it will be cooked enough when it is hot.

To the hot spinach, add *1/4 cup half-and-half* or *whipping cream* and *1/4 cup grated Parmesan* or *Asiago cheese.*

The night before: Put the frozen spinach in the refrigerator to thaw. Leave it wrapped until you're ready to use it. In case the packages leak, thaw them in the dish you will use for cooking.

Variation: Leftover creamed spinach tastes great with poached eggs for breakfast or for an easy lunch or dinner.

PANNED CABBAGE AND CARROTS
For this recipe, you can use the same shredded vegetables that you used for the poppy seed coleslaw.

In a large frying pan with a lid, heat *2 to 3 teaspoons butter* over medium heat. When the butter is hot, add the following ingredients all at once:
8 oz shredded cabbage, red or white
4 oz shredded carrots
*A few drops flavored vinegar: balsamic, wine
   vinegar, or rice vinegar*

Sauté and toss for 3–4 minutes. Cover the frying pan and cook for another 1 to 2 minutes until the vegetables are tender but still a little crisp.

Add *1/4 teaspoon each salt and pepper.* Taste for salt and add more as needed. Another 1/4 teaspoon should do it.

GINGERED BROCCOLI
Sauté *1 pound broccoli florets* in *1 tablespoon toasted sesame oil* at a medium-high temperature until the broccoli is warmed and slightly cooked. Use a frying pan with a tight-fitting lid.

Remove the broccoli from the pan. In the same pan, combine the following ingredients and heat to boiling:
2 Tbsp water
1/4 tsp broth concentrate or bouillon crystals
1 tsp soy sauce
1/8 tsp powdered ginger
1/8 tsp powdered garlic

Put the broccoli back in the pan with the broth and seasoning mixture and cover it with a lid. Cook until the broccoli is crisp-tender but still bright green. It should take about 3 to 4 minutes, but check it as it cooks.

GREENS AND BACON
This is a quick version of traditional salt pork and greens. Once again, even though we use bacon and bacon fat, each serving gives only about 1 teaspoon of fat. The salt in the bacon may do the last-minute salting for you. Taste and decide if you need more.

*16-oz package frozen kale, collards, or chard, or tur-
   nip, beet, or mustard greens*
1/2 tsp salt
4 slices bacon
Freshly grated Parmesan cheese (optional)

Following package directions, cook a *16-ounce package frozen kale, collards, or chard, or turnip, beet, or mustard greens* with *1/2 teaspoon salt.* Be forewarned: Some greens require as much as 35 minutes to cook. When the greens are done, drain them thoroughly in a colander and return them to the pan.

Meanwhile, cook *4 slices bacon* at a low to moderate temperature until they are as crisp as you want and crumble them. *Don't drain!* Add the bacon and bacon fat to the greens, toss, and serve. Add *freshly grated Parmesan cheese* if you like.

Fast tip: Keep bacon in the freezer. When you want a small amount for a recipe like this, saw two or three 1/4-inch slices off the end of the frozen block. Break it apart as it cooks.

Variation: Cook 1/4 cup chopped onion in the bacon fat after you remove the bacon and add it to the dish. Try the bacon and onion trick with yellow beans as well. It adds flavor to an otherwise bland dish.

FIGURE 10.5 FRESH GREENS

Check out your produce section for fresh greens, by which I mean fresh kale, collards, or chard, or turnip, beet, or mustard greens. They are sturdy fresh vegetables that you can generally get year-round. They come as-is in big packages or prewashed and precut. Kale is the mildest-tasting, and rainbow kale in the spring is very tasty. Other greens have various pronounced flavors, so experiment to see what you like. You can use fresh greens instead of frozen greens in the greens and bacon recipe—just put cut-up greens in with the cooked bacon and bacon fat, cover, and cook until the greens are done. You can also use cooked fresh greens instead of the spinach in the spinach-feta frittata. A few fresh greens add color and flavor to soup.

Southerners love their greens and find nothing more comforting than the traditional pork-seasoned dish of turnip greens, kale, collards, or mustard greens served up with freshly baked corn bread to dip into the "pot-likker." The traditional southern method is to "boil them down"—to cook them a long time until they are very tender and even mushy. It might be a method you favor, as well, and the vitamin A and minerals in greens hold up to the rough treatment. You can imitate the southern method—sort of—by cooking greens in chicken or vegetable broth. Include sliced onion—or not. I prefer to stop cooking the greens while they still have their bright-green color. In addition to the frying-pan method, you can cook greens by steaming them until they are as done as you want. Either way, dress them with butter, cream, grated cheese, or salt to make them taste even better and to tone down the strong flavors.

HERBED PEAS

Check out my method on page 171 for microwaving frozen vegetables. Add the salt, sugar, and butter during cooking. The sugar gives the peas a just-picked taste.

Cook according to package directions:
10-oz package frozen peas
1/2 tsp sugar
1/2 tsp salt

After cooking, drain off any liquid and stir in the following:
1 Tbsp butter
1 Tbsp minced fresh herbs of your choice—dill, chives, mint, basil, and parsley all go well with peas

Variations: Combine the cooked peas with pearl onions (you can buy them frozen), cooked carrots, or mushrooms. The added vegetables can be fresh, frozen, or canned. If they are canned, drain them before you add them.

SCALLOPED PEAS

Sauté *2 cloves minced garlic* in 1 tablespoon olive oil. Add the hot cooked peas or peas and onions along with:
1/4 cup freshly grated Parmesan cheese
1 cup flavored croutons

MASHED POTATOES

It is certainly okay to use boxed mashed potatoes. I have gone through many a box of Potato Buds in my life, probably because as a hungry child, when I would whine to my mother, "When is dinner going to be ready?" she would invariably say, "As soon as the potatoes are done." For my children, instant potatoes prevented that trauma, though I undoubtedly traumatized them in other ways.

Even though the boxed varieties are convenient and good-tasting, nothing compares with the taste and texture of mashed potatoes you make from scratch. Mashed potatoes are enjoying a comeback at the finest restaurants. My recipe calls for white potatoes, but you can also try making them with Yukon Gold potatoes—they are yellow and have a buttery flavor.

2 lbs Russet or *other white* or *all-purpose potatoes*
1/2 cup half-and-half
1/4 tsp pepper
1/4–1/2 tsp salt

Peel and quarter or cut into 1-inch slices *2 pounds Russet potatoes* or other white or all-purpose potatoes. Heat salted water (1 teaspoon of salt per quart) until boiling, and put in the potato slices or chunks. Reduce the heat to a moderate boil and cook for about 20 minutes or until the potatoes are fork-tender. Drain off the water by cracking the lid and pouring it through the crack, or use a colander. Put potatoes back into the pan and put the pan on the turned-off-but-still-hot burner to let the extra water evaporate.

Meanwhile, measure out and arrange to have hot when the potatoes are done *1/2 cup half-and-half.* In the cooking pan, mash the potatoes with a hand masher, or put them through a device called a ricer. An electric mixer is also all right, but it will tend to make the potatoes more gluey. When the potatoes are mashed to your liking, mix in the cream a little at a time until the potatoes are the consistency you like. Add more cream if you wish. You may prefer your potatoes more coarsely mashed, with little lumps in them. There are no rules. Taste, add *1/4 teaspoon pepper* and as much *salt* as you need—1/4 to 1/2 teaspoon will probably do it.

Fast tip: Peel the potatoes the night before and let them stand in cold water (so they don't get black). Cook and mash the potatoes ahead of mealtime and put them in a slow cooker, or set the bowl or pan in another pan of simmering water. They will stay warm and you won't have the last-minute rush of getting them ready.

Variations: Mashed potatoes can be prepared in many ways to keep them interesting. Cook the potatoes with the skins on and mash the skins right in; be sure to thoroughly wash them and remove the blemishes and green patches. Make **Garlic Mashed Potatoes** by stirring in 4 to 5 cloves garlic, chopped and sautéed. Or cook the raw garlic cloves in with the potatoes and mash them all together. Try **Portland Potatoes** by substituting milk for some of the cream and stirring in 4 ounces Neufchâtel cheese and a raw beaten egg. The hot potatoes cook the egg. Make **Buttermilk Mashed Potatoes** by using buttermilk instead of cream—it is surprisingly good! Don't heat the buttermilk or it will clump up and separate. When you begin cooking dinner, set the buttermilk on the counter to let it come to room temperature.

Alternate method for mashed potatoes:
If your mashed potatoes get too gluey, consider Shirley Corriher's method from her book *Cookwise.* Corriher recommends cooking the potatoes ahead of time, cooling them, then reheating them in hot water when you are ready to mash and serve them. The cooling sets the starch granules, keeps them from breaking down, and contributes a more mealy texture to the mashed potatoes (see figure 10.4 on page 154). Using this method, you can heat up cold, leftover potatoes and make mashed potatoes.

FIGURE 10.6 POTATOES FOR BOILING OR BAKING
There are two general categories of potatoes: mealy and waxy. The mealy ones have a dry texture and are best for mashing and baking. The waxy ones have a moist texture and are best for boiling, creamed potatoes, and potato salad. Mealy potatoes include Russett Burbanks, also known as Idaho Russetts or just Idahos. Yukon Golds are a cross between mealy and waxy—they can go either way. A relatively new variety of potato on the American market, Yukon Golds have a golden yellow flesh and buttery taste. Waxy potatoes include red potatoes and some round white potatoes. Round reds are also all-purpose potatoes—you can either bake or boil them. Of course, the sky won't fall if you boil a Russett potato, but it will cook apart more than a red potato. If you bake a red potato, the texture will be somewhat soggy rather than dry and mealy.

Actually, there are more than 200 varieties of potatoes, many of them unusual to us, and some of those varieties are showing up in supermarkets and farmers markets. You may see Purple Peruvians, Fingerlings, blue potatoes, and others. These traditional varieties developed in the mountains of South America are relatively high in starch and relatively low in water. They take a long time to cook.

RATATOUILLE

Delicious hot or cold, by itself or in a frittata, ratatouille is nothing more or less than vegetable stew. Reviewer and mother Laurel Henneman warns that, given the children's movie of the same name, you might want to call this dish something else. It looks lots different from the ratatouille in the movie! So why not call it "vegetable stew"? It's certainly easier to say!

This version cooks in 30 to 45 minutes in a pan on the stove top. To set it and forget it, you can also make a slow-cooker version or put it in the oven at a low temperature. It is a wonderful late-summer dish, when the locally grown tomatoes, summer squash, peppers, and eggplant are ready.

Salting the cubed eggplant and letting it sit gets it to "weep" out some of the bitter flavor. There are lots of varieties of eggplant, and some of them are mild enough to let you skip the salting-and-weeping step. Experiment.

Cube:
1 medium eggplant

Salt it in layers in a colander and let it stand for 30 to 60 minutes. Then rinse and squeeze the cubes to get rid of the bitter, salty juice.

In a saucepan, combine the prepared eggplant with:
15-oz can Italian tomatoes
2 small zucchini, sliced
2 small yellow summer squash, sliced
1 medium onion, coarsely chopped
1 large red or yellow bell pepper, cut in thin strips
2 cloves garlic, finely chopped
1 tsp dry basil, finely crushed or *1/4 cup fresh sliced basil*
3 tsp Italian seasoning, crushed
2 Tbsp dried parsley or *4 Tbsp fresh parsley*
1 tsp salt
1/2 tsp pepper
1 Tbsp olive oil

Bring to a boil, reduce heat, and cook on low for 30 to 45 minutes. Check periodically, and when zucchini and yellow squash are almost done (the colors will be bright and the vegetables not quite crisp-tender), put in *8 ounces sliced fresh mushrooms* for the last 10 minutes of cooking.

Taste for seasoning and add more salt and pepper if you think it needs it. For a more zesty flavor, you might try adding some *pitted black olives,* sliced or whole, or a few drops *balsamic vinegar.*

This recipe calls for only *1 tablespoon olive oil,* which isn't very much. I think that's all it needs in order for it to taste good. You may think otherwise. Anything up to 1/4 cup olive oil still qualifies for our definition of moderate fat use.

FIGURE 10.7 BELL PEPPERS
Sweet bell-shaped peppers can be green, red, yellow, orange, brown, or purple, depending on the variety and stage of ripeness. The ratatouille calls for red or yellow bell peppers primarily because of the color, although the sweeter flavor blends well with the other mild-flavored vegetables. Most bell peppers are sold at the mature green stage—fully developed but not ripe. As they ripen on the vine, green bell peppers turn red and become sweeter. Because they lack the capsaicin contained by their hotter cousins, bell peppers have no "bite." All bell peppers are excellent sources of vitamin C, with at least twice as much of the vitamin as citrus fruits.

Oven-Cooked Vegetables

Oven-cooking vegetables offers interesting and appealing tastes and textures as well as a convenient way to cook for a crowd.

BAKED SCALLOPED CORN
This is a reprise of the stove-top **Scalloped Corn** recipe (page 156).

Mix the following ingredients together:
15-oz can cream-style corn
1/2 cup slightly crushed soda crackers (approximately 10)
1 egg, beaten
1/4 cup milk or *half-and-half*
Pinch pepper; salt to taste (you can also put in dried parsley and onions, if you like)

Pour the mixture into an ovenproof baking dish. Bake at 350° F for 45 minutes. Keep this recipe in mind when you have the oven already going for another dish. With the milk and egg, it is almost a meal on its own.

Variation: For **Corn and Broccoli Bake**, add 1 10-oz package frozen chopped broccoli, thawed and drained.

CORN PUDDING
You may have seen this recipe with cornbread mix instead of the dry ingredients. I thought the cornbread-mix version was too sweet, so I created this one. If you don't mind the sweet taste, use the mix in place of the dry ingredients.

Preheat the oven to 350° F or 325° F, depending on what else you are baking (see the next page for cooking times).

Mix together the wet ingredients in a large mixing bowl:
15-oz can cream-style corn
15-oz can whole kernel corn, liquid and all
1 Tbsp butter, melted
1 cup low-fat or regular sour cream(not non-fat)
2 eggs, beaten

Mix together the dry ingredients in a small mixing bowl:
3/4 cup cornmeal
3/4 cup flour
1 tsp sugar
1/4 tsp salt
2 1/2 tsp baking powder

Stir the dry ingredients into the wet ingredients until mixed. Beat with a spoon for 1 minute. Pour into a 2-quart casserole dish. Bake at 350° F for 45 minutes or at 325° F for an hour, until it is golden on top.

OVEN-BAKED MIXED VEGETABLES

I particularly appreciate this recipe when I cook for a crowd. I double it, bake it in a big turkey-roasting pan, and stir it a time or two during the baking. Almost any assortment of vegetables you enjoy works.

Preheat the oven to 425° F.

Mix together the following ingredients:
3 Tbsp olive oil
1 Tbsp lemon juice
1/4 tsp dried rosemary, crushed
1/4 tsp pepper
2 cloves garlic, chopped
1/2 tsp salt

Clean and prepare the following:
2 large onions, coarsely chopped
2 yellow summer squash, cut in slices
1/2 cauliflower, broken or cut into small florets
2 potatoes, cut into wedges

Pour the oil mixture over the vegetables and mix thoroughly with your hands.

Arrange vegetables in a shallow 9 × 13-inch baking pan. Bake for 20 minutes or until vegetables are as tender and browned as you like them. Stir during baking with a pancake turner. Serve hot with grated Parmesan cheese, if desired.

Variations: Instead of the rosemary, use fresh basil. Just before serving, toss with 2 tablespoons slivered fresh basil leaves. You can also try a little garlic or some onion powder. Experiment.

LAYERED ZUCCHINI BAKE

Reviewer and colleague Pam Estes said she knew better, but she planted four zucchini plants this spring. Pam gave me this great recipe that I have made and enjoyed many times. She says she has used all sizes of zucchini except the really big ones, which she shreds for cake and bread. She says, "It is always good, whether I use fresh or canned tomatoes, or American single slices or shredded extra sharp cheddar. The bread crumbs could easily be cracker or potato chip crumbs, too! It is an ideal recipe to just have fun with."

Grease a 10-inch flat casserole dish or frying pan and make 2 layers of the following ingredients in the order they are listed:
3 small zucchini, sliced thinly, about 1 1/2 lb
1 or 2 medium onions, sliced thinly
2 medium tomatoes, sliced or 15-oz can petite diced tomatoes, drained
4 oz shredded or sliced cheese of your preference: sharp cheddar, American, etc.

Cover with the lid or with aluminum foil and bake in a 400-degree oven for 45 minutes. Remove the cover and sprinkle on the following:
1 cup buttered bread crumbs
1/4 cup Parmesan cheese

Bake for another 10–15 minutes until browned. Keep an eye on it, as the butter in the bread crumbs will make them brown quickly.

Variation: Layered Eggplant Bake Substitute an equal amount of eggplant for the zucchini. Treat the eggplant with salt—or not—as in the **Ratatouille** (p. 158). Thinly slice the eggplant and cut large rounds in halves or quarters.

Oven-Roasted Vegetables

Oven-roasting vegetables to the browned stage gives them milder, more toned-down flavor and adds a different flavor that you may enjoy. Browning occurs as a result of the maillard reaction, which is a chemical reaction between protein and sugar in the presence of moderate heat. You can oven-roast vegetables to the texture and degree of browning that you want. In any event, keep a close eye on the roasting, as oven-roasted vegetables can get overdone quickly.

I have specified a 350 to 375° F oven for these recipes. Many recipes call for a 400° F oven, but I find a temperature that high difficult to manage. Before I know it, my vegetables have charred and smoke is pouring out of the oven. If you like the higher temperature and can handle it, you have my blessing.

You will note that I use a lot of zip top bags in these recipes, which offends my commitment to keep plastic-bag usage to a minimum. However, to evenly and gently distribute the oil and seasonings over the vegetables, I find the zip top bags indispensable.

OVEN-ROASTED POTATOES

These are wonderful newly made or reheated. They satisfy the need for French-fried potatoes without having to heat up a large vat of oil.

Preheat the oven to 375° F.

Thoroughly wash *2 1/2 pounds Russet potatoes*, remove blemishes and green patches, cut them into chunks, and blot them with paper towels. Toss them in a large bowl or a big zip top bag with *3–4 tablespoons cooking oil*, coating well.

Mix together seasonings for potatoes and sprinkle into oiled potatoes in the bowl or zip top bag:
5 Tbsp grated Parmesan cheese
1/2 tsp salt
1/2 tsp garlic powder
1/2 tsp onion powder
1/2 tsp paprika
1/4 tsp black pepper

Toss the potatoes well to coat them evenly with the seasonings. Arrange them in a single layer on a jelly roll pan. Bake for 40 to 45 minutes, until potatoes are tender when you push a fork into them. Stir once with a pancake turner during baking.

OVEN-ROASTED ASPARAGUS

1 to 2 lbs asparagus
1 to 2 Tbsp extra-virgin olive oil
Freshly ground black pepper and salt

Preheat oven to 350° F.

Wash the *asparagus* in three changes of water, lifting it out of the water rather than draining it, to remove any dirt particles that may be lodged in the tips or stuck to the stalks. Don't drain through a colander: Draining pours the dirt right back into the vegetable. Snap off the bottoms of the asparagus stalks. Letting the stalk snap at the natural breaking point as close to the cut end as possible preserves the tender stalk but gets rid of the fibrous end. Pat the spears with a towel to dry them as much as you can. Place the washed and snapped asparagus spears in a zip top bag.

Pour 1 to 2 *tablespoons extra virgin olive oil* per pound of asparagus into the bag with the asparagus. Gently move the bag around until the oil evenly coats the asparagus. Lay out the oiled asparagus in single layer on a jelly roll pan. Sprinkle with *salt and freshly ground black pepper*. Add any other spices or herbs that you think you would enjoy.

Roast for 10 to 20 minutes. Keep an eye on the color to roast until the asparagus is done to your liking.

Tender but crisp: Asparagus changes color from a medium green to a dark green.

Mushy and somewhat limp; heightened flavor: Asparagus is lightly browned.

Browned and somewhat crispy with toned-down asparagus flavor: This is a medium brown color and the asparagus stalks are somewhat shriveled. Don't cook beyond this point as blackened asparagus is *not* enjoyable.

OVEN-ROASTED BROCCOLI

1 head broccoli, about 3/4 pound, cut into lengthwise pieces all the way through the stem
2–3 cloves garlic, minced or *1/2 tsp garlic powder*
1 tsp salt
4 Tbsp extra-virgin olive oil
Black pepper

Preheat oven to 350° F.

Cut the *broccoli* into stalks. Wash, drain, and pat with a towel to dry a bit. Peel the stalks—or don't—depending on how chewy you want your final product to be. Put the broccoli in a zip top plastic bag. In a jar, combine the *garlic, 1 teaspoon salt*, and *4 tablespoons extra-virgin olive oil*. Shake it up, pour the oil mixture into the zip top bag with the broccoli, seal it, and shake it until all the pieces of broccoli are well coated with oil. Arrange the broccoli stalks on a jelly roll pan. Bake for 25 to 35 minutes or until the tops are tender when tested with a fork. The stalks will be chewier than the florets unless you have peeled them. Watch closely, as the florets burn easily. Sprinkle with *black pepper* and serve immediately.

OVEN-ROASTED CAULIFLOWER

I don't especially like cooked cauliflower, and for years, the only way I'd eat it was smothered in cheese sauce. But roasting it tones down the strong taste and adds an indefinable flavor that is more to my liking. A sprinkling of Parmesan at the end helps, too.

1 head cauliflower
3 Tbsp olive oil
Salt and pepper
1 cup Parmesan cheese (2 oz)

Preheat oven to 350° F.

Remove the outer green leaves and stem from *1 head cauliflower*, cut the head into florets, and wash in cold water. Pat the florets dry with a towel, place them in a zip top plastic bag, add *3 tablespoons olive oil*, and shake the vegetables and oil until all the pieces of cauliflower are well coated. Arrange the pieces of cauliflower on a jelly roll pan. Sprinkle with *salt and pepper* to taste. Bake for 20–35 minutes until the cauliflower is as tender as you like it when you pierce it with a fork. Sprinkle with *1 cup Parmesan cheese* and bake for an additional 1 or 2 minutes, just until the cheese melts. Serve hot or warm.

Fruit Recipes

Fruit is, of course, perfectly presentable plain. Fresh fruit makes a wonderful dessert or meal accompaniment, as does canned or frozen fruit. It is surprising that although most people like fruit, food consumption surveys say we don't eat much of it. Not only that, but much of the fruit we do consume is in the form of juice.

So it is clear we could use a little enticement. These fruit desserts add little in terms of time, and they add a great deal in terms of taste. We all like our sweets, so why not hook sweets onto something nutritious, like fruit?

PLUM COBBLER
Preheat oven to 375° F.

Wash and cut *20 Italian plums* in quarters or slice *8 purple plums* to yield about 2 lbs of fruit altogether. Spread fruit evenly on a 10 × 6-inch or 8 × 8-inch baking pan. Spread evenly over the fruit:
2 Tbsp sugar
1/4 tsp cinnamon
Butter shavings (the carrot peeler works well for shaving butter)

Mix together the dry ingredients:
1 cup flour (you may use half white and half whole-wheat)
1 cup sugar
1 1/2 tsp baking powder
1/2 tsp salt
2 Tbsp Saco buttermilk powder
1/4 tsp baking soda

Add the following ingredients and stir until evenly blended:
1 egg, beaten
1/2 cup cold water
1/4 cup cooking oil

Pour the mixture evenly over the plums. Be sure to get the topping into the corners. Bake for

45 minutes. The cobbler is done when the top is evenly brown and the plums pierce easily with a toothpick. Check the cobbler toward the end of baking, as it burns easily. Depending on what you have in the oven, you can get away with baking this at 400° F, 350° F, or even 325° F. Adjust the baking time by 10 to 15 minutes for each 25-degree change in oven temperature: Decrease time for the 400° oven, and increase it for the 350° or 325° oven.

Variation: Substitute an equal volume of other fruits for the plums.

Rhubarb Cobbler Sprinkle with 1/4 to 1/2 cup sugar instead of 2 tablespoons.

Peach Cobbler Use 4–5 fresh peaches, peeled and sliced and 2 Tablespoons sugar. Or use a 16-ounce bag frozen peaches, or a 28-ounce can sliced peaches. If the frozen or canned peaches are sweetened, you probably won't need the 2 tablespoons sugar.

Cherry Cobbler Use a 16-ounce package fresh or frozen sour cherries. Add 1/4 to 1/2 cup sugar, unless the cherries are already sweetened. You might enjoy the added flavor of a dash of almond extract.

FIGURE 10.8 BUTTERMILK
Instead of the Saco powder and water, you may use 1/2 cup fluid buttermilk and omit the water. Buttermilk tenderizes baked goods and gives them a pleasant flavor. The acid in the buttermilk plus the soda also leavens the cobbler. If you choose not to use buttermilk or buttermilk powder, substitute milk for the water and leave out the soda. Saco buttermilk powder is a great dried product; it's easy to keep on hand and has the characteristics of "real" buttermilk. In fact, it *is* real buttermilk. Buttermilk you purchase in the dairy case is made by adding a culture to fresh milk to sour it. Saco buttermilk is made primarily from the by-product of the butter-churning process: sweet-cream buttermilk. The word *buttermilk*, in fact, means the fluid remaining after the cream "breaks"—after the fat coalesces into butter in the churning process.

PINEAPPLE UPSIDE-DOWN CAKE
This is a variation of the **Plum Cobbler** recipe (page 162).

Preheat oven to 350° F.

Drain *1 15-ounce can pineapple slices* and lay in the bottom of a 10 × 6-inch or 8 × 8-inch baking pan. Sprinkle with *2 tablespoons brown sugar*. Dot with little shavings of *butter* (the carrot peeler works well for shaving butter). If you want to be fancy, put a *maraschino cherry* in the center of each pineapple ring.

Mix together the dry ingredients:
1 cup flour (you may use half white and half
*   whole-wheat)*
3/4 cup sugar
1 1/2 tsp baking powder
1/2 tsp salt
2 Tbsp Saco buttermilk powder
1/4 tsp baking soda

Add the following ingredients and stir until evenly blended:
1 egg, beaten
1/2 cup cold water
1/4 cup cooking oil

Pour the mixture evenly over the pineapple. Be sure to get the topping into the corners. Bake for 40 minutes. The cake is done when the top is evenly browned and a toothpick inserted near the middle comes out clean. Check the cake toward the end of baking, as it burns easily. After baking, invert onto a serving plate. Serve with ice cream.

Variations: If you like more fruit and less cake, double the fruit or halve the batter.

APPLE CUSTARD

In our family, this is known as "Gross dessert" because I got the recipe from Annette Gross, who put it in a crust and called it "Dutch apple pie." Many of my recipes are named for the person who gave them to me. Cooking connects people and carries sweet memories.

Combine the following ingredients in a blender until the apples are finely chopped:
2 cups milk
4 eggs
2/3 cup sugar
1/4 tsp salt
3/4 tsp cinnamon
4 tsp flour
2 medium apples, washed and cored

Pour the mixture into a 2-quart casserole dish. Bake at 425° F for 10 minutes, then at 350° F for an additional 40 minutes. The custard is done when a clean knife inserted near the center comes out clean.

MICROWAVE CHUNKY APPLESAUCE

Purchased applesauce is good, but fresh home-made applesauce is an event! This applesauce is great as a side dish with pork, as dessert with cream or ice cream, or even with yogurt as a topping for pancakes or over cottage cheese.

Wash, quarter, and core:
6 cooking apples

Cut into bite-sized chunks. Put into a glass dish that can be covered.

Mix the following in with the apples, putting in the sugar before or after cooking, depending on whether you want chunky or mushy applesauce:
1/4 cup water or apple juice
1/8 tsp nutmeg
3 Tbsp brown sugar

Cover and microwave on medium-high for 4 minutes. Stir, then cook 3 minutes more. Check for doneness: Apples will be about half-cooked but still firm. They will soften more and the flavors will blend as they stand. Allow to cool; serve warm or cold.

Fast tip: Cook this the night before or an hour or two ahead of time to let the apples get consistently soft and give the colors and flavors a chance to blend.

Variation: Peel the apples for a softer product. Or, before you cook the apples, add 1/2 package fresh cranberries, halved, and another 3 Tbsp brown sugar. Alternatively add 1/2 cup Craisins and no more sugar. Cranberries give the applesauce a lovely red color.

FIGURE 10.9 COOKING APPLES
The produce manager can tell you which are the cooking apples, and maybe even which ones keep their shape with cooking and which get mushy. Some common cooking apples are McIntosh, Rome Beauty, Golden Delicious, Cortland, and Granny Smith.

Whether your cooked apples are mushy or firm also depends on when you add the sugar. Adding sugar last makes for mushy applesauce. Adding sugar first makes for chunky applesauce. Choosing brown versus white sugar does the same. Brown sugar, which contains calcium, helps to preserve the "glue" between cells and keeps the chunks firmer. Tomato processors use the trick of adding calcium to canned tomatoes to preserve their texture.

PEACH CRISP

3 cups sliced fresh, frozen, or canned peaches
  (drained)
1/2 cup brown sugar, packed
1/2 cup flour
1/2 cup oatmeal
1 1/2 tsp cinnamon
1/4 cup (1/2 stick) butter, softened

Preheat oven to 375° F.

Put *3 cups sliced fresh, frozen, or canned peaches (drained)* in the bottom of a 10 × 6-inch or 8 × 8-inch baking pan.

Mix in a large mixing bowl *1/2 cup brown sugar, packed, 1/2 cup flour, 1/2 cup oatmeal,* and *1 1/2 teaspoons cinnamon.*

Using an electric mixer, cut *1/4 cup (1/2 stick) room-temperature butter* evenly into the dry ingredients. If you have a food processor, you can use refrigerator-temperature butter. Sprinkle the mixture evenly over the fruit. If you like more topping, make two thin layers of fruit with two layers of topping.

Bake around 40 minutes. The crisp is done when the top is lightly browned and the fruit feels tender when you stick in a toothpick. As with the **Plum Cobbler** (page 162), you can adjust the temperature and time depending on what else you are baking.

Serve warm or cool, plain or with cream, ice cream, or **Brown Cream Sauce** (page 164).

Fast tip: Double or triple this topping recipe, label, and keep the extra in a glass jar in the refrigerator. Then when you want to make a crisp, all you have to do is prepare the fruit and sprinkle on the topping.

Variation: An equal volume of other fruit can be substituted for the peaches. You can start out making these crisps rather sweet, then gradually cut down on the sugar as your family develops a taste for more tart fruit. If fruit is very sour, sprinkle on a tablespoon or two of sugar per cup of fruit. Alternative fruits for this recipe could be—

Apples: peeled or unpeeled, cored and sliced

Pears and blueberries; pears and blackberries
Fresh plums, pitted and sliced

OLD-FASHIONED BREAD PUDDING

Bread pudding gives you a handy way of using up those bits and scraps of bread you have left over. Cube them and let them accumulate in a zip top bag in the freezer. Then when you get enough, make a bread pudding. This is a delicious, nutritious dessert that can double as breakfast.

Distribute the following ingredients evenly in a 9 x 13 inch baking pan:
6 cups cubed bread: white, whole wheat, raisin,
  cinnamon—whatever you have
1 1/2 cups freshly grated apple or *1/2 cup raisins* or
  1/2 cup Craisins or *no fruit at all*
1/2 cup chopped walnuts or *other nuts* or *no*
  nuts—your choice

Mix together the following and beat well:
3 cups milk
3 eggs
1/2 cup brown sugar
1 tsp cinnamon
1/4 tsp nutmeg
2 tsp vanilla extract
1/4 tsp salt
1 Tbsp lemon juice

Pour the milk/egg mixture over the bread mixture. Let soak a few minutes before baking. Bake at 350° F for 35 minutes or until the bread pudding is lightly browned and a knife inserted near the center comes out clean.

Serve warm or cool with cream, ice cream, fresh fruit, applesauce, or nothing at all! If you were in New Orleans, you could get this with whiskey sauce. For that, you are on your own.

Variations: One of my variations on this recipe is to leave out the fruit, but then if I did that I would have no excuse to include it in this chapter! You can also serve it topped with fresh strawberries or raspberries, which tastes wonderful.

FRUIT WITH BROWN CREAM SAUCE

Mix the following ingredients together:
1 Tbsp light brown sugar
1/2 cup sour cream
1/4 tsp vanilla or other flavored extract

Pour the sauce over 3 to 4 cups cut-up fruit:
oranges
apples
bananas
berries or nuts

The Generics of Fruits and Vegetables

I have given you many recipes for fruits and vegetables. You don't have to use them. You do not have to be fancy. If you cook vegetables properly, they will be tasty and appealing. If you open a can of fruit and put it in a nice bowl, it will become an attractive part of the meal. In fact, if you make a main dish that requires time and energy, it would be better if you *didn't* go to a lot of trouble with the other parts of the menu. Putting too much on yourself with food preparation will just defeat you, later if not sooner. Many experienced cooks plan vegetables and fruits for a meal by leaning on the pantry door or peering into the freezer.

On the other hand, my daughter-in-law Laurie loves fresh fruits and vegetables. She makes vegetables the backbone of her meals and plans the protein course around the vegetables she has available.

Whichever way you do it, the vegetables must be properly cooked, and you do need to add some salt and fat for them to taste their best. To me, a moderate amount is about 1/8 teaspoon of salt and 1 to 2 teaspoons of butter or fat equivalent (see page 142) per 1/2-cup serving of vegetable. In my recipes, I recommend starting with 1/4 teaspoon of salt before cooking, and then adding salt carefully after cooking, tasting after each addition. The amounts of salt and fat in each of my recipes are reasonable and moderate; they enhance flavor without drowning it. Use these amounts as rules of thumb for evaluating recipes in other cookbooks as well.

A child will enjoy "coloring" the hot vegetables with the opened end of a stick of butter. The lightly buttered result will give about 1 teaspoon per serving—and a *lot* of flavor. You might like bottled cheese spreads, like Cheez Whiz, on your vegetables. Or you can make your own **Cheese Sauce** (page 149) to put over broccoli, cauliflower, or any other vegetable you like.

Use a variety of vegetables and fruits. Use fresh, frozen, canned, and dried fruits and vegetables. Your children are more likely to learn to appreciate them if you offer many different choices over time. Processed varieties are at least as nutritious as fresh.

FRESH VEGETABLES AND FRUITS
Some fresh vegetables and fruits are standbys of many menus: potatoes, onions, carrots, celery, greens for salads, bananas, apples, oranges. Other fresh vegetables and fruits are available in a more limited way, but they come canned, frozen, or even dried, so you have a choice: Consider corn, peas, green beans, beans, peaches, apricots and plums. Most times, it is a matter of choice. Some people emphasize fresh produce over other kinds because they prefer the taste, texture, and look.

When vegetables are in season, why not buy and use fresh? There is nothing like an August meal of fresh sliced tomatoes, corn on the cob, and cucumbers in sour cream or a **Sweet-Sour Dilled Cucumber Salad**. When fruits and vegetables first come to market, they taste so good, you don't even miss the main dish. Ah, the luxury of a bowl of fresh strawberries in June! Makes your mouth water, doesn't it?

Fresh vegetables and fruits carry memories in a way that no other food does. I got hives the spring I was 4 years old from eating too many strawberries. A coven of aunts, feeling sorry for me because my mother was away for a few days, had plied me with strawberries. Every June, I get nostalgic about the time we were in the Yakima Valley in Washington State when the Bing cherries were ripe. We ate Bing cherries by the carton. Luckily, no one got hives. I'm sure you have your own memories. To make more, consult the discussion about seasonal fresh vegetables and fruits in chapter 12, "Shopping to Get You Cooking," pages 195–196.

Fresh vegetables and fruits are not necessarily the most nutritious. It depends on how they have been handled between the farm and your plate. Produce loses nutrients every day it travels from the farm to the supermarket to your table. Losses become even more dramatic if the produce is mishandled in any way, say, if it is transported in a hot truck or stored unrefrigerated. Even if "fresh" food is refrigerated, if it sits for a few days before you eat it, nutrients can decrease significantly.

I'm not saying that you should stop eating fresh vegetables and fruits. Even if the quality has degenerated a bit, you can make up for nutritional losses by eating a variety. Eat fresh, frozen, canned, and even dried vegetables and fruits. What one lacks the other will offer.

CANNED VEGETABLES AND FRUITS
Now you know better, but if you thought fresh produce was best, you had lots of company. Eight out of 10 consumers believe that fresh is superior to processed and that frozen foods are

more nutritious than canned foods. Some believe that canned vegetables contain less fiber than fresh. The fact is that canned vegetables and fruits provide the same fiber and nutrients as their fresh or frozen counterparts. Most nutrients survive the canning process well and are stable during the 1-year shelf life of canned foods. Some vitamin C, folate, and other water-soluble nutrients dissolve into the cooking liquid and can be recovered by using the liquid to make soups, sauces, and gravies.

Canned produce can be nutritionally superior to fresh because produce for canning is picked at the peak of ripeness, when nutrient content is at its highest, and rushed through processing immediately after harvest. Packers strive for the best-tasting, best-looking food that will arrive in your kitchen as appetizing as possible. With vegetables and fruits, being tasty and appetizing goes right along with preserving vitamins and minerals.

Canned vegetables and fruits have a distinctive taste and texture, and they are wonderfully easy to keep on hand and convenient to use. I know a food scientist who loves canned peas and prefers them to the frozen or fresh variety. I love canned corn, both the whole kernel and cream-style variety, and I appreciate the convenience of opening a can and warming it up. I could not live without canned tomatoes and appreciate the variety of canned-tomato products. Canning methods are being refined, and the resulting products are crisper and have less water in them than those canned using traditional methods. As I write this, you can buy Del Monte Freshcut corn and green beans, and they are wonderful. You can buy diced, petite-diced and crushed tomatoes and tomatoes with Mexican, Italian, and Cajun flavorings.

If you hesitate to use canned vegetables and fruits, it may be because you have heard they are not good for you. Bosh. All the nutrients of vegetables and fruits are in the can. Canned vegetables do have added salt, but it isn't that much and it is better to eat vegetables than to avoid salt. The added salt is strictly for taste. The amount is modest and reasonable: about 200 to 300 milligrams per 1/2 cup. In the prologue to "How to Cook," I suggest that about 250 milligrams of sodium per 1/2 cup of food is standard and tastes right to most people. The main problem with canned vegetables and fruits has been political, not nutritional. The difficulty arose when one bureaucracy tried to talk to another. The U.S. Food and Drug Administration (FDA)

set out to do its labeling job. The task was to define the word *healthy* so as to conform to the Dietary Guidelines. The FDA decided that the word *healthy* could appear on a food label only if certain conditions were met: (1) the food had to be low in sugar, fat, and saturated fat; (2) it had to meet limits for sodium and cholesterol; and (3) it had to contain at least 10 percent of certain vitamins and minerals. Such standards ruled out scallions, iceberg lettuce, mushrooms, and a host of other foods.

More recently, the FDA recognized that vegetables and fruits in general have a place in a healthy diet and allowed all produce as well as canned fruit to be called healthy. However, because they contain the dreaded sodium, canned vegetables still can't be called healthy. Despite their considerable nutritional value, and despite the greater nutritional importance of eating vegetables than avoiding sodium, canned vegetables are still condemned by the nutrition enthusiasts as being too high in sodium. For more about the sodium debate, see appendix O, "Sodium in Your Diet."

These convoluted standards are bad, particularly for low-income people, who are most likely to use canned vegetables and fruits. Like the rest of the population, low-income people have learned their nutrition lessons. They have learned that what they can afford to feed their families, keep on hand, and *prefer* is inferior. In an article about hunger and food insecurity, a Cornell University researcher quoted a low-income mother who lamented, "I buy canned vegetables to substitute for a vegetable. You can get them cheaper, but I don't like them. I rinse them, but I still don't like the thought of it." Making people feel this way is not good nutritional policy, it is nutritional bullying.

It bothers me enormously when nutritional politics undermine people's relationship with food and make it hard for them to enjoy their eating. You wouldn't think anybody could get so worked up about canned vegetables, would you? I am a little surprised myself. But getting down off my soapbox and back to the issue at hand, I recommend that you use canned vegetables and fruits if you like them. Use them, secure in the knowledge that you are doing something good for your family.

You can buy canned fruits that are packed in light syrup or in fruit juice, but it isn't necessary, and they generally cost extra. The fruit juice in canned fruit is generally concentrated grape juice; it has doubtful nutritional value and is actually high in sugar. It isn't necessary to avoid regular sugar syrup. The syrup makes the fruit taste good and preserves its shape and texture. Sugar helps fruits and vegetables retain their texture longer by slowing down the breakdown of what are known as pectic substances, the glue that holds cell walls together. A canned peach has about the same calories as a fresh peach. The syrup is extra. A tablespoon of syrup on canned fruits gives about 50 calories. If that 50 calories worries you, you don't have to eat the syrup.

Packers use sugar and salt the way good cooks have always used sugar and salt—to make food taste good, to improve the texture, and to make it appealing. Most of us, and children especially, are not on such nutritional tightropes that we can't afford a little extra salt and sugar.

FROZEN VEGETABLES AND FRUIT
Like their canned counterparts, frozen vegetables and fruits are processed at the peak of ripeness, freshness, and nutritional value. As long as they are held throughout the storage period at zero degrees Fahrenheit or below, the food stays nutritious and maintains high quality.

In most cases, vegetables are frozen without added salt. The exception to that rule is that lima beans, peas, mixed vegetables, and corn have a light salt brine to keep them from sticking together during freezing.

Frozen vegetables taste more like their fresh counterparts and are a breeze to cook and serve—there is no cleaning or sorting. Just put them in a covered pot, boil or microwave, doctor them up however you want to, and *voilà*! Dinner is served.

There are lots of products in the frozen vegetable case that producers call "value-added." That is, they have something done to them that will make you willing to part with more money to buy them. Potatoes are a helpful value-added frozen vegetable that let you make fried potatoes or hash browns in your own oven. Some stores carry frozen chopped onions, which taste pretty good and save time and tears. With other value-added vegetables, the helpfulness is less clear. Vegetables with sauces save you the time of *making* the sauce, but often you get more sauce and less vegetable than if you made your own sauce and bought the vegetable plain. Mixed vegetables with added pasta give you the idea and assemble the ingredients for you, but often the combination is a simple one and you pay extra for it. Meal starters, both with and without

pasta, have you "just" add the protein, which is the most expensive ingredient. Only you can decide if the value-added feature is valuable to you. Periodically, when you have a little extra time, it is worth exploring the frozen vegetable case to find any new products that can help you—for a price you are willing to pay.

Keep in mind that if you know the rudiments of planning and cooking, many of the products will be unnecessary. Manufacturers are increasingly catering to people who don't know the first thing about cooking. Many people plan dinner by pulling something out of the freezer. There is nothing wrong with that, but when you know how to plan and cook, you have more choices.

DRIED VEGETABLES AND FRUITS
Ah, now you put me to the test! What are some dried vegetables? Well, potatoes, of course. Mashed potatoes are dried, and so are scalloped potato mixes. Most dried vegetables are freeze-dried—you can tell because they are paper-thin and lightweight. Freeze-drying is vacuum-drying at temperatures far lower than those used for standard freezing. Ice crystals in the food go directly into a vapor, which keeps the cell membranes from rupturing. Reconstituted freeze-dried products have the taste, texture, and nutritional value of frozen foods. As long as products are stored dry, are reasonably cool, and are protected from crushing, they hold up well. You can find freeze-dried fruit chips and vegetable chips in the produce section. Freeze-dried vegetables are often included in dry soup mixes—in the little packages or in soup starters that cook up to hearty soups with significant amounts of vegetables. Spices are freeze-dried—consider dried onions, garlic, chives, and parsley. Camping and backpacking outfitters offer a whole array of freeze-dried foods. They are expensive but lightweight versions of dinner for you to take with you into the wild.

Drying at air temperature or in the sun is done to make dried tomatoes, which are generally lightly salted and dried in the sun. Roma tomatoes, or Italian plum tomatoes, are usually used for drying because their solids content is two to three times that of regular tomatoes. Some of the more familiar air-dried fruits are raisins (dried grapes), prunes (dried plums), dates, figs, and apricots. Unless you live in a tropical area, you may not eat fresh figs, but almost everybody knows about figs in the form of Fig Newtons. Some vitamin C may be lost in drying, but other nutrients are relatively unaffected.

You can find air-dried apples, peaches, pears, and mangos in the produce section, the bulk foods case, or the baking aisle. The cranberry people are on to a good thing with their new dried snack Craisins. These good-tasting fruits are wonderful for both eating and cooking, and they extend the short fresh-cranberries season. Other dried fruits also make great snacks and wonderful ingredients for baking.

Prune puree is showing up on the market and being touted by nutrition enthusiasts as a low-fat baking ingredient. Pureed prunes are used as a substitute for fat in recipes because prunes hold moisture and presumably mimic the tenderness and moistness that the product usually gets from fat. It won't surprise you that I think those products are unnecessary. You *can* tell the difference; baked products that substitute prune puree for shortening are *not* as good. In my view, if you are going to bake, it makes more sense to make something truly delicious and enjoy it to the maximum. You can't trick your eaters into thinking they are getting something they are not. If you want to use prunes in baking, ask me for the wonderful prune cake recipe I got from my mother!

Enlisting Your Children's Help

In chapter 8, "How to Get Cooking," and chapter 9, "How to Keep Cooking," many of the suggestions for how children can help with meal preparation have to do with fresh fruits and vegetables. Your child can wash apples, peel bananas, and spin salad fixings. If you give her a plastic picnic knife to work with, and if you can tolerate the results, even a young child can cut up apples for applesauce or chunk watermelon for a salad. Children can help a lot with making salads: They can spin and tear the greens, peel oranges, and break apart onion rings. Here are some other ways children can help:

- Empty canned fruit into a serving bowl.
- Paint vegetables with butter.
- Separate broccoli florets.
- Mix up simple vegetable and fruit recipes.
- Shave butter with a carrot peeler (e.g., see the **Plum Cobbler** recipe on page 162).

Wash all your produce carefully before anyone handles it. Teach your children to wash their hands before *and* after they handle fresh produce. Even fresh vegetables can have harmful microorganisms on them. Particularly if those germs get

on other foods and are allowed to grow and multiply, bacteria can reach high enough levels to make someone ill. Read more about food safety in figure 11.4, "Food Safety," on page 183.

Preparation of Fresh Vegetables

Wash vegetables well before you cook them. Unless they are clearly labeled "prewashed," assume there is something on them that you would rather not eat. Even then, you may want to wash them. See figure 10.2, "Prepackaged Salad Greens or Do-It-Yourself?" on page 151.

Here is a bit of do-as-I-say-not-as-I-do advice: When cooking vegetables, especially the low-starch varieties, pay attention to be sure they don't cook too long. I tend to be a put-it-on-then-do-something-else cook. In my own defense, I was raising children during my most intense cooking years, and children have a way of *seeing to it* that you do something else. Statistics show that with a toddler around, a parent is interrupted about every 6 minutes! Back to the point. Pay attention, and take the vegetables off as soon as they are done. Other dishes can wait and can get overcooked without hurting them too much. Vegetables suffer, though, especially the green ones. Yellow, orange, and red fruits and vegetables can tolerate longer cooking times than green vegetables can.

When green vegetables are cooked, the cells break down so that the chlorophyll in the cells comes in contact with natural acids in the vegetables. The chlorophyll breaks down, and the color turns from bright green to olive green and, eventually, to brown. Generally, this color change takes place after about 7 minutes of heating, but the time varies because some vegetables have tougher cells than others; some have more or less acid. To get your vegetables done in the critical 7 minutes, cut them into small pieces. With cabbage family vegetables like broccoli, cauliflower, brussels sprouts, and, of course, cabbage, to preserve the mild, sweet taste, keep the cooking time even shorter: closer to 5 minutes if you can. The extra 2 minutes *doubles* the amount of hydrogen sulfide gas—the rotten-egg smell—that the vegetable produces.

Cooking methods that dilute out the acids also help to keep vegetables green. Steaming lets the volatile acids evaporate or drip to the bottom of the cooking pan. Cooking uncovered in a large amount of rapidly boiling salted water lets the acids evaporate as well as dilutes them as they cook out. Salting the cooking water helps preserve the pectic substances, or "glue," between the cells and protects the vegetables' texture.

Because they are blanched before freezing, frozen vegetables are easier than fresh to keep green. Blanching removes some of the acids in the vegetables that change the color to olive drab. Microwaving creates fewer volatile compounds than other methods. A microwaved whole artichoke or an unpeeled onion, turnip, or beet is delicious. Check your microwave handbook for directions.

An iron skillet or tin-lined pan makes green vegetables turn brown. Copper pans turn green vegetables a vivid green from the formation of a copper-chlorophyll compound, but it may not be safe to eat that much copper.

SLOW-COOKING AND FAST-COOKING VEGETABLES

To plan your cooking strategy with fresh vegetables, it is helpful to know that they break down roughly into two categories: slow-cooking and fast-cooking. Food scientist and reviewer Yvonne Bushland educated me that the difference *isn't* starch content, as I had believed—and written—in the previous edition. In fact, food chemists haven't fully identified the characteristics that distinguish slow-cooking from fast-cooking vegetables.

Both slow-cooking and fast-cooking vegetables can be prepared by boiling, microwaving, or baking. Both need to be cooked with moisture to hydrate the starch and/or soften the cell walls. There the similarities end. Depending on how small you cut the pieces, slow-cooking vegetables take 10 to 15 minutes to cook, and some, such as chard and fresh green beans, take 20 minutes or more. Artichokes take 45 minutes to cook. Kale and other greens can take less time if they are young and tender. Slow-cooking vegetables require water to hydrate and cook the starch and fiber. For boiling and steaming, you add water. For baking or microwaving, there is enough water retained in the vegetable to cook the starch and the tough cell walls.

Fast-cooking vegetables are relatively high in water and have tender cell walls. It is easy to break cell walls and make the vegetables mushy with too much heat or too much handling. Again, depending on how small you cut the pieces, they take 7 minutes or less to cook and some, such as spinach and mushrooms, cook in a minute or two. (Remember the 7-minute

cooking rule from the previous section.) Boil or microwave fast-cooking vegetables in a small amount of water. You can also bake them, but put a lid on the dish to retain the moisture.

Slow-Cooking Vegetables
Artichokes
Beets
Carrots
Corn
Green beans
Greens: Collards, kale, chard, beet greens, mustard greens, turnip greens
Parsnips
Potatoes
Rutabagas
Squash
Sweet potatoes
Turnips

Fast-Cooking Vegetables
Asparagus
Broccoli
Brussels sprouts
Cabbage
Cauliflower
Celery
Mushrooms
Onions, mature and green
Peas
Spinach
Zucchini

PREPARING FRESH SLOW-COOKING VEGETABLES

Boiling Slow-Cooking Vegetables
Peel or scrub the vegetables and remove blemishes. Cut them into similarly sized pieces—the smaller the piece, the quicker the cooking. Rinse the vegetables with cold water. To keep them from blackening, cover potatoes with cold water until you are ready to cook them. Choose a pan with a lid that is large enough to leave head room for boiling water. To preserve nutrients, the best method is to start the water boiling first (add 1 teaspoon of salt per quart) and then add the vegetables. Boiling water immediately inactivates the vegetables' enzymes that would otherwise break down the nutrients. Reduce the heat to keep the water boiling rapidly but not boiling over.

Boil until the vegetables are as done as you like them. Drain them, put them back in the pan, and put the pan back on the turned-off burner to let the rest of the water evaporate. Boiling vegetables generally takes about 10 to 15 minutes.

Baking Slow-Cooking Vegetables

Heat the oven to 425° F. Prepare the vegetables as you would for boiling. Put them on a baking sheet to catch drips (squash will drip). Line the sheet with aluminum foil or parchment paper for easy cleanup. Bake until done. A medium baked potato will take about an hour. So will half a medium squash, a beet, a turnip, or a rutabaga. Since parsnips and carrots are more slender and are subject to drying out, watch them during baking or put them in a covered dish to bake.

Microwaving Slow-Cooking Vegetables

Prepare vegetables as you would for the other methods. If you are leaving the vegetables whole, puncture several times with a fork to let out steam and to keep them from exploding. Check your microwave book for directions about cooking times, power settings, and standing times. As with everything else you prepare in the microwave, the more food you cook, the longer it takes.

Corn on the cob can be microwaved without even shucking it. Four ears of corn can be cooked in 8 to 10 minutes, plus 5 minutes of standing time. As with anything you microwave, to cook the food evenly it is a good idea to stop halfway through to rearrange it. To prepare corn for microwaving, peek inside to be sure no worms are riding along, cut off the silk end down to the level of the corn, leave part of the stem end on to give something to grab onto when you eat it, and microwave away. You don't have to add water because the husk retains the moisture. Once the corn is cooked, the silk comes off easily when you peel back the husk.

PREPARING FRESH FAST-COOKING VEGETABLES

To retain nutrients, flavor, and texture, be fast and conservative about water when cooking most fast-cooking vegetables. Use as little water as you can, and get the vegetables done as quickly as you can.

Clean fresh vegetables well. With all their little blossoms and wrinkles, fast-cooking vegetables are hard to clean. Sort the vegetables by removing tough stems and damaged areas. Soak them in a pan of cold water to loosen up the dirt and sand. Swish them around, and then lift them out and place them in a second and

then a third pan of water, being careful to swish all the areas where sand might be hiding. There is nothing worse than getting a gritty mouthful of sand when you are trying to enjoy your spinach or asparagus.

Steaming or Boiling Fast-Cooking Vegetables

Vegetables are done when they are crisp-tender; green vegetables are done when they are bright green, not gray-green or olive green. Generally, when people think of steaming, they think of using a vegetable steaming rack or a special insert in a pan to get the vegetables up and out of the water. The more finely divided the vegetables, the more quickly they will get done. To keep times below the 5- or 7-minute limit, make the pieces small and uniform.

Some nutrients, like carotene and minerals, hold up well with cooking. Others, like vitamin C and B vitamins, migrate into the cooking water or are broken down somewhat. Consequently, the less water you use, the less you throw away, and thus the fewer nutrients you lose. That principle makes my next bit of advice seem pretty strange.

To introduce children to the strong flavors of cruciferous vegetables, such as cabbage, cauliflower, broccoli, and brussels sprouts, tone them down by cooking them with extra rapidly boiling salted water and leaving the lid off the pan during cooking. Cut them small enough to get the cooking done within 5 minutes. Cruciferous vegetables contain sulfur, but the word *crucifer* comes from the Latin word meaning "cross," because these vegetables bear a cross-shaped flower. Some research indicates that these vegetables may be helpful in protecting against certain forms of cancer.

Despite their presumed health-giving qualities, learning to like these cabbage-family vegetables is challenging because of their strong taste and smell. Cooking them in lots of water with the lid off the pan helps to cook off the sulfur and dilute the flavor. But even with expert cooking, some children are particularly sensitive to the flavors in cruciferous vegetables and at first don't like them at all. Studies of taste show that this aversion is *real* and it is *unpleasant*. With any food, but with cruciferous vegetables in particular, don't try to get your child to eat if she doesn't want to. If you respect her wishes and enjoy those vegetables yourself, eventually she is likely to learn to enjoy them, too.

Microwaving Fast-Cooking Vegetables

Often, the water from washing is enough to cook fast-cooking vegetables in the microwave. At the very most, put in 1/4 cup of water per pound of vegetables. Use a glass dish with a cover for cooking. Depending on how much you are cooking, 3 to 4 minutes cooking time plus 2 to 3 minutes standing time may be enough. Stir the vegetables halfway through cooking.

Baking Fast-Cooking Vegetables

You hardly ever bake fast-cooking vegetables. If you do, the principle is to keep the vegetable moist. Cabbage wedges taste great in a pot roast, and they cook slowly enough so they can be put in with the other vegetables. On the other hand, to include zucchini or mushrooms in a stew, it would be better to wait and add them toward the end of cooking.

Cooking Frozen Vegetables

Cooking frozen vegetables is a snap. Keep them frozen until you put them in the pan. Use minimal water and minimal time, and *attend*. Stop cooking the vegetables the instant they are done. As I said earlier, it is easier to keep the color bright in frozen vegetables because they are blanched before they are frozen. Blanching gets rid of some of the color-destroying acids.

MICROWAVE COOKING

Quite by accident and through some benign neglect, I discovered an easy method for microwaving frozen vegetables that gives a wonderfully fresh taste. I started some vegetables cooking for the usual first 5 minutes, then forgot all about them. When I went back a half-hour later, the vegetables were perfectly cooked, but a little cool. After I warmed them up for a minute or two, the vegetables tasted great and had a just-picked flavor.

Place the desired amount of frozen vegetables in a covered glass casserole dish. Do not add water, even if the package says to (with the exception of lima beans). Add 1/4 teaspoon of salt per 10 ounces of vegetables and dot with butter. Use the method above, or cook as usual by microwaving on high 4 to 6 minutes, stirring, then microwaving an additional 3 to 5 minutes. The stirring is to ensure even heating.

You can even prepare frozen vegetables (10 ounces) in the original package. Pierce the top of package and set it on a glass plate. If vegetables are frozen in pouches, pierce the top of the pouch also. If packages are foil wrapped, remove the foil, or you will get fireworks along with your vegetables.

STOVE-TOP COOKING

Place the amount of frozen vegetables you want (blocks of vegetables are usually 10 ounces; bags are usually 14 to 16 ounces) in a covered pan. Add the amount of water called for on the package or *less*. Experiment to see how little water you can use. Extra water just gets thrown away, and along with it, a few nutrients.

Begin by adding 1/4 teaspoon of salt per 10 ounces of vegetables. Cook on medium-high for 3 to 4 minutes or for as long as it says to on the package. Check during cooking and stop when vegetables are crisp-tender, even a little underdone. They will continue cooking in the hot pan or serving bowl. Add butter or other seasoning. Check the taste, and add pepper and more salt if you think it needs it. Another 1/2 teaspoon or less should do it.

Cooking Commercially Canned Vegetables

Don't boil canned vegetables. They are already cooked and just need to be warmed up. Canned vegetables are very tender. To keep them from breaking apart and getting mushy, stir and heat as little as you can.

To prepare canned vegetables, drain the liquid into a saucepan and bring it to a boil. Add the vegetables, turn down to the heat to medium high, and heat through for about 2 minutes without boiling. When preparing dishes that involve combining them with other ingredients, add the canned vegetables last.

Some of the nutrients from canned vegetables are in the liquid. Most canned vegetables have more liquid than you would generally consume. There are, however, some varieties of canned vegetables, packaged in 13-ounce cans, that contain considerably less liquid. They are good-tasting and well worth looking for, but they aren't available everywhere.

To keep from having to throw away water-soluble nutrients (vitamin C and folic acid) with the liquid, you can boil the liquid down a bit before you put in the vegetables. If there is less liquid, you'll be more likely to eat it rather than throw it away. Of course, the boiling breaks down the nutrients some, but otherwise you would throw them away. Boiling down also concentrates the flavor, which is a plus.

To cook canned vegetables in the microwave, do the same thing as with stove-top cooking. Heat up or boil down the liquid first in a glass dish, add the vegetables, and heat as little as possible. Don't stir. Let stand for a minute or two to equalize the temperatures. You won't need any more salt, but you might enjoy the taste of a little pepper.

There you have it: fruits and vegetables. You can use them to round out your meals or you can use them for the backbone of your meals. Either way, eat them because you enjoy them, not because you feel obligated.

Chapter
11
Planning to Get You Cooking

Planning is good. You can use planning to save time, simplify feeding your family, and lower your stress level. Planning can save you from the daunting late-afternoon lack of ideas and energy as you wonder, "What's for dinner?" Done kindly, planning can provide its own reward in making cooking and eating enjoyable and rewarding. However, planning can be *abused*. Unrealistic planning can cost you time, complicate feeding your family, and raise your stress level.

You are *using* planning when you rough out a menu for the next few days, then take 5 minutes the night before to check the menu, put the spinach in the refrigerator to thaw, and get the canned goods lined up for the next night's dinner. You are *using* planning when you take shortcuts and use leftovers to provide PPMs (pre-prepared meals, if you recall).

But you are *abusing* planning if you let your enthusiasm or your conscience get the better of you. You are *abusing* planning when you use working ahead to make everything from scratch, add super-fancy touches, and do advanced preparation to turn out a meal that is so stunningly elegant that your family doesn't dare eat it. Whereupon you will be furious because you worked your fingers to the bone to make something nice for them. You are also *abusing* planning when you say, "Oh, we shouldn't eat that; it isn't good for us." Whereupon you turn out a meal that is so drab that nobody is interested in eating it.

Either way, you will get discouraged and say, "What's the use, anyway?" and take everybody

out to have hamburgers with eight slices of bacon. Remember, planning is your servant, not your master.

Given today's punitive, conscience-ridden attitudes about food, many people depend on impulse in order to be able to feed themselves at all. Certainly, it is easier to eat "forbidden" food if you don't think about it too much. You'll recall from earlier chapters that in fact *there is no forbidden food*.

If you must be rigid about something, be rigid about *structure*. If you can hang on to the structure of meals and planned snacks, nutrition has a way of falling into place. In order for food to work well, you have to make it a priority. However, it doesn't have to be *such* a priority that it overshadows everything else. The trick is to think about food a lot when you plan it, cook it, and eat it. Then forget about it between times. If you do your planning and feed yourself well, you *will* be able to forget about it between times.

Plan Your Escape

In this chapter, we are going to get organized. That will take time and focused attention. We are going to talk about cycle menus (3 weeks of menus that you use over and over again), inventories, planned shopping trips, storage, and equipment. However, because there is a lot to this topic and because I worry that you will become overwhelmed and give up—or, worse, get overzealous—we will start by planning your escape. The all-important escape is a little deliberate vacation from cooking. An escape comes in handy when your planning has run amok (or was amok in the first place), when the tire goes flat, when the computer crashes or when your appointment runs overtime. You also need an escape when you are just so tired you can't stand to think about cooking. Here are some suggestions to jump-start your ideas.

- Plan meals that in the past your food conscience wouldn't let you think of (assuming that your food conscience is less hyperactive after reading this book). How about hot dogs, beans, and potato chips—with ice cream for dessert? Macaroni and cheese and canned green beans? Bologna sandwiches on bread with mayonnaise, canned peaches, and store-bought cookies for dessert? For more ideas, see "Grab-and-Dump Meals" or "Fast Meals for One" in chapter 9, "How to Keep Cooking."
- Order in, go out, or hit the deli for an HMR (you know, a Home Meal Replacement). You might get some ideas for meals you can make at home.
- Pull out the leftovers. Put them on the table cold. Let everyone fill their own plate, pile up the plates by inverting an empty plate over a full one, and nuke them in the microwave. You can still have a meal together, even if everyone is eating something different.
- Have breakfast food for dinner: toaster waffles, pancakes and eggs, or cereal and milk.
- Have popcorn and cocoa on Sunday nights in front of the television.
- Have some nutritionally worthless meals. I am hard-pressed to think of one—let's see— gum drops and Kool-Aid? Even Kool-Aid is fortified with vitamin C. I guess your toddler shouldn't have the gum drops—choking hazard. How about potato chips and soda? But even potato chips have potato nutrients. Hmmm …

Manage Your Day So You Can Manage Dinner

If your planning works well, you will spend 20 to 30 minutes right before dinner preparing the meal and getting it on the table. At that time, I promise, you will be tired and touchy and your child will be, too. If you are just home from work, you will be trying to do two things at once: connecting with your child and getting dinner on the table. If you count connecting with yourself, you have *three* priorities. "Mom

chef" reviewer and registered dietitian Joy Lenz calls this the *bewitching hour.*

If you are a typical young woman, you will also be hungry because you will not have eaten well all day. If you are a typical young man, you may have eaten better, but all the rest will be the same. In other words, you will be feeling *stress* and *conflict.* Little wonder that 78 percent of households eat out at least once a week.

CONSIDER THE RESTAURANT MEAL
You will have lots of company if you decide to go out to eat. In 2006, restaurant meals accounted for 49 percent of our total food expenditures.[1] One fantasizes about the advantages of a restaurant meal: sitting calmly, resting, giving the other family members your full attention, munching on something to keep your strength up, waiting serenely for the dinner that someone else has prepared. Ah, but the fantasy has dark edges. You have to get *back* in the car to go there and you have to keep the kids entertained while you wait for the meal to be served (and when they finish eating before you do). The restaurant commotion makes it difficult to connect with other family members. You have to pay two to three times more for it— at least—than if you purchase the food and cook it at home. And you have to settle for restaurant food. Believe it or not, you will get to the point that you enjoy what you make at home more than what you get at a restaurant.

Certainly a restaurant meal now and again is a worthwhile investment in time and money. Going out for something that you wouldn't prepare at home makes it even better. For strategies to help your child order in restaurants, see figure 7.3, "Choosing Food in Restaurants," on page 84.

PREPARE FOR THE BEWITCHING HOUR
But most of the time, there is a better way. Perhaps there is a way of neutralizing the spell cast by the end of the day, at least in part. How can you manage your day so you have energy for the end of the day? How can you get a little rest before you start working on dinner? How can you connect with your child so that you don't have to keep putting him off while you prepare dinner?

Begin by considering the way you feed and take care of yourself throughout the day. Do you have breakfast? Do you have a decent lunch that lets you take a break and relax? Do you have a snack in the afternoon to tide you over during that long stretch between lunch and dinner? Do you use snack time as a way of relaxing and recharging? If you consistently answer "no," you will pay for it at the end of the day. You will be exhausted, cranky, and depleted. You will likely pay for it *during* the day, as well. Efficiency experts tell us that long, unrelieved work days don't pay: productivity drops.

You won't be able to give to your child and family unless you first give to yourself. In fact, taking care of yourself teaches children an important lesson: Others have needs, too. A major toddler task is learning to respect others' needs. Unlike the young infant, the toddler no longer benefits from being made the center of the universe. The same, of course, is true for older children. Presumably, though, these older children have already learned to respect others' needs as well as their own. If your children have not, teach them.

How do you apply that bit of developmental psychology to the end of the day? First of all, arrange to have some energy left by giving yourself food and rest during the day. Then make some choices. How do you want to use that first half-hour when you get home from work? Having some time to yourself? Connecting with your child? Cooking dinner? Put the emphasis on *want*. Any of the answers is right, as long as you work it out with your child so he knows what to expect and how to be helpful to you.

Then you have to take your child's needs into account. Until he can tell you otherwise, it is safe to assume that his list is short: He wants to be with you. So how are you both going to get what you want? Talk about it. Say, "I want to spend some time with you, but first I want to change my clothes and check the mail. How would it be if I do that, and then we can play blocks for a while?" So what if he says, "I want to play blocks first"? Why not say (if you feel like it), "OK, but first I want to change clothes."

Also consider your child's need for food. He has had a long day, too, and it may have been hours since he had his afternoon snack. Consider giving him a little pick-me-up snack, such as a piece of fruit or a small glass of juice and a couple of crackers. This is the one time I recommend putting limits on amounts. The idea is to take the edge off his hunger, but not to have him eat so much that it spoils dinner.

PAY ATTENTION WISELY
Here is a secret about playing with your child: With playing, as with eating, children like to take the lead and want you to be a supportive

presence. You don't have to pile up blocks for him to knock down or make elaborate houses or teach about the laws of shapes and sizes and proportions. All you have to do is be there, pay attention, ask about what your child is doing, and make little comments like, "That's a big wall." You can even do all this in a prone position, as long as you truly pay attention and take an interest.

Playing together doesn't have to go on forever for you and your child to connect. In fact, if you really tune in, after 15 or 20 minutes you both will feel better and you can go on with what comes next. Set a timer, if it will free you to take this time. You may even feel energized enough by then that you won't need your break. But if you do, take it. A few minutes of putting your feet up could make all the difference between food preparation being pleasant and rewarding and being a real drag.

Another routine might be to get dinner started, and then sit down and play. A few of the menus will allow you to do that: the **Swiss Steak** (pages 106) can be warming up and the potatoes can be cooking while you rest on the floor. Not every day has to be the same. What has to happen, however, is that you deliver on your promise of time with your child. Then let him know he has done a good job when he lives up to his agreements with you.

Cooking together is also a fine way of connecting with your child. I have made lots of suggestions in the cooking chapters about what your child can do to help prepare the meal. That early help will turn into real help in a few years, so be patient. Be friendly, companionable, and appreciative while you cook. Don't be gushy in your praise, or your clever child will decide, "She must think I am really a baby to get so excited that I can do *that*." Or, he might conclude, "If she is making such a fuss about this, it must be I'm not supposed to like it." You really can't fool a child. He may not be able to put it in words, but his feelings tell him what is going on.

When you start cooking, you and your child will likely be somewhat hungry, but not so famished that you just can't wait. To help him learn to wait for dinner, teach him about distraction. "Let's just think about cutting up these mushrooms for now, and dinner will be ready before we know it." "Tell me about your day; that will make it easier to think about something else." "Let me tell you about something funny I heard on the radio today."

Logistics for Peaceful Mealtimes

Put everything on the table at the same time (including something to mop up spills), announce the last call for table service, sit down, and don't get up until you are finished. I often work with young mothers who are trying to get a grip on their eating. Too often, they complain that they can't pay attention to their *own* meal and enjoy it because they are running after their children.

Such attentiveness is not necessary. Children behave exactly as their adults teach them to behave. If you hover and jump up and chase after and respond to every little demand for attention, your child will ask for it all and more besides. If, however, you help your child get served, serve yourself, and refuse to be distracted from your own meal, your child will attend to his own meal rather than try to get you to perform.

For the most part, put the food in serving bowls and let children serve themselves. Put a pitcher of milk on the table. Teach children to pass food to other people and to say "yes, please" and "no, thank you." To make the presentation more interesting, have a variety of big and little serving bowls, some colorful and crazy and interesting. The bowls don't have to match. Give some thought to your serving spoons, tongs, and forks, as well. These have to work for small hands if your child is to be successful serving himself.

If your child finishes his meal before you do, let him get down. Arrange to have toys nearby so your young child can entertain himself. Don't pick him up to let him keep you company and *don't* let him eat off your plate. By the time he was a year old, Sebastian, our office baby, had learned to entertain himself and let Clio and me finish our lunches. He comes around and talks, and we talk to him or pat him on the head, then he goes back to playing. Now that he is a toddler, he has his relapses and will even have tantrums when we don't stop what we are doing to play with him. He gets over it, because we hold the line. Encourage your older child to read a book. Keep the television and the computer off during meals and snack time. They are enticing enough that they can interfere with children's attention to their eating.

Develop a Pattern

Now that we have some of the logistics in place, let's consider the big picture—how do you put it all together to allow you to come up with a pattern of day-in-day-out food preparation? These suggestions will streamline your planning and cooking and even allow you to keep serious food preparation down to 3 or 4 times a week.

- Consider putting together a list of 20 main-dish recipes that you can make in a hurry. Use that list when you rough out your menus and make your weekly shopping list.
- Make another list of more time-consuming recipes. Use those recipes on weekends or when you have more time.
- Plan to cook ahead on weekends or days off and have leftovers for one or two dinners during the week.
- Consider having Monday or some other night regularly be "grab-and-dump" night. Read though the suggestions on page 138 and highlight the ones that would work for you. Read through "fast meals for one" on page 139 and add any that sound appealing and doable to your grab-and-dump list.
- Consider having one night be a "clean-out-the-refrigerator" night.

The Cycle Menu

A more planned-out way of considering the big picture is the cycle menu in Figure 11.1.

You work the cycle menu by going through the 3 weeks, starting with **Beef Stew** on the first Sunday, ending with **Braised Pork Chops with Sweet Potatoes** on the last Saturday, then starting all over again. Or you can start on the first Wednesday with **Mostaccioli with Spinach and Feta** and end with a pre-prepared meal: stew on the first Tuesday. To get started, however, you might want to confine yourself to your favorite week. That works best if you start with Wednesday or after, because Tuesday often uses something from the previous Saturday or Sunday. When you get comfortable with one week, add another.

For a young family and a beginning cook, a 2-week cycle menu is long enough to give a lot of variety. I decided on 3 weeks to help you keep your customers from getting tired of the food. I also needed the extra week to make use of the recipes for a few more main dishes and side dishes and increase the chances that you would find foods that appeal to you.

The main entrée dishes form the backbone of the cycle, and the vegetables, fruits, salads, and desserts provide the rest. I have filled in all the blanks by providing suggestions for quick and easy "meal accompaniments": vegetables, fruits, salads, and desserts. I hope some of these accompaniments become standbys for you. For home planning, it is typical to preplan only the main entrée dishes and rely on standbys for the accompaniments. A certain salad may be easy to throw together and sure to please. It is easy to send an older child to the freezer to pick out the veggie for dinner. Put it in the microwave for 5 or 10 minutes, color on some butter, and

you are done. Open a can of peaches, put it in a bowl, and dessert is served.

Some fruit or vegetable recipes are appealing enough to turn them from being an accompaniment into being the star of the menu. Examples of such special recipes for me are **Layered Zucchini Bake**, **Tomato and Fresh Mozzarella Salad, Mashed Potatoes** (or any kind of potatoes), and **Ratatouille**. You undoubtedly have others. Seasonal fruits and vegetables can often raise your meal from ordinary to outstanding— when fresh corn and tomatoes are available, when the strawberries or cantaloupe make your mouth water, or when the winter squash is at the roadside markets and you *have* to have some. Let the produce section provide you with inspiration.

FIGURE 11.1 THE CYCLE MENU

Sunday	*Monday*	*Tuesday*	*Wednesday*	*Thursday*	*Friday*	*Saturday*
Beef Stew Baking powder biscuits or Yorkshire Pudding Canned peaches or fruit in season Cucumber slices or bread and butter Pumpkin Custard	**Tuna Noodle** Casserole Poppy Seed Coleslaw Celery sticks Dill pickles Toasted bagels and butter More Pumpkin Custard	**PPM: Beef Stew** Apple wedges Orange slices or fruit in season Green salad Toasted bagels and butter Ice cream	**Mostaccioli with Spinach and Feta** Scalloped Corn Toasted English muffins and butter Plum dessert or fruit in season	**Hamburgers on buns** Potato chips Celery sticks and pickles Canned fruit or fruit in season	**PPM, eat out, or** *last-resort dinner* Spaghetti Carbonara Green salad Any appealing leftover fruits and vegetables	**Chicken and Rice** Glazed Carrots or vegetables in season French bread in the oven Apple Custard or fruit in season
Swiss Steak Mashed Potatoes Gravy Gingered Broccoli or vegetables in season Bread and butter More Apple Custard	**Wisconsin Fish Boil** Melted butter Bread and butter Cherry Cobbler Ice cream	**PPM: Beefy Shortcut Stroganoff** Mashed Potatoes or noodles Green salad Ice cream, cookies	**Lemon Chicken** Oven-Roasted Potatoes Creamed Spinach or vegetables in season Green salad Bread and butter Peach Cobbler or Peach Crisp Fruit in season	**Broccoli Chowder** Homemade bread with peanut butter Fruit in season More Peach Cobbler or Peach Crisp	**PPM, eat out, or** *last-resort dinner* Frittata Fruit in seaZson Any appealing leftover fruits and vegetables	**Meat Loaf** Boxed scalloped potatoes Carrot and celery sticks Herbed peas or vegetables in season Bread pudding with raisins or fruit in season
Savory Black Beans and Rice Corn pudding Orange rounds with parsley snips or fruit in season Ice cream	**Marinated Chicken Stir-Fry** Rice Fruit in season Bread and butter More bread pudding	**PPM: Spaghetti and Meatballs** Green salad French bread Apple and orange wedges or fruit in season	**PPM: Black Bean Soup** Variety of crackers, including oyster crackers Cheese on toast Fruit with brown cream sauce	**Herb-Baked Fish** Boxed scalloped potatoes Green salad Bread and butter Pineapple upside-down cake or fruit in season	**PPM, eat out, or** *last-resort dinner* Macaroni-tomato-Hamburger Casserole Any appealing leftover fruits and vegetables	**Braised Pork Chops with Sweet Potatoes** Microwave Chunky Applesauce Bread and butterå Ice cream

STRATEGIES FOR PLANNING THE CYCLE MENU

Here are the strategies I used for putting together these menus:

- Cook some days, not others. The cycle menu calls for you to cook five days a week—both weekend days and Monday, Wednesday and Thursday—and use PPMs the other two days. If that is too much cooking for you, double the recipes on more cooking days and increase the number of PPM days.
- A variety of main dishes. I used meat, poultry and fish, cooked dried beans, cheese, and eggs. I have planned meatless meals 2 days a week, and I used red meat 2 to 3 days per week. I have used cooked dried beans for main dishes and as salads. If you want to adapt the cycle to make it a lacto-ovo-vegetarian one, figure 11.2 gives suggestions for combining plant proteins to provide complete protein. If you want to follow a *vegan* diet—that is, to avoid milk, eggs, and cheese—then I can't help you. I don't recommend vegan diets for children. If you are determined to follow a vegan diet, see a registered dietitian.
- Flexibility. Menu planning can foster both order and flexibility. For example, with fruits and vegetables, I used fresh, canned, and frozen. For most days' menus, I have made suggestions for fruits and vegetables, but I have also reminded you to consider "seasonal fruit" and "seasonal vegetables." For a list of those seasonal foods, see chapter 12, "Shopping to Get You Cooking," pages 187–200. I have also planned PPM nights and last-resort dinners. The last-resort nights are generally on Fridays, when I assume you are tired and ready for a break from cooking. Those menus are especially easy.
- Weekdays versus weekend. Weekday menus can be prepared in about 30 minutes, start to finish. Weekend meals are equally quick to put together but take longer to cook. I am assuming you can put weekend meals in the oven or slow cooker and then peek at them from time to time. For instance, the **Chicken and Rice** on the first Saturday bakes in an hour or two, but you can get it ready to go in the oven in 10 or 15 minutes.
- Down time. On Tuesdays and Fridays you take it easy. Meals those days give you a break from cooking. Tuesday is PPM day, when a meal makes a repeat performance (as with the **Beef Stew** in week 1) or gets a face-lift (as with **Swiss Steak's** transformation into **Beefy Shortcut Stroganoff in** week 2). Friday is "clean out the refrigerator" day. If what's left in the refrigerator is unthinkable, dump it and make a grab-and-dump meal. Or order in. You deserve it.

FIGURE 11.2 COMPLEMENTARY PLANT PROTEINS

Plant proteins, in contrast to animal proteins, are incomplete: They don't have all the components (amino acids) needed to build and repair muscle and other body tissue. Since plants vary in their amino acid contribution—and limitation—a plant from one food group can combine with a plant from another food group to make a complete protein. We used to think we had to have these combinations at the same meal. Newer research shows that we have a day or more to consume the combinations. That means you can be more casual about combining plant proteins: If you prepare a variety of legumes and grains, and if you regularly use eggs and milk, chances are you are balancing things out.

It seems to me, however, that half the fun of cooking vegetarian is making use of complementary proteins and cooking traditional dishes. Centuries of eating—and surviving—have demonstrated the nutritional utility—and the taste appeal—of these dishes. Here are some combinations of plant proteins that add up to make a complete protein.

Legumes + Grains
- Split pea soup and crackers
- Peanut butter on wheat bread
- Black beans and rice
- Corn tortillas and refried beans
- Tofu and bulgur (wheat)

Legumes + Seeds
- Hummus (chickpea and sesame seed dip)
- Sunflower seeds sprinkled on navy bean soup
- Falafel patties with tahini (sesame butter)
- Snack mix of roasted soy beans and seeds

Grains + Milk
- Macaroni and cheese
- Cheese and crackers
- Rice or bread pudding
- Cereal and milk

Grains + Egg
- Fried egg sandwich
- French toast

- Equipment use. To find the most efficient method for each meal, I have used baking, slow cooking, stewing, microwaving, stir-frying, and even—gasp!—frying. When I have used the oven, I have tried to bake an additional menu item at the same time, such as potatoes or a dessert, to take advantage of the hot oven. Each cooking method has something to offer in your overall strategy for getting a meal on the table. More important, I want to give you experience with all of these cooking approaches.

- Pre-prepared ingredients. I have made heavy use of pre-prepared ingredients, such as portion-cut or already-cubed meats, pre-washed or preshredded vegetables and cheese, and canned and frozen meats, fish, vegetables, sauces, and broth bases. For a more detailed list of pre-prepared

ingredients and suggestions for how to use them, see figure 11.3 on this page.

Protecting Children in the Kitchen

Having children in the kitchen when you are cooking can be dangerous. The solution to the problem is not to keep children out, but rather to give some time and thought to keeping it safe for them. *You* are in the kitchen and you are doing all these intriguing things. What child wouldn't be eager to see and hear and touch and smell? Your toddler will tug at your pant leg, wanting to get up and see. Pick him up to show him, then put him down again. In between times, let him sit by your feet. Having young children in the house teaches you to look down before you move your feet.

FIGURE 11.3 GROCERY LIST OF CONVENIENT FOODS AND INGREDIENTS

Grocers and food manufacturers know that your time is limited and that you want to cook at home. They cater to your needs by taking care of some of the preparation for you. Prepared foods may cost more money, but think of the extra expense as "help" cost, not as food cost. In fact, the extra cost may not be as much as you think, when you consider that what you buy is all edible. You don't have to pay for anything that gets peeled off or cut away. Convenient foods and ingredients may or may not be worth the extra expense depending on what you have more of: time or money. Using them certainly is cheaper than eating out.

Meat, poultry, fish, dry beans, eggs, and nuts: Chicken thighs, boned chicken breasts or stir-fry, canned chicken; frozen fish fillets, canned tuna or salmon; boneless pork chops, cutlets, or stir-fry; pork tenderloin; beef tri-tip (see "Two Amazingly Fast and Tasty Roasts," page 193), small ham roasts and slices; stew meat (needs to be cooked slowly); breakfast steaks (thin, quick-cooking steaks); prepared meat patties; regular and low-fat luncheon meats, sausages, and hot dogs. Canned baked beans, cans or jars of pre-cooked navy beans, garbanzos, black beans, and refried beans. Eggs. Peanut butter.

Milk, yogurt, and cheese: Preshredded cheese, cheese slices, cheese spread in jars. Milk to drink. Instant and prepared puddings and custards. Plain and flavored yogurt. Canned cream soups to reconstitute with milk.

Vegetables: Frozen potatoes, instant mashed potatoes, boxed scalloped potatoes, canned or frozen vegetables, fresh cleaned and chopped vegetables from the produce section, shredded coleslaw mix, shredded carrots, peeled baby carrots, cleaned salad fixings by the pound. Vegetable juices, such as tomato juice and vegetable juice cocktail. Flavored canned tomatoes, such as Italian, Mexican, Cajun.

Fruits: Fresh, canned, or frozen fruits and fruit juices. Cleaned and portioned fruits from the produce section. Fruit nectars (apricot nectar is a good source of vitamin A). Dried fruits such as raisins, prunes, apricots, apples, peaches, mangos. Fig Newtons, raisin cookies.

Breads, cereal, rice, and pasta: Enriched or whole-grain bread. Noodles, macaroni, spaghetti. Rolls, frozen bread dough, corn bread mix, muffin mix, Bisquick, pita bread, tortillas. Twist-can biscuits, roll dough. Instant plain or brown rice. Pizza bread. English muffins, bagels. Pancake mix. Foccacia.

Convenient ingredients: Sauces and seasonings let you put together quick and tasty meals from ready-to-go foods. Ingredients you can keep on hand include prepared sauces such as spaghetti or pizza sauce, cream soups, and seasonings to sprinkle on (like lemon pepper), to mix in (like taco mix), or to serve on the side (like picante, tartar, or cocktail sauce).

Your older child will hang around, hungry and wanting to help. It is worth the trouble to think through your work spaces to let your child be in the kitchen with you. The first and all-important safety rule is to protect your child from anything hot or sharp. Turn the handles of pans to the back of the range or cook on the back burner so your child can't grab them and pull them over. Put your child in a safe place and teach him to stay there while you take pans off the range or out of the oven. Let him move around again immediately after you finish moving it, whatever it is, and tell him he did a good job. Put sharp knives at the back of the counter where your child can't reach them.

Organize your kitchen into functional work areas, so you can pretty much plant your feet (or your child) and not move while you assemble whatever it is. Have a baking area, where you put all your measuring cups and spoons, bowls, and canisters. Store your sugar, flour, and salt in canisters that are easy to dip into. Find dippers that double as quarter- or half-cup measures and leave one in each canister so you can scoop out and measure at the same time. If you have space, consider storing your baking utensils in a crock or large jar on the countertop. Get a little crock for your measuring spoons. You will be able to find utensils quickly, without pawing through a cluttered drawer. Have a separate crock by the stove with pancake turners, stirring spoons, and strainers. A pot and pan rack is great if you have the ceiling space for it. Have a fruit and vegetable preparation area near the sink, where you put your peelers, knives (including plastic knives for your child to use), scrubbers, and cutting boards.

If it just doesn't work in your kitchen to organize your storage in logical areas, assemble everything you need before you start to prepare food.

Designate an area where your child can "cook." For the toddler, this might be the sink, where he can pour water around. Let the faucet dribble and give him some measuring cups to fill and empty. Give him some sturdy vegetables, like potatoes or carrots, to "wash." Put him up to the table with a pan of rice and let him feel and measure. Whatever you give him to do, know that it won't last long. You are developing his cooking habit, not expecting much from him except—probably—a mess. But an older child can actually be of some help. If you organize his place and equipment, an older child can open cans, wash celery, put pickles on the plate, and cube watermelon—the list can go on and on. Make use of the suggestions given with the recipes in the cooking chapters for how children can help with meal preparation.

Organizing Your Storage

Figure 12.2, "Staples List," on page 198, includes both staples and perishables. Staples are foods like flour, sugar, canned goods, and frozen foods. These are foods you can keep around a while. The strategy I recommend is that you do a big staples shopping trip once every 3 weeks, and then run to the store once or twice a week for perishables, like produce, milk, and possibly bread.

Keeping staples on hand saves trips to the store for the one item missing in a recipe. It allows you to make the in-between grocery stops very quick, thus saving on time and impulse purchases. But keeping staples on hand means you need a way of storing them so you can find them.

If you have room in your kitchen for 3 weeks' storage, that's great. If not, build a pantry and keep only the most-used foods in the kitchen. For the backup inventory, hang a set of plastic shelves behind a door or put some shelves in a closet or in the back part of the basement. To keep the canned goods as cool as possible, place the shelves away from the refrigerator and stove. Foods are easier to find if the shelves are shallow.

Having extra freezer space is great. If you have a big freezer on your refrigerator, that might be enough. Otherwise, consider buying a little chest-type freezer. These sell for less than $300 and run for about the cost of powering a 50-watt lightbulb. In your little freezer, you can keep a 3-week inventory of meat, poultry, and fish. You can also keep on hand an assorted supply of frozen vegetables, fruits, and extra bread that you can pull out as needed.

Upright freezers are easier to organize and get food into and out of, but they are generally bigger and not as energy-efficient. Because they are harder to fill up, they frost up more easily. Organization was a problem for me with my chest-type freezer until I hit on my bag method. I sort the food into cloth bags—you know, the type you get with some business name written on it or canvas grocery bags. I have a bag for red meat, one for chicken and fish, one for vegetables and fruit, and one for breads. I label the handle of each bag using a permanent marker. I pull out the bag and rummage through it for the food I want, rather than rummaging through the whole freezer.

Keeping Food Safe

When raising children, it is generally better not to get compulsive. Food safety and sanitation, however, are exceptions to that rule. Be compulsive about sanitation. Since I think you can't emphasize this topic too much, I am going to be compulsive by repeating some things I have said before. You can be compulsive by attending to some basic rules of food handling, storage, cooking, and shopping. As long as you are compulsive about sanitation, you have nothing to worry about.

Bacteria are always with us. By handling food properly, you keep bacteria from growing to the dangerous levels where they can do harm. Food safety experts rank food-borne disease as the greatest health risk from the food supply. Part of learning to cook is developing lifelong methods that you (and your children) can use for staying clean and handling food. Certainly food manufacturers and government regulators have an obligation to keep our food as safe as can be. However, what happens to food in the home, when it is stored and cooked and served and stored again, has a major impact on food safety. We have to do our part to ensure a safe food supply.

Because their immune systems are immature, preschool children are particularly vulnerable to food-borne diseases. Young children also bring their own hazard to the food safety issue because of their diapers, their awkward and inexperienced toileting, and their tendency to play in the dirt. When you live with children— changing their pants, helping them go to the bathroom, and pulling them out of the dirt— you have to be super careful about washing your hands. In the tragic outbreak of *E. coli* 0157 in 1993, an infant in a Washington State child care center became ill even though he hadn't eaten the contaminated ground beef that caused the outbreak. He got infected when the provider failed to wash her hands thoroughly after she changed an infected child's diapers.

HAND WASHING

Keep hands clean. To wash hands thoroughly, the International Food Safety Council says to wet your hands, soap them thoroughly, and rub them together, fronts, backs, and forearms, for 20 seconds before you rinse. This is long enough to sing "Happy Birthday" twice. Given the quick, soapless rinse that most of us give our hands, I would happily settle for "Happy Birthday" once and consider it a huge improvement. Lace your fingers together and rub them up and down to wash between them. Curl your fingers and hook your hands together to soap the fingertips. If you give them credit for good hand-washing technique, your children will take it seriously and be proud of doing a good job. Wash hands after going to the bathroom or changing diapers; before handling food; after handling any meat, poultry, fish, or fresh produce; and before eating.

Also be sure to keep clean towels around for wiping your hands, and find a place to hang the towel so it can dry. Change your towel daily— more often than that if it gets so much use that it is always damp. Consider using paper towels.

Since hand cleanliness is so important, antibacterial hand cleaners, detergents, and soaps would seem to be a good idea. Not so. Antibacterial cleaners tend to be antibiotic, and routine use of antibiotics leads to antibiotic-resistant bacteria. The problem with cleaners is the same as with medicine: Using antibiotics when you don't really need them can make them useless when you do. Using soap is enough to clean thoroughly, and, for really tough disinfecting jobs, chlorine-type bleach is a good choice.

Preventing Food Contamination

Keep your work area and equipment clean and dry. Bacteria require three conditions to multiply: nutrients, heat, and moisture. That is, they need smears or quantities of food, they need moisture (dried smears don't culture germs), and they need the proper temperature to grow. Again, bacteria are always with us. Your task is to deprive them of any or all of their requirements for growing and thriving. You do that by keeping your tools and work surfaces clean and dry and by refrigerating foods promptly.

Plastic containers, dishes and baby bottles represent a particular challenge because they don't hold the heat from dishwashing and consequently don't dry well. Be sure plastic equipment is thoroughly dry before you stack it or cover it. Moisture left on surfaces gives bacteria a perfect place to multiply.

Keeping cutting boards clean presents a special challenge, because their grooves and slashes hide moisture and bacteria and because the boards come in such direct contact with food. As with many of the issues we have grappled with, the research and the press releases have gone back and forth about whether it is better to use wooden or synthetic cutting boards. Even though you can put synthetics in the dishwasher, they still seem to harbor more germs than wooden boards. Or maybe not. At latest report, the recommendation is to have separate cutting boards for produce and for raw meats, poultry, and fish. I think it would be a good idea to have a third cutting board for carving cooked meats. Do what you can stand, but if you use only one cutting board, wash it thoroughly, bleach it, and let it dry after you use it for raw meats or produce.

COMMON FOOD BACTERIA

For more important ways to be compulsive about food safety, see figure 11.4 on the next page. For more motivation to be compulsive, read on. Some bacteria cause infections when they grow and multiply to levels high enough to make us sick. *E. coli* and *Salmonella*, which are potentially present in all raw and fresh foods, and *Clostridium perfringens*, which is present everywhere, are examples of infective organisms. Other bacteria cause food poisoning when they produce toxins that make us sick. *Clostridium botulinum*, which causes botulism, is a toxin produced by spores that grow in improperly processed, low-acid canned foods, like the cold potato soup that caused an outbreak some years back.

Although any microorganism can find its way into a kitchen, four pathogens are particularly significant when cooking for children. *Shigella* is a bacterium that causes diarrhea, fever, abdominal pain, and bloody stools. It is transmitted through fecal contamination on food or hands or through contaminated food and water.

E. coli 0157 causes bloody diarrhea, severe abdominal cramps, and vomiting and is particularly dangerous because *E. coli 0157* infection can progress to kidney failure. *E. coli 0157* outbreaks come from any food that has been contaminated by the feces of a ruminant animal, like a cow or deer. Outbreaks have been caused by contaminated, undercooked ground beef; raw milk; unpasteurized apple juice (made from windfall apples that come in contact with cow or deer feces); contaminated water; poorly washed lettuce; and bagged, ready-to-eat spinach.

Salmonella causes headache, abdominal pain, diarrhea, fever, and nausea, which usually begin 8 to 48 hours after eating the contaminated food. Symptoms can last from 1 to 8 days. Even though poultry processing methods are being improved, so much poultry—including organically-raised poultry—continues to be contaminated with *Salmonella* that we must assume that it is contaminated and handle it with care. *Salmonella* outbreaks come from raw or undercooked foods such as poultry and eggs, unpasteurized milk, and unwashed fresh fruits and vegetables. In recent years, outbreaks of *Salmonella* have been caused by the contaminated skins of cantaloupe, watermelon, and tomatoes.

Clostridium perfringens is present in all food, and given the opportunity, it will grow and cause diarrhea and gas pains that begin 6 to 24 hours after ingestion and last 24 hours. Symptoms are usually mild. *Perfringens* multiplies where there is little or no oxygen and especially likes growing in the center of casseroles, stews, and gravies that are held for extended times in the danger zone between 40° F and 140° F.

To protect yourself and your family from contaminated produce, follow the directions in figure 11.4. In conclusion, let me give you a word of encouragement: Worrying about sanitation is a drag, but once mastered, these techniques will become easy and automatic.

Equipment and Appliances

An important part of planning is choosing your equipment. Think this through carefully, get what you need, but don't clutter up your kitchen with a lot of unnecessary stuff. If you are willing to forgo the brand-name appeal and aesthetics of the high-end, gourmet cooking equipment, you can find moderately priced, high quality, serviceable equipment. On the other hand, if you can afford it and appreciate the aesthetics of beautiful, expensive pans, why deprive yourself? Good-quality pans will be with you for a long time. But be sure they *are* good quality, and not just hype and marketing. Check *Consumer Reports* for ratings on equipment and appliances. You might also check the *America's Test Kitchen Equipment Corner*.

FIGURE 11.4 FOOD SAFETY

- Keep hot foods hot and cold foods cold. Bacteria grow most rapidly at temperatures between 40° F and 140° F. Adjust your refrigerator to keep it at 40° F or below. When you keep food hot, maintain the temperature above 140° F.

- Never leave perishable food out of the refrigerator for more than 2 hours, including preparation and standing time. At room temperature, bacteria grow quickly and the food can become unsafe. If you can't go home right after you shop, take along an ice chest to keep your food cold.

- Freeze fresh meat, poultry, or fish immediately if you can't use it within a couple of days after you buy it. Freezing food doesn't destroy bacteria. If food is contaminated going into the freezer, it will be contaminated coming out.

- Thaw food in the refrigerator, not on the kitchen counter. Most fresh vegetables, opened canned foods, meat, eggs, and dairy products should be kept in the refrigerator. It is all right to cover the can and put it in the refrigerator. Ketchup, mayonnaise, and mustard go in the refrigerator after opening.

- Thoroughly wash your hands—and the hands of anyone who will help—before starting to prepare food. Use soap and follow the 20-second rule.

- Bacteria live in kitchen towels, sponges, and cloths. Change your dish towel and cloth every day, and wash them in hot, soapy water. Sanitize sponges, kitchen brushes, and nylon scrubbers every day. Washing them in the dishwasher doesn't sanitize them—the temperature isn't high enough, long enough. Wet them and microwave on full power for 2 minutes[2] or soak them for 5 minutes in a solution of 1 teaspoon of chlorine bleach (like Clorox)

per cup of water. Rinse them out with clear water. Be careful not to get bleach on your clothes or it will take out the color.

- Keep raw meat, poultry, and fish (and their juices) away from other food when you shop, store, and cook. Bag raw meats separately in an extra plastic bag. Wash your hands, cutting board, and knife in hot, soapy water after cutting up raw meat, before handling other foods. Get a clean dishcloth or sanitize your sponge after washing up from working with chicken. See figure 8.5, "Keeping Clean When You Cook Chicken," on page 101, for special precautions.

- Cook meat, poultry, fish, and eggs thoroughly to kill bacteria. For temperatures, see figure 8.11, "Purchasing and Using a Meat Thermometer."

- Reheat food to 165° F. This would apply to PPMs and to bread dressing.

- Rinse all fresh fruits and vegetables thoroughly with cold water before you start working with them, even the rinds and peels you plan to throw away. Assume the rinds have bacteria on them and realize that as a knife slices through a contaminated rind, it carries bacteria into the fruit. Wash mushrooms, even though the gourmets say not to.

- Refrigerate produce after you slice it.

- Don't use detergent to wash produce. It can soak into the produce, and detergent ingredients have not been deemed safe for consumption.

- Avoid any fruit or vegetable juice that hasn't been pasteurized.

- Don't use raw sprouts, especially for children. The temperature and humidity necessary for sprouting seeds is also ideal for culturing bacteria, and some alfalfa sprouts have been contaminated.

BUYING AND USING KNIVES

Knives deserve special mention. Get good knives, and learn how to store them and keep them sharp. To protect both your fingers and the edges of the knives, rig up a knife block or a drawer with knife slots in it for holding your knives securely in place. Your knives don't have to be the best ones in the world, as long as you know how to use a knife sharpener or a steel. The basic four knives are:

- The chef's knife (for vegetables)
- The slicing knife (for meat)
- The utility knife (a long paring knife or a short slicing knife)

- The paring knife (for peeling and cutting small pieces of food)

The santoku knife is being touted on some cooking shows as an all-purpose knife. *America's Test Kitchen* found that while the santoku is better at precision slicing—thinly slicing carrots or chicken breasts—the chef's knife is a better all-around knife for tackling more substantial tasks. The chef knife's curved blade lends itself to a fluid rocking motion that allows rapid slicing, mincing and chopping.

While there are other variables, like the handle shape, materials, color, and type of attachment, the blade is the most important consideration. Blades vary in method of production and in the grind on the blade. Forged knives are shaped from a single piece of steel and are heavier; stamped knives are cut out of a sheet of steel and are lighter. Relative to the cutting edge, knives can be taper-grind, hollow-grind, or flat-grind. Pictures of these grinds, and their descriptions, are in figure 11.5. For more information about knives in general, and brand and price recommendations in particular, go to www.ConsumerReports.org for the most recent information. Currently, forged-steel knives are the highest rated—and the most expensive. However, Consumer Reports also found some very good stamped-steel knives that cost one-fifth the price of the best forged-steel knives. For ease and safety, keep your knives sharp with a steel or a knife sharpener. It is as easy as it is flashy to give your knife a few strokes with the steel each time you use it. Ask your butcher to demonstrate. You will make a friend for life, and he will remember you when you call up to ask for your specially cut pieces of meat. The steel doesn't actually sharpen the knife blade but only lines up the little metal burrs on the blade edge that weave around and stick out (minutely) and make the knife seem dull. Steels vary in hardness and are matched by manufacturers to their knives, so it's best to purchase the steel that is intended for your knives.

If you let your knives get so dull that a sharpening steel doesn't help, you will need to use a knife sharpener to grind off the little burrs. Consumer Reports recommends an electric sharpener, Chef's Choice for $140, that has magnets to hold the blade at a proper angle as you guide the knife through. I use a hand sharpener that I got for $10, but the angle is up to me.

Do be mindful of your personal safety with knives. Surprisingly, sharp knives are safer than dull ones. A sharp knife cuts easily through food. Because you don't have to saw away, a sharp knife isn't as likely to slip. Use a cutting board. Don't let sharp knives lie around. After you use a knife, wipe it off and put it away. If knives need washing, put them in soapy water one at a time and wash immediately so you don't plunge your hands onto a sharp knife. Dry immediately and put away. Don't put knives in the dishwasher; it dulls the edge and is dangerous for whoever unloads the dishwasher. Grabbing the blade of a sharp knife is not fun.

FIGURE 11.5 GRINDS OF KNIFE EDGES

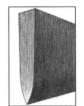

Taper Grind: The most expensive knives, these are thick at the back of the blade and taper down to a fine edge. These are generally hefty, strong knives with a durable edge. They keep an edge longer, but they are also more difficult to sharpen once they lose their edge. The Henckels and Sabatier brands are generally taper-grind.

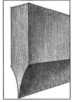

Hollow-grind: These knives are the same thickness from the back of the blade to the cutting edge. The edge is beveled down to a sharp point, and then it is hollowed out to bring it to a very sharp cutting edge. This type of blade can be very sharp because the cutting edge is quite thin. However, the hollowed-out area can be weak and vulnerable to breakage. It loses its sharpness more easily than a taper-grind knife, but the sharpness can be easily restored with a steel or sharpener. With the exception of the chef's knife, Chicago Cutlery knives are hollow ground.

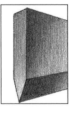

Flat-grind: These knives are like the hollow-grind, except the blade is sharpened flat rather than hollowed out. It isn't as sharp as the hollow-grind, nor does it keep an edge as long as the taper-ground. This type is the least expensive to produce, but it isn't necessarily a low-quality product.

POTS AND PANS

Buy the best pans you can afford. They will be with you for a long time, and they hold memories. When your children start to cook more, you will say, "Take the big pan with the black handles and fill it half full of water." For the rest of your life, you will remember those young hands on those handles.

Good pans are not necessarily the most expensive. In fact, a lot of pricey gourmet pans offer improved looks more than improved function. Read what *America's Test Kitchen Equipment Corner* has to say about high-end cooking equipment. But you don't need to spend top dollar to get good pans. Read *Consumer Reports* to help you decide what you want and to get an idea about prices. Do your research, and once you figure out what you want, you can go to discount stores, hardware stores, and even garage sales to get the best price.

The main consideration with buying pans is the cooking quality of the materials. Aluminum pans heat quickly and evenly, but bare aluminum is hard to clean. And unless they are heavyweight, aluminum pans lose their shape and develop uneven bottoms that don't sit flat on the burner. Stainless steel pans are easy to clean and are even dishwasher safe, but they get hot spots. Aluminum lined with stainless steel combines the best of both. Nonstick coatings (such as Teflon or Silverstone) are wonderful for cooking particular foods such as eggs, and they are easy to clean. However, they require plastic or wooden utensils, they don't brown as well as nonstick pans and they shouldn't be used with very high heat. There is a big variation in the durability of nonstick coatings, so if you plan to pay a lot for a nonstick pan, check *Consumer Reports* or *America's Test Kitchen* to find out which one will last. I find it handy to have one or two nonstick pans, but I buy less expensive ones and plan to replace them when the nonstick coating begins to peel off.

Enamel (also called porcelain) is pretty and heats well, but it chips. Copper heats and cools quickly and looks great if you keep it polished, but even thin solid copper cookware is expensive. Glass pans require a special little rack on an electric burner. They are heavy, and of course, they can break. Cast iron is heavy, heats evenly, and can handle high temperatures. It has to be seasoned before you use it for the first time, but that isn't difficult. Rub the pan inside and out with shortening (not butter) or cooking oil and bake it in a 350° F oven for an hour. Wipe off the excess oil and store. Wash it by hand using a plastic scrubber, not a scouring pad. Cast-iron pan aficionados say not to use soap for washing, but I just can't stand it, so I wash mine along with the other dishes and reseason them when they begin to rust or develop sticky spots. A deep-sided, covered cast iron skillet makes a great Dutch oven, and it can be used on top of the stove or in the oven. Be sure to get one with a lid.

My recommendation? If you are just starting out, get a good cook set with two frying pans, one large and one small, and four saucepan sizes: 1, 1 1/2, 3 1/2, and 4 1/2 quarts (the larger one benefits from two handles). Get a lid for each pan. Then supplement the cook set with a cast iron Dutch oven with a lid, one or two nonstick frying pans, and an 8-quart soup pot. Casserole dishes, bread pans, and so forth are listed in figure 11.6 on the next page.

UTENSILS AND SMALL APPLIANCES

I assume you have the basics: a cooktop, oven, and microwave. After that, it gets complicated. Utensils are highly personal and can either make or break you. I love gadgets, and I have to resist them. Looking at gadgets gives me the hopeful notion that I can buy a garlic peeler or a lemon juicer and my life will fall beautifully into place, organized and serene. I have yet to find that gadget. Some tools I use over and over again, like a potato peeler or an immersion mixer (electric hand mixer). Other tools I use occasionally but can't get along without, like a grater. I put a food processor on the list even though I have just a small one and use it only occasionally. Other cooks can't get along without their food processors. They use them for everything from slicing carrots to baking bread.

Listed in figure 11.6 are the tools I have recommended in the recipes in this book. I consider this list to be adequate for a modestly well-equipped kitchen.

A Word of Encouragement

Getting yourself organized to cook will be time well spent. It will pay huge dividends in pleasure and achievement. You can be a good cook, and you can help your children grow up to be good and healthy eaters. You can give them—and yourself—the security they need to know they will be well- and happily fed.

FIGURE 11.6 A STARTER LIST OF UTENSILS AND EQUIPMENT

Pots and Pans
Large frying pan
Small frying pan
Saucepans: 1-, 1 1/2-, 3 1/2-, 4 1/2-quart sizes with lids (the 4 1/2-quart size should have two handles)
One or two nonstick frying pans
Dutch oven with lid
8-quart pan (soup pot) with lid

Baking Dishes and Bowls
Covered ovenproof casseroles: 1-quart, 2-quart
9 × 13-inch glass or aluminum cake pan
10 × 6- or 8 × 8-inch baking dish
Loaf pan
Muffin tin
Jelly roll pan (10 × 15-inch pan with 1-inch-high sides)
Assorted glass mixing bowls
Salad bowl

Small Appliances
Toaster oven
Electric hand mixer
Blender or food processor
Slow cooker

Utensils and Gadgets
Colander
Measuring cups and spoons
Long-handled slotted spoon
Wooden spoons
Ladle
Serving spoons
Tongs

Wire whip or whisk
Plastic knives for children to help in kitchen
Plastic dishwashing pan
Knives: chef's knife (8- to 14-inch blade), slicing knife (10-inch blade), utility knife (5- to 6-inch blade), paring knife (3-inch blade)
10-inch butcher's steel or other sharpener
Three cutting boards: one for produce, one for raw meat, and one for cooked meat, poultry, and fish
Cheese grater
Pastry brush
Food thermometer (see figure 8.11, "Buying a Meat Thermometer," on page 113)
Carrot peeler
Potato masher
Can opener
Pancake turner
Plastic freezer zip top bags
Assorted jars with lids (for storing chopped onions, etc.)
Clear oven cooking bags, medium size
Aluminum foil

Optional
Platter
Ice cream scoops: size 30 (2 tablespoons), size 60 (1 tablespoon)
Salad spinner
Soup tureen
Wok
Garlic press
Roller-style pizza cutter
Timer (not essential if you have a kitchen clock, but handy)
Vegetable steaming rack

References

1. U.S. Department of Agriculture. Briefing rooms: food CPI, prices, and expenditures [Web page]. http://www.ers.usda.gov/Briefing/CPIFoodAndExpenditures/. Accessed December 14, 2007.
2. Park DK, Bitton G, Melker R. Microbial inactivation by microwave radiation in the home environment. *J Environ Health.* 2006;69:17-24; quiz 39-40.

Chapter
12
Shopping to Get You Cooking

To feed a healthy family, you have to have food in the house. To position yourself to plan and cook a meal—or to grab the ingredients to throw together a meal—you have to have tools to work with. You have to shop. It is not always fun.

As a matter of fact, it occurs to me that the amount of difficulty I am having getting to work writing this chapter is an exact reflection of the difficulty many of us have getting to work writing the shopping list and going out for groceries. It is as time-consuming—and empowering—as it can be. I don't like to do it. For me, the only thing worse than conducting my grocery-shopping campaign is *not* conducting it. But my chief operations officer (and tester of recipes) Clio Bushland reminds me that she *likes* shopping lists and shopping. Perhaps it is in your frame of mind. Clio is relaxed and interested in shopping and uses her shopping trips as an inspiration for her cooking. I am impatient and pragmatic. However you feel about it, it is an important chore that goes best if done carefully and thoughtfully.

Paulette Sharkey, my developmental editor, feels the way I do. Paulette says, "Even though it's painful at the time, you'll feel better later if you do it. Every weekend I just hate having to sit down and write the list and then do the shopping. But if I don't do it, I feel mad all week. I don't have the ingredients I need, and cooking is a real hassle."

Having admitted our negative feelings to ourselves and each other, Paulette and I came up with a way to *get organized*, and we offer our system to you. You may think our scheme is really nifty, or you might not like it at all. Your scheme may be totally different, and that's okay. The important thing is that you *think* about it and come up with a method that works for you. Random grocery shopping wastes time, energy, and money and defeats your cooking endeavors.

The P&E (Paulette and Ellyn) Shopping System

Our strategy is to shop at three different levels:
- Every 3 to 4 weeks: Big staples shopping. This is a major shopping excursion at a grocery emporium to stock up on foods that keep, such as frozen, canned, bottled, and dry foods, cleaning supplies, and paper goods.
- Weekly: Produce, dairy, and fresh meat for the week.
- Quick-stop: Milk, maybe bread or bananas.

Consumer research says that on the average we make 2.2 trips per week to the grocery store. Using the P&E method, you will make about 2.2 trips per week. We hope, however, these strategies will help you make these trips *count* and cut down on time, expense, and frustration.

Do you like shopping trivia? Here is more. Consumers tend to shop consistently all week. Half of consumers working full-time shop on weekends. Most shopping trips are done in the morning, followed by afternoon and then evening. Only 5 percent of shopping trips are done late at night.

Picking Out the Grocery Store

You can pick out a different grocery store for each of your three levels of food shopping. For the big staples shopping, it is worth traveling a distance. For the weekly shopping and the quick-stop shopping, it will save time and transportation expense to shop at a store closer to home. It's best to pick out particular stores and stay with them. Going back to the same store time after time lets you become thoroughly familiar with the layout so you can finish your shopping and get out as quickly as possible. You can even arrange your shopping list to lead you through the store. It may be too much to ask for in today's impersonal world, but you might even get to know some of the people there, which always adds a note of comfort and connectedness.

Food Is Cheap, but Don't Waste Money

As a nation, we don't spend that much on food. On the average we spend 10 percent of our income on food. That percentage, of course, varies enormously depending on income level. People in the lowest income bracket spend about 37.3 percent; those in the highest bracket spend 6.6 percent or less. We spend about $1,769 to $2,737 per person per year on food. Several-person households have lower per-person food costs, and single-person households have higher.[1]

To find out how you are doing with your food costs, do a web search on "cost of food at home" and click on "www.cnpp.usda.gov/USDAFoodCost-Home.htm" Official USDA Food Plans: Cost of Food at Home at Four Levels, U.S. Average. This website publishes the average food cost at four levels: thrifty, low-cost, moderate-cost, and liberal.

We expect ample, low-cost, safe, and wholesome food. In the past, we have been spoiled. With increased energy costs and competition for food crops by ethanol production, it is hard to say if that spoiling will continue. Since 1997, the Consumer Price Index (CPI) for food has increased 2.5 percent annually. The CPI is forecast to increase to 4 to 5 percent in 2008 as retailers pass higher commodity and energy costs to consumers.[2]

Even though prices are going up, we still have reasonably priced food. We would benefit from appreciating and celebrating our bounty. However, that does not mean we have to throw away our food dollars.

It's tough to do comparison shopping between grocery stores. Do try to do some price checking so you can get an idea of whether you have chosen a store that is competitive, but don't drive yourself crazy with it. Other considerations, such as convenience and a positive shopping atmosphere, may be important enough to you that you are willing to pay more for groceries. Consider whether it's the produce section that is most important to you, the meat section, the frozen-food section, or some section I haven't thought of, such as the greeting card section! Keep in mind that for the big staples shopping trip, the primary considerations are quality and variety of frozen and canned goods and staples. To get good canned goods and staples, you might have to settle for a more limited selection of produce or meat. Then you can choose a different weekly produce store, and the milk-stop store might be the gas station on the way home.

In addition to the standard supermarket, today's grocery-shopping world offers magnificent food emporiums such as no-frills warehouse clubs and supercenters. At warehouse clubs you can find big bargains, if you don't mind big bottles and boxes, although the food is not always cheaper. The downsides are that there is little service, brands are mostly limited to best sellers, there is an annual membership fee, and the checkout lines tend to be long. Supercenters are inexpensive and offer everything you'd find at a drug and mass-merchandise store, plus banks, hair salons, and maybe even eyeglasses stores. But their typically five-times-larger size can use up your time and energy.

Limited-assortment stores such as Aldi's and Trader Joe's are small in size and have relatively low prices, but they offer about 5 percent the amount of items the typical supermarket does, focus on private-label brands, and have a limited number of perishable foods.

Do your own research to choose your store. The best big staples shopping store is not necessarily the biggest store. A supersized store may just wear you out. A smaller store makes for less walking and faster shopping and may offer a bigger selection of the food you want.

Read the grocery store ads to get some idea of stores that feature price as their calling card. They are in the newspaper, but most stores also post their specials online. Your store may e-mail you their specials. Tempting as it may be, it's generally not a good idea to run from store to store to pick up the bargain of the week. It is time-consuming and gas-consuming and will make food buying more complicated, laborious, and possibly more expensive than it needs to be.

The ads will entice you with appealing "loss leaders." These are foods that are priced so low that the grocer makes little or no money on them, in hopes that when you are in the store to buy the bargains, you will do the rest of your shopping as well. If you need them, loss-leader foods represent savings. Oftentimes milk, produce that is just coming in season, chicken, or ground beef are used as loss leaders. Quick-stop stores may routinely offer low-priced milk or bananas as a loss leader.

However, be aware that sometimes food featured in grocery store ads is not bargain priced at all. Regular-priced products may be prominent in ads, on grocery store shelves or on the end-caps of aisles because they are overstocks or because their manufacturers have paid the store to feature them.

KNOWING THE STORE SAVES MONEY
Being familiar with the grocery store can save you money. This may just be an urban myth, but I understand there is a formula that says for every minute you spend in the store, you spend $5 on groceries. Whether it's true or not, the idea has merit. The more things you walk by, the more you'll throw in your cart. That is why many grocery stores put their "quick run-in" items like milk in the far back corner of the store, way behind all the other enticements that they hope you will pick up as you go by. But that appears to be changing. Some big stores realize they have to compete with the convenience markets and are putting their milk and bread at the front of the store, near the express checkout.

I do not mean to say that grocers are rapacious money-grubbers who are out to spoil your food budget. They do attend to merchandising and they do keep a careful eye on what you, the consumer, want. They do not have a big profit margin. Most grocery stores hope to make a profit of about 1 to 1.5 percent. That's not a lot to play around with, especially since stores work with potentially disastrous variables like food spoilage, equipment breakdown, crop failures all over the world, and the labor market. Food stores and departments that have the bigger profit margins are those that offer a lot of value-added services (see the "Value Adding" section on p. 190) such as Home Meal Replacements and other pre-prepared dishes.

Supermarket Organization and Marketing Strategies

To save time and frustration in any market, it is helpful to have a general organizational plan in your head. In almost every market, the produce, meats, dairy, and—to a certain extent—frozen foods are arranged on or near the perimeter. Canned, bottled, and dry foods, cleaning supplies, and paper goods are in the aisles in the middle.

The practicalities of food storage and production dictate supermarket layout. Refrigerated and frozen foods require large coolers. Meat departments and bakeries require both refrigerated storage areas and production areas. Behind-the-scenes equipment takes up a lot of space, so putting these departments on the perimeter of the store is simply practical. Of course, these are marketing considerations as well. Smelling the aroma of fresh-baked bread when you first come into a store can't help but excite your interest in buying food!

Arrangement on the *shelf* is primarily a *marketing*, not a *practical* consideration. Prime retail space is the space at eye level. (Prime retail space for sugar-coated breakfast cereals is your child's eye level.) Less-prime space is that above or below eye level. Grocers tend to position the major-markup foods at eye level and the foods you will buy anyway or that have a lower profit margin above or below eye level. Think about it. Which shelf usually holds the salt? Why, the one down by your ankles, of course.

Positioning products on the end of the aisles—the endcap—and on islands in the aisles suggests bargain pricing. It doesn't follow. Check prices on those foods carefully. The endcaps might just contain products that the grocer wants to move quickly—overstocks or foods nearing their expiration dates.

Within the shelves, stockers are supposed to rotate their stock. If they don't and they have an alert boss, they don't last long. Stockers move the product already on the shelf to the front and put the products being unpacked in the back. I suppose if you wanted the freshest cans possible you could reach back and get them. However, food stays fresh in cans for a year, so fishing for the cans in back isn't really necessary.

Value Adding

Earlier I mentioned *value-added* foods. Plain rice in a box or bag is a food. Rice with flavoring and bits of herbs and seasonings is a *value-added* food. Something has been done to the rice in manufacturing to increase the consumer appeal. It also increases the price. I found a package of herbed rice—a value-added product—to be eight times more expensive for a 2-cup serving than regular, converted rice. If you make your own herbed rice, the herbs and spices and extra time add to the time and cost. Is it worth it? You decide.

While some value-added foods are pricey, some value-added foods are not that expensive. The boxed tuna noodle casserole, including the cost of the tuna that you have to buy separately, is only about 10 percent more expensive than the noodles, soup, and canned tuna for the **Tuna Noodle Casserole** we made in chapter 8, "How to Get Cooking."

The value-adding chain goes all the way back to the farm. Wheat is the original food, noodles and macaroni are value-added products, and boxed tuna noodle casserole is value-added again. The farmer doesn't get much of the money for a food. The value-adding comes later. North Dakota farmers got tired of settling for their small portion of the food dollar, so they built a noodle manufacturing plant, Dakota Growers Pasta Company. They now process their own fine semolina wheat into pasta and keep the value-added profits closer to the grower.

The value-added issue has an impact on how shelf space is assigned in stores. High-markup items tend to be assigned more shelf space. Both my supermarkets devote a full aisle to chips and snacks, and another aisle, or even two, to soft drinks. All supermarkets have *lots* of breakfast cereals, most of them featuring value-added gimmicks like flavoring, sugar, shapes, or large amounts of added nutrients. As I tell you in chapter 13, "Choosing Food," you don't need

cereal to contribute "100 percent of total daily requirements," and your child will learn to prefer the cereal you regularly purchase. My staples market has a full aisle of canned fruits and vegetables, my produce market only about a fourth of an aisle. My produce market has a full aisle of candy and two full aisles of cleaning products. Very strange. If they didn't have such good produce, I wouldn't bother.

Manufacturers compete for prime positioning in supermarkets—or for any position at all. If an item doesn't sell, it loses its space on the shelf. Many new products come on the market every year, are test-marketed regionally, and then are sold nationwide. To make it, a new product has to sell fast and sell consistently. Products that don't sell are discontinued.

The Big Staples Shopping Trip

I assume that when you do the big, occasional staples shopping you will pick up your produce and meat for the week and your dairy for the next few days. The staples shopping trip is serious shopping. It is on the order of a campaign. To make a list that is as complete as possible, check your menu, consider anything special or extra you want to make, unearth your running list of "things we need," and get the master list ready. Then check the inventory to see what you have on hand and what you have to restock, and get your money lined up. Don't forget the money! It is darned aggravating to have all the groceries gathered and checked out, only to find that the checkbook is empty and the debit card is at home on the counter.

THE STAPLES LIST
The "Staples List" in figure 12.2 at the end of this chapter is a roll call of all the foods I used in all the recipes on the 3-week cycle menu. Some foods on the list (like salsa) I didn't use, but I've included them to give you a well-stocked kitchen. Still other foods are on the list to help you get ideas of nutritious foods you might enjoy, like the list of canned juices or the partial list of breakfast cereals that are nutritious and moderate in sugar. To help you when you get to the store, I have grouped the staples list the way foods are often grouped in grocery stores.

Like a lot of the issues we deal with on this project, the staples list is daunting but manageable. Make some photocopies of the list or download a copy from www.EllynSatter.com and highlight the items you need for the recipes you plan to make. I leave it to you to edit the list to fit the way you plan to shop and cook. I thought it would be easier for you to *eliminate* foods than to try to remember to include them. You may already have many of these foods on hand. Other foods are very occasional purchases, like spices and baking powder. Still other items on the list aren't foods at all, but things you still need to remember to buy, like paper products, cleaning supplies, and plastic bags.

The staples list works as an inventory list, as well. After you decide what to cook and highlight those ingredients on the staples list, check the pantry and all the hiding places to see what you have. Go on an excavation through the refrigerator and throw out anything questionable. Make a mental note that you really *didn't* use the eggplant you bought last time.

ORGANIZING THE STAPLES LIST
I take my staples shopping one step further. I hesitate to recommend it to you for fear it will make you tear your hair. But it helps me so much that I will tell you. I keep printed copies of my staples list, arranged to match the path I follow through my staples grocery store. I enter my list on the computer, arrange it, and print copies. To remind myself or anyone else who helps me with shopping, I even write down brand names, sizes and other specifications. Then when I get ready for my monthly shopping, I take a copy of my list and highlight what I need. I keep a running list of things I need on a handy scrap of paper, and then transfer it to the staples list when I get ready to go shopping.

I map my path through the grocery store so I end up with refrigerated and frozen foods last. That shortens up as much as possible the time cold or frozen foods have to sit in my cart at room temperature.

But you know, being compulsive is not all bad. It lets me organize and write books and even keeps me going when the task is writing a chapter on shopping. Like with planning, being compulsive is bad only when it becomes your master rather than your servant.

TAKE CARE OF YOURSELF
Get all the help you can. If you are organized, it will be easier for other people to take on part of the chores of food shopping and preparation. Taking a tip from Tom Sawyer, who persuaded his friends to do his chore by telling them how much fun it was to white-wash the fence, maybe you could interest your school-age child in taking your well-organized list and conducting the food inventory. In fact, she might even *like* doing it, especially if you make sure to say how much it helps you.

The staples trip is big. Try to be rested for it, and don't be hungry. Consider whether you really want your child along for this trip. It will take a lot of energy to tend a child and shop as well. Not only that, but you will have to unpack and put away the groceries once you get home, so preserving yourself is your first priority. Do recruit other family members to help carry in groceries and put them away once you get home. It will help a lot, and if they know what comes in, they will feel more capable of helping to cook it.

You might find that another family member is willing to do the shopping, at least on an occasional basis. With a complete shopping list, having someone else take over is much easier.

COUPONS
In today's world you can download coupons from the Web. I do not use coupons because I can't stand the fussing and the time it takes, no matter *what* it saves me. I do enjoy reading the coupon fliers, because they give me an idea of what is new, weird, and wonderful on the market. If you make good use of coupons, I congratulate you. Shoppers who make a science of coupons can save money if they don't let themselves be enticed into buying food they don't need in order to make use of the coupon. As I have asked before, is your time or your money in shorter supply? If your money is in shorter supply, you can use your time well by clipping and organizing coupons.

IN-STORE SHOPPER'S CLUBS
As a member of an in-store shopper's club, you receive a card that entitles you to automatic discounts on products without having to clip coupons. Consumer Reports says it is wise to use such cards. You may also receive access to unadvertised specials. Stores may also use the information they receive when you use their card to target you for particular promotions. For instance, new parents who buy disposable diapers may be mailed coupons for baby food.

SHOPPING FOR CANNED GOODS
Choose clean cans without bulges, rust, or gouges. Pick out cans that are not dented to

decrease the chances that the seal on the can will have been damaged. A broken seal allows spoilage. However, if you get home with a dented can, it's still likely to be all right as long as the seal is intact. If you can't tell by looking, you will be able to tell when you open it. If a can is intact and still properly sealed, it will make a whooshing or spitting sound when you cut into it with the can opener. Never buy—or use—a can that bulges.

Canned goods have packing dates and even times on them, but the dates are written in codes that most of us can't figure out. The grocer can figure it out and uses the packing dates for tracking inventory, rotating food on shelves, and locating items in case of recall.

Make use of unit pricing. The unit price label on the shelf shows both the retail price (the total price you pay) and the price per pound, ounce, quart, or other unit. The unit price will tell you that the biggest package is not necessarily the best buy, especially if you don't use it all. Keep in mind the use you are intending for the product. You don't need premium tomatoes to make **Macaroni-Tomato-Hamburger Casserole** and you don't need fancy peaches to make **Peach Crisp**.

BAKED GOODS

You can buy bread periodically and freeze it, get it once a week on your produce-shopping trips, or pick it up at the quick-trip store. It depends on where you can find the bread that you and your family like. Some communities have great bakeries, and it may be worthwhile for you to make a special trip to stock up—and to pay the extra price those breads command. They are no more nutritious than other breads, just more interesting.

If you want whole grain, read the ingredients label to be sure that is what you are really getting. For whole-wheat bread, the first listed ingredient should be *whole-wheat flour.* If the label simply says "wheat flour," it doesn't tell you anything. It might be whole-wheat or it might be white—which is "wheat flour" as well. The key word to look for on the ingredients list is *whole.*

Sometimes breads are made to look like whole grain with the addition of caramel coloring or flecks of bran. Those breads can taste good and be interesting, but they are not whole grain.

RICE, BARLEY, BULGUR, COUSCOUS, AND OTHER CEREAL GRAINS

Other cereal grains add interest and variety to the menu, and when you feel like experimenting, this is a good place to start. You can buy other grains prepackaged or in bulk. Many times the more unusual grains are available only in bulk, often called the "organic" section. Consider short- and long-grain brown rice. Barley is a wonderful grain to include in beef vegetable soup. Bulgur is a coarsely cracked and toasted whole wheat product used mostly in the Middle East. Tabbouli, a salad side dish that you are likely to find at Middle Eastern restaurants, uses bulgur. Couscous is coarsely ground semolina pasta that is a staple in many North African countries. You can use it instead of rice as a side dish. Pre-cooked couscous (which it mostly is) cooks quickly and easily: Just pour an equal volume of boiling water over the couscous, add salt to taste, let it stand 5 minutes, fluff, and serve.

From time to time other cereal grains are touted by "health foods" people as being particularly nutritious. Quinoa ("keen-wah") comes to mind. This is a grain used by the Incas that is touted as being highly nutritious. Quinoa adds an interesting flavor and texture to soups, and I recently was served a wonderful salad with quinoa, chickpeas, vegetables, and balsamic vinegar. However, in my nutritional comparison of quinoa and whole wheat, whole wheat came out ahead in everything except for vitamin E and iron. While quinoa has something to offer, being exotic doesn't give it any unique nutritional properties.

STORAGE OF STAPLES

In chapter 11, "Planning to Get You Cooking," I suggested supplementing kitchen storage space with a pantry in the basement or an out-of-the-way closet. This storage space should be clean and dry and as cool as possible, with shelves that keep food and supplies up off the floor.

Unless you can refrigerate them to keep them from getting stale, plan to keep whole grains just a month or two before you use them. For other dry products and canned goods, plan to use your stock within 6 months. While canned goods and packaged and bottled products keep up to a year, unless you are buying in bulk from a canner, there is nothing to be gained from letting your inventory sit in your home for so long. Move the older foods to the front of the shelf and put the newer ones behind, or mark the date of purchase on the can.

Fish, Poultry, and Meat

For a list of cuts of meat, poultry, and fish categorized by fat content, see figure 12.1 on the next page.

BUYING PORK
In the past, pork was high in fat and often contaminated with a parasite called *trichina*. Today's pork is far lower in fat and is free of *trichina*. Pork makes an enjoyable and worthwhile addition to your cycle menus because of its distinctive and enjoyable taste. Pork is high in B vitamins, especially thiamin, which is necessary for nerve health.

BUYING CHICKEN
To make chicken preparation easier, I have used boneless chicken breasts and/or thighs in my recipes. I visualize you purchasing them fresh, but you may also find it convenient to purchase the individually frozen chicken breasts in zip top bags. Because they don't stick together, you can take out as many or as few as you need. You can get them bone-in or boneless, with or without skin. Fresh or frozen, you pay for the convenience, but you don't have to mess with cutting up the chicken and discarding extra fat and pieces you don't use. When you buy chicken whole, quartered, or packaged in some other way, such as best of fryer, you may have to do some dissecting, and you may or may not know how to do that. It is also messy, and you have to be excruciatingly careful about contamination.

TWO AMAZINGLY FAST AND TASTY ROASTS
Have you discovered **Pork Tenderloin**? This roast is tender and small (about 1 1/2 to 2 pounds, 3 inches in diameter, and 10 to 12 inches long) so it cooks fast—in as little as 45 minutes in a 325° F oven. Roast in an open pan with a rack to an internal temperature of 155 to 160° F. (it will gain another 5 degrees with standing.) Remove from the oven and let stand for 10 minutes. Slice across the grain. You can purchase pork tenderloin with marinade, or you can mix up your own marinade. Look on the Web to find recipes.

Beef Tri-Tip is another marvelous discovery. The "tri" stands for triangle, a shape the roast takes from being cut from the upper, most tender tip of the sirloin. It generally weighs from 1 1/2 to 2 pounds. Roast in an open pan to an internal temperature of 140 to 165° F, depending on whether you like your meat medium rare, medium, or well-done (it will gain an additional 5 degrees with standing). Remove from the oven and let stand for 10 minutes. Slice across the grain.

Even though harmful bacteria are usually only on the surface of whole beef cuts, there is growing concern that bacteria may be present in the internal portions of the meat as well. That's why it is now recommended that whole beef cuts be cooked to an internal temperature of no less than 145°F. If you hate this idea and long to cook your beef—even your hamburgers—rare, look for irradiated beef. Irradiation reduces or eliminates pathogenic bacteria, insects, and parasites. It does not make food radioactive, compromise nutritional quality, or noticeably change food taste, texture, or appearance.

BUYING FISH
Your butcher may be able to help you learn what fresh fish really looks like, or you may get better information by going to a dedicated fish shop to do your learning. Such places generally pride themselves on *really* fresh fish, and they go to special trouble to buy it fresh, ship it fast, and store it properly.

When you buy frozen fish, look for the freshness date. Make sure the packages are undamaged. Be sure the fish does not have freezer burn (off-color patches and dried-out edges) and is not partially thawed or covered with ice crystals. Ice crystals mean the fish was thawed and refrozen, so the quality and bacterial safety will be lower. Use frozen fish within 3 to 6 months. The longer you keep it, the more likely it will be to develop off color, texture, and odor.

Canned fish is convenient and readily available. Most canned tuna is packed in water, broth, olive oil, or canola oil. The price varies widely and depends upon the kind and cut of fish, fishing method, and canning process. Albacore is the most expensive canned tuna and is labeled "white." It has such a mild flavor that you can substitute it for canned chicken in many recipes. Yellowfin tuna and other varieties are labeled "light" on cans. Bonita and skipjack tuna have the strongest flavor and highest fat content. If the can doesn't say "white" or "light," it's probably bonita or skipjack tuna. Within each type of tuna, solid pack is the most expensive and contains large chunks of meat. Chunk tuna has smaller pieces and is less expensive. Flaked or grated tuna is least expensive, but it is mushy.

There are three main types of canned salmon: pink, sockeye, and king (chinook). Pink salmon has the lightest color and mildest flavor. Sockeye has brighter salmon color and flavor. King salmon, a premium fish, also called chinook, is prized for its succulent texture and supreme flavor. The label should also indicate if the salmon is wild. Wild salmon has a pure, pronounced salmon flavor.

Weekly Shopping: Produce and Dairy Products

For the produce and dairy trip, you can shop the perimeter of the grocery store. As you recall from the organizational section in this chapter, produce and dairy cases tend to be on the outside border of the market primarily for the grocer's convenience. Now you can capitalize on that bit of information to cut down on time, distraction, and money.

Having a weekly produce and dairy shopping trip gives you the flexibility of buying perishable foods and filling in the blanks left after the big staples trip. This weekly produce and dairy venture might also help keep you from doing the time- and gas-consuming last-minute run to buy one or two items to finish a recipe. If you know the produce and dairy trip is coming up, you can save the recipe for a day or two. This shopping trip is manageable enough that it can become an outing in which you include the children. You can explore the vegetables together and see what takes your fancy, and you can stay away from the cereal aisle.

This trip also helps you make productive use of the farmers market, if you are lucky enough to have one. Our cycle menu has plenty of places where seasonal fruits and vegetables are suggested. At the farmers market, you can fill in those gaps and have a good time besides. But stay realistic about when you will *use* all of that luscious food, or your budget will suffer.

FIGURE 12.1 FAT IN MEAT, POULTRY, AND FISH

Lean choices: Lean meat has about 3 grams of fat per ounce. With the exception of sirloin and tenderloin, which have less connective tissue and therefore are more tender, beef cuts on this list need to be tenderized or cooked with moist heat. Pork, poultry, and fish are tender because they don't have much connective tissue. If you are careful not to dry them out with too much cooking, they will be tasty using any cooking method.

To better understand meat cuts and what affects tenderness and flavor, check the Cook's Thesaurus at www.foodsubs.com. Click on "Meats" and follow the links to poultry, beef, pork, lamb, and so forth. This reliable and award-winning Web site is worth keeping on your resources list for when you have questions about ingredients, kitchen tools, and substitutions.

Beef: Round, sirloin, chuck arm, tenderloin, flank, ground round, ground chuck
Pork: Boneless or bone-in center loin roast or chops, tenderloin, Canadian bacon, ham
Chicken and turkey cooked without skin
Wild game

All veal cuts except ground or cubed cutlets
All fresh and frozen fish (even "fatty" fish like salmon), fish canned in water

Not-quite-so lean choices: Not-quite-so lean meats have about 5 grams of fat per ounce, still a modest amount. Fresh meat cuts on this list are tender and good for grilling and roasting, especially if you avoid cooking them to the well-done stage.

Beef: Rib roast and steak, chuck blade, regular ground beef
Pork: Shoulder roast and steak, loin rib chop
Veal cutlets
Chicken and turkey with skin
Duck, goose
Fish canned in oil
86 percent fat-free luncheon meats

Higher-fat choices: Higher-fat meats have 6 or 7 grams of fat per ounce.
Beef: Short ribs
Pork: Sausage
Regular luncheon meats

AVOID WASTING PRODUCE

Almost everybody throws away fresh fruits and vegetables that get spoiled before they can use them. I do it. Alison Lockridge, one of my helpers, jokes with herself by saying, "I can have fresh produce when I become more responsible." If this sounds like you, you have a lot of company. Try your best to break this bad habit. Waste of this sort is the enemy of the family food budget. Some kinds of waste can't be helped, like plate waste when kids are around or having to throw away the rest of the casserole that's already been reheated once. But it's best to avoid wasting fresh produce if you can.

How can you avoid it? Don't buy impulsively. Buy produce only when you have specific plans for it. Since fresh fruits and vegetables deteriorate in quality and nutritional value the longer you store them, use them early in the week; don't save them. Clean salad greens before you store them, so it is easy to throw together a salad at the last minute.

CHOOSING PRODUCE

You choose most produce by color, shape, and size. Choose oranges and grapefruit by hefting them. A relatively light fruit means that a lot of the volume is skin. Press the blossom end of a cantaloupe. It should give slightly, indicating it is ripe. Nobody really knows how to tell if a watermelon is ripe, short of cutting into it. Smelling it may be the most accurate method, but then you have to know what a ripe watermelon smells like. Honeydews are mystery to most everyone—good luck!

Pears and bananas are generally picked and sold green, then you ripen them on the counter. Someone once said you have to sit up all night waiting for a pear to get to just the correct ripeness so you can eat it! Pineapples are picked and shipped ripe. Look for the wonderful "gold" pineapples. They are very tender and sweet; the flesh has a yellow-orange color to it. Pineapple is likely to be ripe if the top one or two leaves pluck out easily. Pineapple experts say to put a pineapple upside-down for a couple of hours before you slice it to distribute the sweetness. Is this true? I do not know. Try it and see what you think.

KEEPING SALAD GREENS FRESH

To keep delicate produce like salad greens very crisp, you must keep it moist but avoid having water on the surface, which can make it rot. Make sure the cells of greens are filled with water before you store them. Soak the salad greens in very cold water for a few minutes, shake or spin off the moisture, wrap in a paper towel to wick off the moisture, place in a zip top plastic bag, squeeze out the air, seal (to limit oxygen exposure), and refrigerate. The dry paper towels will help to keep your greens fresh for a longer time.

You will be justified in decreasing your salad complications by using prepackaged, prewashed greens. These last longer in the refrigerator because manufacturers know the secrets of hydrating fresh greens, then removing the surface water. I have wondered how to get greens dry, so I have been doing my own little survey of the vendors at the farmers market. One vendor said she simply washed and drained her greens, then spread them out to dry for a while. She recommended putting a paper towel or two in the plastic bag to wick off the moisture. Another didn't have much to offer—he said he simply drained his greens in strainers. But I knew still another would be my favorite from the sheepish expression he got when I asked. He told me he used net bags and an old washing machine. He hand-washed the greens in the bags in a tub, put bags and all into the washing machine, and then spun them dry!

It makes sense to me. However, most of us don't have an old washing machine sitting around to use for spinning salads. You might prefer a salad spinner, and I certainly recommend one. Or put the greens in a net bag to wash them, and then send one of the children outside with the bag on a string and have her spin them dry for you. She'll think it's a hoot! In years to come when she learns about centrifugal force, she will have her own, odd little mental example to think about.

SEASONAL FRUITS AND VEGETABLES

In years past, the availability of fresh fruits and vegetables in grocery stores was limited to what was grown seasonally and locally. With modern systems of storing and shipping, you can buy almost any fresh fruit or vegetable at any time of the year.

For those of us living in the north, buying nationally or globally is the only way we can get some fruits and vegetables, like bananas, oranges, pineapples, and artichokes. Wherever we live, most us of eat fall crops year-round, like apples, squash, and potatoes. The price and quality of these foods, and others like them, are generally good because they are sturdy and they store and travel well.

There are still seasons for fresh produce, and quality and price reflect those seasons. Apples and squash are best and lowest-priced in the fall. New potatoes are harvested when the vines are still growing and green. They come on the market in mid- to late summer, and they are delicious. Citrus is best and lowest-priced in the early months of the year, when the Florida and California trees are producing. Pineapple is best in late summer.

For other out-of-season fruits and vegetables, like raspberries and tomatoes, you will pay a premium, and the quality won't be as good as when they are in season. Raspberries that are grown in the South American summer, for instance, are flown to us to be available during our North American winter. However, to make them more durable during shipping, raspberries are picked relatively unripe. They soften during transit, but they don't really ripen. As a consequence, they lack the flavor and texture of locally grown raspberries that ripen on the bush.

For your own region, the two best ways to know when vegetables and fruits are in season are by visiting the farmers market and watching the produce section: They will be plentiful, reasonably priced, and of good quality. Asparagus and rhubarb are spring produce. Cherries and berries appear early to mid-summer. Melons, tomatoes, corn on the cob, green beans, cucumbers, peaches, nectarines, plums, and grapes are mid- to late summer crops.

The truth is, if you are willing to pay for it, you can have what you want at any time of the year. However, eating locally and respecting the local rhythms of crop production tastes better and costs less. It also saves resources. More and more consumers are becoming concerned about *food miles*: the distance their food travels from the location of its production.

BUYING LOCALLY

Many fine restaurants make their calling card fresh, locally grown meats and produce. Some favor food that has been raised with respect for the land. The concept of *sustainability* in food production is important to many consumers, and they act on their conviction by patronizing local growers who use minimally invasive methods of food production. You may have access to community-supported agriculture programs, where you can contract with local growers for produce in season. The Madison Area Community Supported Agriculture Coalition puts out a *great* cookbook, *From Asparagus to Zucchini: A Guide to Farm-Fresh, Seasonal Produce*, which is available on Amazon.com.

Whether you buy it in the supermarket or direct from the farmer, fresh, recently picked produce *does* taste better. Depending on how it is handled and stored, it may or may not be more nutritious than what you buy frozen or in cans. Holding produce in the fresh state makes it vulnerable to losses in nutrients and quality. However, there is a certain grounding (no pun intended) that comes from honoring agriculture as a part of eating. Making a connection with the land on which food is grown and with the people who grow it dignifies and enriches shopping, cooking, and eating.

You may or may not want to get that involved. If you do, you may not want to be slavish about it. You can still make some trips to the farmers market or to local farms. There is certainly an excitement of discovery and a broadening, for parents as well as for children, in discovering how food is grown and how it gets to your table. There is no doubt that a trip to such a place is an inspiration for the cook.

DAIRY AND EGGS

Buy the biggest container of milk that you will use by the end date on the package. Buy plain yogurt and add your own fruit (you will be nutrients ahead) and sweetening, or learn to enjoy yogurt without sweetening. Choose ultra-pasteurized half-and-half. Unopened ultra-pasteurized dairy products keep a long time; the end date on packages usually gives you a month or two. After you open the package, ultra-pasteurized dairy products have the same shelf life as regularly pasteurized products.

Consider purchasing dry milk and mixing it up for drinking. I did this when my children were young because they drank so much milk I couldn't keep it in the house. It tastes good if you reconstitute it and refrigerate it for several hours before you drink it. In fact, I did a blind taste test with my husband, and he couldn't tell the difference between fluid skim milk and reconstituted dry skim milk. Of course, if you use *non-fat* dry milk, you have to be sure to provide other good sources of fat with your meals. Some dry milk now has at least some fat in it, and that is better for children. If using reconstituted powdered milk for drinking seems a little daring to you, just use it for cooking.

Open the package of eggs in the store and examine them to see if they are cracked or broken. Shift each one around to see if any are cracked and stuck to the carton.

Check the date on packages and buy dairy products and eggs with the latest dates possible. The "sell by" date on milk indicates the last day the product should appear on a supermarket shelf. Depending on how well it is stored, most milk is safe to drink for about a week after the "sell by" date.

Eggs, yogurt, and cottage cheese generally have a "use by" or expiration date, which indicates when the quality of the product will have deteriorated. Don't buy eggs, yogurt, and cottage cheese that are past their "use by" dates.

Get grade AA eggs if you can. Many markets have only grade A eggs, which are all right but of somewhat lower quality, although equally as nutritious as grade AA eggs. Even when the "use by" date is okay, the only way you can tell how fresh eggs *really* are is by the way they behave when you fry or poach them. A fresh egg stands up. The yolk makes a high, rounded dome and so does the white. The white surrounds the yolk and keeps it well centered. There is only a small amount of watery white around the outside edge. A not-so-fresh egg flattens out, and a *really* less-than-fresh egg lets the yolk wander off to the side and even break. In my experience, some markets have fresher-performing eggs than others, no matter what their "use by" dates say.

STORAGE OF PRODUCE AND DAIRY

Generally, fresh produce has to be refrigerated, although there are exceptions. For example, one of the critical flavor components of tomatoes disappears when tomatoes are chilled. Tomatoes taste best when they are stored on the counter and eaten at room temperature. Bananas have to be stored at room temperature or they get black. To ripen fruit, put it in a loosely closed paper bag on the counter until it is as ripe as you want, then refrigerate it. For faster ripening, put an apple in with the fruit. The apple gives off ethylene, which aids the ripening process. Wash fruit just before you use it, even if you will discard the peel. Harmful bacteria from the peel can get on your hands and contaminate the fruit.

Refrigerate celery, carrots, and greens in airtight bags so they don't get wilted. Keep strawberries and mushrooms dry and in the refrigerator until you are ready to wash and use them.

Store dairy products covered, and use the oldest supplies first. If you are willing to risk dumping the contents, turn opened cottage cheese and yogurt containers upside down to store them. That makes a tighter air seal so they keep fresher longer.

To keep produce and dairy products fresh as long as possible, maintain your refrigerator temperature somewhere between 35° and 40° F. Don't store eggs and dairy products in the door of the refrigerator, because the temperature varies and can cut down significantly on shelf life. Put your ketchup, mustard, and jellies in the door.

Quick-Stop Shopping

Convenience stores that sell gasoline have become our neighborhood grocery stores. They provide a great service and deserve to be patronized. The economics of convenience stores means that selection is limited, most food costs more, and package sizes are small. However, it is worth paying for the convenience of the regular milk stop and for the occasional purchase of other items. Actually, many convenience stores have milk prices that are quite competitive, which makes convenience stores even better for milk stops. Milk sells quickly and is likely to be fresh. But since convenience stores are generally gas stations, not grocery stores, standards of cleanliness may be a little spotty. Take a look at sanitation. Are the floors and shelves clean? Are food spills wiped up promptly? Are the end-dates on cartons and packages current?

Online Shopping

Reviewer and parent Nancy Pekar says she shops online and *loves it*! Some stores let you order ahead for pickup. Others compile your order and deliver it *to your door*! Of course, there is likely to be a delivery charge, and groceries at that particular store may be relatively high in price. It comes down to whether you have more time or more money. You can make good financial use of your time by identifying the store with the lowest prices and picking up the groceries yourself. Of course, you have to factor in your transportation expense. On the other hand, you can save time by letting someone else do it for you. But it doesn't have to be all one or the other. It seems to me that online shopping would work great for the big staples trip, and going to the store yourself would work best for the shorter list of the weekly, fill-in-the-blanks shopping trip. Going to the store yourself has the advantage of letting you see what is new and giving you ideas to spark your cooking.

To search for a grocery store that delivers, I first checked the Web—searching on "online grocery" brought up some hits for me, although it didn't help me find a store that delivers. The Yellow Pages weren't much help, either. So I asked around and called a store that I heard delivered and they directed me to their Web site.

The most difficult part with online shopping is compiling your shopping list for the first time. That involves searching, one at a time, for the items you want, then marking your preference on a detailed list of choices. Consider shopping for canned tomatoes. First you get a list of *type*: whole, stewed, diced, sauce, puree. If

you happen to choose *diced* you get a list of brands, can sizes, added flavorings, petite diced. Each listing gives specific price information: total price and unit price. You might even be able to insert comments, such as "Please choose the bag with the most uniformly small onions." After that first time, you can save your shopping list, which streamlines the process, and your list can also act as an inventory. Telephone shopping is a bit more complicated. In my area, you call a service that takes your order and does the computer work for you.

That does it. If you have more ideas for shopping, let me know. I wish you the best on your shopping campaign. I hope you find a way to make it gratifying and rewarding. If you don't, I can only tell you that the *product* is well worth the effort. Being orderly and planning your shopping carefully can improve the quality of your mealtimes and can save you a *lot* of time, money, and frustration.

FIGURE 12.2 STAPLES LIST
With this list, you can make all the recipes in this book—and be ready for quick cooking on many other occasions. You can also find this list at www.EllynSatter.com.

Baking Supplies
Baking powder
Baking soda
Bisquick
Bread crumbs
Buttermilk powder
Cake mixes
Canned pumpkin
Chocolate chips
Corn meal
Cracker crumbs
Dried fruit: dates, pitted prunes, raisins, Craisins, etc.
Flour: white, whole-wheat, quick-mixing (e.g., Wondra)
Muffin mix
Nuts: almonds, pecans, walnuts, etc.
Pudding mix
Sugar: white, brown
Vanilla extract
Yeast

Crackers
Oyster
Saltines

Sociables
Triscuits
Wheat Thins
Your choice

Cereal
Oatmeal
Cheerios
Cornflakes
Kix
Rice Chex
Rice Krispies
Wheat Chex
Wheaties

Condiments and Seasonings
In addition to the ones here, stock what you like.
Chiles: canned, dried
Herbs and spices: basil, chives, cinnamon, cloves, dill weed, garlic powder, ginger, Italian seasoning, lemon pepper, mint, Montreal Seasoning, mustard (dry), nutmeg, onion flakes, onion powder, oregano, paprika, parsley, pepper, poppy seeds, rosemary, sage, salt, thyme, turmeric
Jam or jelly
Ketchup
Mayonnaise
Miracle Whip
Mustard: yellow and Dijon
Oil: olive, peanut or canola, vegetable, toasted sesame

Olives: black, green
Peanut butter
Pickle relish: sweet, dill
Pickles: sweet, dill
Salad dressing
Salsa
Sauce mixes
Soy sauce
Taco seasoning mix
Vinegar: white, balsamic, rice, wine, flavored
    (e.g., raspberry)
Worcestershire sauce

Pasta, Rice, and Other Boxed Grains
Barley
Bulgur
Couscous
Macaroni and cheese (boxed mix)
Pasta: noodles, macaroni, spaghetti, fettuccini,
    etc, mostaccioli (or other tube-shaped pasta)
Potatoes: instant mashed, boxed scalloped
Rice: brown, white, seasoned
Stuffing mix, dried

Soup
Bouillon: paste, crystals or cubes
Broth (stock): canned chicken, vegetable, beef
Chicken rice
Cream of mushroom
Cream of potato
Golden mushroom
"Hearty" style (with at least 5–7 grams of
    protein per serving)
Onion soup mix, dried
Tomato
Vegetable soup mix, dried

Canned Vegetables and Sauces
Artichoke hearts, marinated
Corn (whole kernel and cream-style)
Green beans
Mixed Vegetables
Mushrooms
Peas
Potatoes, small whole
Spaghetti sauce
Three-bean salad
Tomato paste
Tomato sauce
Tomatoes: stewed, diced, petite diced (with and
    without seasonings)

Beans
Canned or dried beans: black, garbanzo, kidney,
    navy, cannelloni
Canned pork and beans
Canned refried beans

Canned Meat and Fish
Beef stew
Chicken, canned deboned
Salmon
Tuna

Canned Fruit and Juices
Apple juice
Apricot nectar
Apricots
Cherries
Cranberry juice
Mandarin oranges
Maraschino cherries
Peach nectar
Peaches
Pears
Pineapple: rings, chunks, crushed
Tomato juice
Vegetable juice

Cleaning Supplies and Paper Products
Aluminum foil
Bar soap or liquid hand soap
Chlorine bleach
Dish washing detergent
Fabric softener
Freezer zip top bags
Garbage bags
Laundry detergent
Napkins
Oven cooking bags
Paper handkerchiefs
Paper towels
Plastic wrap

Baked Goods
Bread
Croutons
English muffins
Hamburger buns
Pita bread
Tortillas: corn, flour, crisp

Fresh Produce
Apples
Bananas
Basil
Bean sprouts
Berries: blueberries, strawberries,
    raspberries, etc.
Broccoli: whole, florettes, chopped, broccoli
    coleslaw mix
Brussels sprouts
Cabbage: whole, shredded
Carrots: whole, baby peeled, shredded
Cauliflower: whole, florettes, prewashed florettes
Celery: whole, celery hearts

Chard
Chives
Cranberries
Cucumbers
Dill
Eggplant
Garlic (fresh bulbs or bottled minced garlic)
Ginger (fresh ginger root or bottled chopped ginger)
Greens: kale, collards, chard, turnip, beet, mustard
Green beans
Lemons (or lemon juice)
Mushrooms
Onions: green, white, red
Oranges
Parsley
Peaches
Pears
Peppers: green, red, yellow
Plums
Potatoes: baking, boiling, sweet
Salad greens (prewashed or not): lettuce, romaine, spinach, mixed
Snow peas
Summer squash: zucchini, yellow straightneck
Tomatoes: regular, Roma, cherry, grape
Winter squash: acorn, buttercup, butternut, hubbard

Meat and Fish
Bacon
Beef chuck roast
Breakfast sausage
Chicken: boneless breasts
Fish: cod, halibut, etc.

Ground beef
Ham
Roast: beef, pork, lamb, ham
Steaks and chops: beef, pork, lamb
Stew beef

Frozen Vegetables and Fruit
Broccoli
Brussels sprouts
Combination vegetables: Mixed Vegetables (corn, peas, carrots and possibly lima beans), other combinations
Fruits: cherries, raspberries, strawberries, etc.
Greens: mustard, turnip, beet, etc.
Juice concentrate
Onions: chopped, pearl
Peas
Potatoes: French fries, hash brown, nuggets, mashed
Snow peas
Spinach: chopped, cut-leaf, creamed
Stir-fry vegetables

Other Frozen Foods
Breads: Bagels, bread dough, waffles
Ice cream
Pizza
Pre-prepared meals or main dishes

Dairy and Other Refrigerated Foods
Dairy: butter (or margarine), half-and-half, milk, sour cream, yogurt
Cheese: blue, cottage, cream (or Neufchâtel), feta, Parmesan (or Asiago), ricotta, sharp cheddar, Swiss
Other: eggs, fresh pasta, juice, refrigerated biscuits, tortillas

References

1. Blisard N, Stewart H. Food spending in American households, 2003-4. Economic Information Bulletin No. (EIB-23) [Web page]. U.S. Department of Agriculture Web site. http://www.ers.usda.gov/Publications/EIB23/. Accessed December 14, 2007.

2. U.S. Department of Agriculture. Briefing rooms: food CPI, prices, and expenditures [Web page]. http://www.ers.usda.gov/Briefing/CPIFoodAndExpenditures/. Accessed December 14, 2007.

Chapter
13
Choosing Food

We have spent the previous 12 chapters discussing the *how* of eating, feeding, and cooking. This chapter addresses the *what* of eating. Knowing more about nutrition and food composition will reassure you that you can eat what you enjoy, including foods such as red meat, eggs, starchy and salty foods, and fats and sweets. Essentially, I spend this chapter blessing the food. Your task is to make practical use of this information without becoming wary about food. I have done as much as I can to shield you from wariness by taking great care to discuss nutrition and food composition without turning the discussion into a lot of rules-that-must-be-obeyed. My intent is to continue to give you permission rather than taking it away. The rest is up to you.

Getting caught in the rules is the antithesis of being a competent eater. If I were working with you clinically, I would wait to introduce this information until I was sure you were ready. You would be ready when you could do most of the behaviors on the checklist in Epilogue I, "How to Eat." You would have developed the meal habit and built up patterns of food selection that worked for you. At that point, nutrition and food selection information would reinforce what you were doing and answer questions that have occurred to you, rather than loading you up with shoulds and oughts. Why am I being so cautious? Because almost without exception, even though I bend over backwards to be positive and accepting, my patients decode a discussion of nutrition principles as a set of shoulds and oughts that ends up looking

a lot like a diet. That sends them off on a cycle of restraint and disinhibition, first restricting themselves to some personal definition of a virtuous diet, then disinhibiting to eat all the foods they think they should avoid. It takes a while to settle them back down again.

That negative reaction is so predicable that I am often tempted to forget about teaching nutrition and food selection altogether. In fact, many eating therapists stay completely away from such lessons and even avoid encouraging their patients to eat meals. I always decide to address both; ignorance and avoidance do not add up to bliss. Not knowing the nutrition and food composition facts will give you less freedom with food selection than you would have otherwise. For instance, many people avoid perfectly acceptable food because they think it is bad for them, or too fattening, or "forbidden" for some other vague reason. Addressing those concerns gives greater choice. So I am giving you the information, but it is up to you to settle yourself down.

Because this chapter is a food-selection survival guide, it is detailed, and it is long. You will find lists of foods in the major food groups, lists of foods-that-contribute-certain-nutrients, and tables of nutritional requirements. I find it all very interesting. You might, too. On the other hand, you might find it boring beyond belief. Read it if you enjoy it, flip through it if you don't so you know what it contains. Either way, think of it as a reference chapter, and pick it up when you have questions. The information is indexed, and the figures are listed in the front of the book.

If you start to feel overwhelmed by the information, put it down. Eat a little, cook a little, feed a little, wonder a little. Your curiosity will lead you back to this chapter, and you will read it when you need it.

You Need Food Facts

You need not go by rigid guidelines of what and how much to eat to take good care of yourself with nutrition and food selection. You do, however, need to know the basics. There are pitfalls. Those pitfalls, ironically, are created by our wonderfully rich and varied food supply and our wonderfully rich and varied access to information. In times past, we could fall back on food and mealtime traditions that not only taught us what to eat but dignified our eating it. Every culture that has survived has invested millennia of trial and error in picking and choosing from what is available and putting together food combinations that support life and allow reproduction. If they didn't, their descendents wouldn't be around to talk about it! As illustrated by the variety of ethnic and regional cuisines, few cultures have settled for basic survival and have, instead, found ingenious ways to prepare food that increase the pleasure of eating.

Instead of food tradition, today's eaters often seem to be ruled by food fashion. That fashion is made up of contradictory nutrition and health claims, a marketplace that generates and promotes umpteen dozen new food products a *week*, and an attitudinal milieu that cultivates at one and the same time wariness and suspicion about food, food preoccupation, food asceticism, food-as-medicine, food-as-status-symbol, food-as-guilty-pleasure, and food-avoidance-as-fashion-accessory. Some foods are glorified as magic bullets that will protect us from medical malady; other foods are vilified as causes of those very same medical maladies. Food manufacturers, nutrition activist groups, authors, and even nutrition professionals regularly alert us to a food or food component that we are to become hysterical about. Little wonder that we are paranoid about our food!

The upshot of it all is that we no longer can settle for survival of the nutritional fittest or for following nutrition fashion. Our available food is too complex and ever-changing for us to evolve ways of coping with it. There are far too many self-styled experts who tell us what to eat and don't give a care about the evidence. Instead, we have to use our heads. Some dietary patterns sustain life and support vitality; others do not. A basic knowledge of nutrition will empower you to know the difference. While you are entitled, if you wish, to experiment with the Mediterranean or the Palm Beach or the blood-type or the vegan diets, in order to preserve your health you must also evaluate whether that diet is nutritionally adequate. According to the principles of nutritional science, all diets are *not* created equal. *If you are feeding a child, you don't get to experiment.* You must use reliable information about nutrition and food selection to make sure you are offering your child a nutritionally adequate diet.

All Foods Are Important

Our shared understanding of the basic food groups represents what little we have left of a trustworthy cultural tradition surrounding food. As a nutrition moderate, I was far happier with the Basic Four Food Plan—which was discontinued about 15 years ago—than with the Food Guide Pyramid (now MyPyramid), which replaced it. The Basic Four Food Plan told us to consume meat or other protein, grains, fruits and vegetables, and dairy. It also drives home several important points:

> - No one food has all the nutrients you need.
> - All the basic food groups combine to give a nutritious diet.
> - Any diet that lacks one or more food groups is likely to be nutritionally inadequate and even dangerous.
> - Each food group contributes certain essential nutrients and is lacking in others.

For instance, grains—breads and cereals—give B vitamins and iron; fruits and vegetables give vitamins A and C, phytochemicals, and antioxidants; meat, fish, poultry, eggs, and cooked dried beans give protein, iron, zinc, and other trace elements; dairy products give calcium and vitamin D; and fats and oils give vitamin E and essential fatty acids. On the other hand, each of the food groups is devoid—or almost devoid—of the nutrients not attributed to it.

As you can see from figure 13.1, a list of the basic foods groups is easy to remember and to follow and accentuates the positive. It tells you what to eat rather than what to avoid.

These food guidelines are based on the nutritional requirements established by the Food and Nutrition Board of the National Research Council.[1] Figure 13.1 puts a floor under your food selection. If you have regular meals that include choices from all four food groups, you will put up your own walls and ceiling and satisfy your nutritional requirements. You do not have to count and total what you eat, and everything you eat doesn't have to be nutritious. You have a fudge factor.

Enjoy Bread, Cereal, Rice, and Pasta

Four or five servings from the enriched and whole-grain bread, cereal, rice, and pasta group are enough to give you the complex carbohydrate, B vitamins, and iron you depend on these foods to provide. In fact, enriched and whole-grain breads and cereals give us about half of our dietary iron.[2] Whole grains give significant amounts of fiber. Despite the claims of the fad diets, there is nothing inherently fattening about high-carbohydrate foods, nor is there anything inherently slimming. High-carbohydrate foods support satiety because they are relatively bulky and taste good. If they are chewy, they help even more. Chewy choices include bagels, corn tortillas, and shredded wheat.

There is no need to purchase breakfast cereals with cost-increasing gimmicks such as flavorings, extra sugar, or cute shapes. Children prefer the cereal they grow up on. Interesting and appealing cereals that are made with enriched or whole-grain flour and are not encrusted with sugar and flavorings include Cheerios, Wheaties, and Kix. Before you spend extra for a cereal with "100 percent of your total daily requirement," consider that you don't need cereal to contribute "100 percent," and paying extra for vitamins, minerals and protein is unnecessary. Each food contributes something to your diet. You count on cereal to give you B vitamins and iron. Added together with all the other food choices you eat in a day, it will give you what you need. If it is whole grain, you also get a wide range of other vitamins and minerals in moderate quantities.

The Mother Principle of meal planning on page 90 encourages you to include bread and one other complex carbohydrate—like rice, pasta, or potatoes—at every meal. Figure 13.2 on the next page shows you foods that belong on this list.

Enriched grains give B vitamins and iron as well as added folic acid that is more easily absorbed than the natural folic acid in whole grains or even in leafy green vegetables. Whole grains give fiber as well as other trace elements not added back to refined grains. Get the benefits of both by serving whole grains about half the time, but only if you enjoy them. Eating all whole grain is not necessary and isn't good for children—too much fiber and phytate can interfere with iron and zinc absorption. Many labels imply whole grain, but don't really deliver it, by using terms such as wheat flour, rye flour, or unbleached flour. Read the label: The first ingredient in a truly whole-grain product will be a whole grain, such as whole-wheat flour or whole-grain cornmeal. Other whole grains include brown rice, wild rice, bulgur, buckwheat, and oatmeal.

Generally, children have no trouble eating what they need from this group. Starchy foods are easy to like because their taste and texture are not too challenging and because we often serve starchy foods with butter or other fats. Pay attention to your appetite. Seek out good-tasting breads; eat rice and noodles if you like them. Use butter or a sauce to make starchy foods more interesting.

Every culture has a particular starchy food that *has* to show up on the table, such as rice, spaghetti, grits, potatoes, plantain, or refried beans. Of course, potatoes and refried beans aren't grains, but they do serve as the starchy anchor for the meal in many cultures. I am still amused when I remember the menu listings in a wonderful small-town Iowa restaurant: "Spaghetti and meat balls—no potatoes," "Chicken

FIGURE 13.2 BREADS AND CEREALS
This list includes anything that is made with grain such as wheat, rye, or corn meal. Arranged in the order of more to less common, this amazing and rewarding array of relatively easy-to-like foods adds variety and pleasure to menus. Read ingredients labels and choose products made with enriched or whole-grain flour. If you choose to increase the whole grain in your menus, having whole grain about half the time is enough.

Bread
Buns
Biscuits
Bagels
Corn bread
Corn tortillas
Flour tortillas
Chapattis
Pancakes
Pita bread
Waffles
Crackers
Snacks made with flour: Bugles, Cheetos, Goldfish, pretzels
Pasta: noodles, spaghetti, macaroni, lasagna, pasta shells such as manicotti, tortellini, ravioli
Rice
Breakfast cereal, cooked or dry
Popcorn
Oatmeal
Couscous
Wild rice
Buckwheat
Bulgur
Barley
Grits
Flaxseed meal
Millet
Quinoa
Sorghum
Spelt
Amaranth
Triticale

chow mein and rice—no potatoes," "Enchiladas, rice, and refried beans—no potatoes." I expect those Iowans are as attached to their potatoes as the diners were to their rice and bread in the story told to me by Yvonne Bushland, food scientist, reviewer, and former Peace Corps volunteer: "I served a 'traditional American' pot roast [beef roast, potatoes, carrots, onions] and apple pie meal to a Malaysian headmaster. After the meal, he told me it was delicious, but since there wasn't any rice, he was still hungry. When I got back home, I lovingly served my parents a grand Malaysian meal. My father looked at all the food on the table and gently asked, 'Where's the bread, Yvonne?'"

If they taste good to you, you can emphasize the complex carbohydrates in your diet by making those the foods you and your family fill up on. Fill-up food is a concept worth bringing back. The traditional strategy for stretching food dollars is to fill up on starch. People who do hard physical labor need to leave the table feeling fully satisfied in order to have energy for their active lives. Many times they have extra servings of rice or potatoes with plenty of gravy or butter.

To satisfy everyone's need for pleasure at a ho-hum meal, include a bread that tastes really good, such as muffins, biscuits, toasted bagels, or English muffins.

Enjoy Fruits and Vegetables

You need five fruits and vegetables a day to get what you need of vitamins A and C, B vitamins, fiber, phytochemicals, antioxidants, and other still unidentified, possibly protective substances. Surveys show that adults eat, on the average, 1 to 1 1/2 fruits and 2 1/2 to 3 vegetables a day, for an average total of 4.7 a day.[2] That's remarkably good. There is room for improvement with respect to variety, however, because white potatoes in French fries and chips and tomatoes in spaghetti sauce, pizza sauce, and salsa make up most of our vegetable choices. There is nothing wrong with potatoes and tomatoes. Potatoes are rich in vitamin C and even contribute some protein. Tomatoes are rich in vitamins A and C and in lycopene; research goes back and forth about whether this is a protective nutrient. Despite the fact that the humble potato protected the Irish against scurvy and starvation, potatoes are currently vilified by often-sensible nutritionists as having a high glycemic index. That means the starch in potatoes rapidly digests and gets into the bloodstream as blood glucose. That is apparently true, but who eats unadorned potatoes? Are you in the habit of munching on a boiled or baked potato? Of course not. You eat them French fried, made into mashed potatoes, or incorporated into meals. As I explain in chapter 5, "Feed Yourself Faithfully," and in appendix G, "Select Foods That Help Regulation," a mixed meal or snack providing protein, fat, and carbohydrate gives a sustained release of glucose.

But, I rant. The low fruit consumption is a surprise. Most people say they like fruit and find vegetables more challenging. Most children find fruit easier to like than vegetables. They *certainly* like juice. In fact, today's children drink too much juice and not enough milk.

Fruits and vegetables are important nutritionally, but no more important than foods from the other food groups. Experiment with cooking them, cultivate your enjoyment by sneaking up on them and learning to like them, and eat them if you enjoy them. Best intentions aside, you will continue eating fruits and vegetables only if they give you pleasure. Forcing them down out of duty will work for a while, but eventually you will give it up.

Five fruits and vegetables a day, combined, are enough. You likely eat more fruits and vegetables than you think you do, if you consider juices, potatoes, and foods such as mixed dishes, pizza, and tacos. Reviewer and dietitian Edie Applegate told of a mother who lamented her dislike of vegetables and her difficulty eating them. Come to find out, the mother loved peppers and used them in great quantities. Because she liked them so much, it hadn't occurred to her that peppers were vegetables!

Fruits and vegetables don't have to be fresh to be nutritious. Use canned and frozen vegetables and fruit to cut down on preparation time and to vary the taste. Keep cans of fruit and vegetable juice around; reach for them rather than soda, and include them with snacks. Apricot and peach nectar are wonderfully tasty and nutritious and are simply fruits in a different form. Raisins, dried apricots, and prunes give vitamin A and iron and make a nutritious, sweet snack.

Don't forget about breakfast as an opportunity to include fruit and vegetables: An omelet with spinach or a dish of peaches can add to the day's offerings. Depending on how big it is, the daily glass of orange juice can add up to one or two servings. Snacks also may include a fruit or vegetable: a banana; a few slices of dried apple; raw vegetables with dip; a pear with some peanut butter; frozen peas, corn, or blueberries eaten frozen like little ice cubes—all can add to the day's offerings.

Use fat and salt to prepare fruits and vegetables so you enjoy them. In chapter 8, "How to Get Cooking," and chapter 9, "How to Keep Cooking," I give tasty recipes for casseroles and soups that have vegetables in them. In chapter 10, "Enjoy Vegetables and Fruits," I dress vegetables up with butter and sauces and give you dip recipes to use with raw vegetables. For the true vegetable novice, I give a section of "vegetables in disguise," which is not at all the same as sneaking vegetables into other dishes. I include recipes for fruit cobblers and crisps, and I remind you to consider including canned and dried fruit in your menus.

GIVE YOURSELF AN OUT

Even though the fruit or vegetable sounds delicious when you are planning the meal, give yourself and your child an out. Stay in touch with your appetite—how the food tastes at the moment you eat it—and trust your child to do the same. Eat it if it tastes good to you; don't eat it if it doesn't. Another time, it will taste good. If you pay attention to whether you really enjoy the food, you—like your child—will be more interested in eating it the next time you have the opportunity. If the food is new, allow time for it to catch on. Experiment the way your child does: Look but don't taste; taste but don't swallow; swallow but don't force yourself to take another bite. Remember, research with children shows that they need 10 or 15 or 20 tastes, in as many meals, before they like a new food. You are likely to need the same. Experience says it can take more—many more. Increase your vegetable and fruit use slowly— don't shoot for a 5-a-day goal right away. Start, for instance, by trying to offer two fruits a day, perhaps juice at breakfast and fresh or canned fruit later on. When you are consistent about that, nudge it up.

Lumping the fruit and vegetable lists together and trying for five altogether helps when planning meals for children. Sometimes children eat fruits, sometimes vegetables, and there is no predicting which it will be! When you get so you regularly include fruits and vegetables in your menus, consider offering two at each of your main meals to increase the chances your child (and you) will find one of them appealing enough to eat. This might be a fruit and a vegetable, like corn and peaches; two fruits, like a big fruit salad; or two vegetables, like tomatoes in the lasagna and a vegetable salad.

Fruits and vegetables prepared interestingly and well are tasty and rewarding. However, as any experienced dieter knows, trying to fill up on them—particularly when they are *unadorned*—is quite another matter. I have worked with far too many recovering dieters who have tried to do just that, and simply can't *look* at another pile of vegetables.

THE FOOD COMPOSITION LESSON

Figure 13.3 lists excellent and good food sources of natural vitamin C. While all fruits and vegetables provide some vitamin C, some are better sources than others. Some juices, such as apple juice, grape juice, and non-citrus juice blends, may be fortified with vitamin C. Check the label. Other juices have protective nutrients besides vitamin C. Juice *drinks*, which have a very small proportion of real juice, have little to offer except sugar and added nutrients.

Children seem to love their juice, and your child may drink too much of it if you let him. The problem is that he will fill up on it and not eat the other nutritious foods he needs. In general, let your child have juice only once a day.

FIGURE 13.3 VITAMIN C IN FRUITS AND VEGETABLES

Choose one excellent or two good sources per day if you can. However, almost all fruits and vegetables have some vitamin C, so eating a variety will keep you from being vitamin C deficient. Because the body doesn't store vitamin C very well, you need to consume it every day.

Excellent Sources
Broccoli
Brussels sprouts
Cabbage
Cantaloupe
Cauliflower
Grapefruit, grapefruit juice
Kiwi
Kohlrabi
Mango
Oranges, orange juice
Papaya
Peppers
Spinach
Strawberries
Vitamin-C-fortified infant juices

Good Sources
Asparagus
Bean sprouts, raw
Chard
Honeydew melon
Potatoes
Pureed baby fruits
Tangerines
Tomatoes, tomato juice

Vitamin C is a water-soluble vitamin, which means the body can't store it. In contrast, vitamin A is a fat-soluble vitamin, which means that it can be stored in the body. As a consequence, you don't have to consume a vitamin A source every day. Figure 13.4 lists excellent, good, and fair sources of vitamin A.

FIGURE 13.4 VITAMIN A IN FRUITS AND VEGETABLES

Choose one excellent or a combination of two good sources every other day or a fair source every day. Notice that some fruits are good vitamin A sources. Also keep in mind that pasteurized milk has vitamin A in it, so if your child drinks milk, he will get a fair amount of vitamin A. Vegetables and fruits that aren't on the list contribute other nutrients.

Excellent sources
Apricots, dried
Cantaloupe
Carrots
Mango
Mixed Vegetables
Pumpkin
Spinach, other greens
Sweet potatoes
Winter squash

Good Sources
Apricot nectar
Asparagus
Broccoli
Nectarines
Purple plums

Fair Sources
Apricots, fresh or canned
Brussels sprouts
Peaches
Peach nectar
Prunes, prune juice
Tomatoes, tomato juice
V8 juice
Watermelon

Enjoy Meat, Poultry, Fish, Eggs, Dry Beans, and Nuts

You need 5 to 7 ounces a day of cooked meat, poultry, or fish or their high-protein equivalent. Figure 13.5 lists foods that belong on this list.

FIGURE 13.5 MEAT, POULTRY, FISH, EGGS, DRY BEANS, AND NUTS

The following satisfy your mealtime requirement for a high-protein food. The foods may be purchased fresh, frozen, canned, dried, pickled, or smoked. Milk and cheese are good sources of protein as well. They appear on the milk list.

Meats: beef, ham, lamb, pork, veal
Poultry: chicken, turkey, duck, goose
Fish and shellfish
Eggs
Game meats: venison, bison, bear, rabbit, squirrel
Luncheon and deli meats, hot dogs, sausages
Organ meats: liver, giblets, heart, kidneys, sweetbreads
Dry beans and peas (legumes): lima, navy, pinto, kidney, soy, white, black, chickpeas (garbanzo beans), lentils, split peas, dahl
Bean-based foods: tofu, tempeh, falafel, texturized vegetable protein (TVP), bean burgers, sausage substitutes, tofurkey
Nuts: almonds, cashews, hazelnuts, mixed nuts, peanuts, nut butters, pecans, pistachios, walnuts
Seeds: pumpkin, sesame, sunflower

Meat, fish, and poultry can be baked, fried, sautéed, roasted, broiled, simmered. They can be ground or served as roasts, chops, or steaks. Cooked dried beans and peas can be eaten as a side dish as well as made into soups, incorporated into salads, and purchased fabricated into other foods, such as tofu, tempeh, textured vegetable protein, and meat imitations such as veggie burgers and soy sausages and hot dogs. Nuts and seeds are good protein sources, as well.

Politically correct protein foods right now, in order of the virtue attributed to them, are dried beans and peas (especially soybeans), nuts, fish, and poultry. In last place, and, in fact, generally considered *not* to be virtuous at all, is red meat.

ENJOY RED MEAT

Meat's sad fate is based on urban myth. (An example of an urban myth is the idea that your eyeballs will pop out if you sneeze with your eyes open.) The urban myth is that red meat is bad for you. It is not. Even MyPyramid, that guidepost of cautious eating, says to eat 5 to 7 ounces a day from the meat group, and it assigns lean meat equal importance and virtue with other foods in the group. Red meat is

good for you and, in fact, carries more than its nutritional weight. National statistics indicate that from beef alone, which accounts for only about 7 percent of the calories we consume, we get 18 percent of our protein, over 25 percent of our vitamin B12 and zinc, 10 percent of our vitamin B6 and niacin,[2,3] and over 20% of our dietary iron.[2] The iron in meat, fish and poultry is in the form of well-absorbed *heme* iron, in contrast to *non-heme* iron, in breads and cereals, fruits and vegetables, which is not nearly as well absorbed. In addition, red meat—and poultry and fish, to a lesser extent—contains *meat factor*, an important food component that helps the body to absorb iron. For more information, see appendix K, "Iron in Your Child's Diet."

The framers of nutrition policy urge caution in red meat consumption based on its saturated fat content. In my view, the caution is misplaced. Compared with the 18 percent of protein and all the other nutrients it gives, beef contributes only 11 percent of the saturated fat we eat. In reality, about a fourth of the saturated fat in red meat is stearic acid, which has been clearly shown to neither raise nor lower total blood cholesterol or LDL cholesterol.[4] Not only that, but beef contributes 13 percent of our monounsaturated fat intake and 2 percent of polyunsaturated fat, both considered "good" fats by the policy makers. (For more detail about fat composition, see appendix N, "A Primer on Dietary Fat.")

In truth, the fat content of red meat really isn't worth quibbling about. Most of today's meat is low in fat, as indicated by figure 12.1, "Fat in Meat, Poultry, and Fish," on page 194. Some people avoid meat, fish, and poultry for religious reasons, or out of concern for animal welfare. Those reasons are personal, and I won't quibble with them. Keep in mind, however, that avoiding any category of food increases the difficulty of eating a nutritionally adequate diet.

Others avoid meat out of concern for the environment, a concern that raises complicated issues. Producing enough nutritious, reasonably priced food for all of us is a challenging business that has led to some agricultural practices that are troubling. Animal production raises particularly difficult issues with no right or wrong answers—only choices. Animals raised for meat are high on the food chain—they eat the same food people do. The argument is that raising animals represents an inefficient use of land—it requires several times the amount of acreage to grow grain and soybeans to feed the animals than it would if we just ate the grain and soybeans in the first place. But beef animals don't eat only grain. They are raised by grazing on grassland pastures and are fed grain only in the last few weeks before they are slaughtered. Sixty percent of the earth's cropland is grassland. Without grazing animals, that land could not be responsibly or efficiently used for agriculture. Moreover, because of the way pastureland is managed, grazing does not deplete or destroy the land.

Of course, many animals such as pigs and chickens spend their whole lives in CAFOs—concentrated animal feeding operations—and those facilities have a huge environmental impact. Then there is the issue of safety in meat-packing plants, both for workers in this dangerous occupation and for consumers: Bacterial contamination is a problem, especially with large-scale production of ground meat. These are issues that have been surfacing in the media in the last several years and can only be addressed by increased consumer awareness, political pressure to improve conditions in food production industries, enforcement of stringent sanitation rules, and careful and clean management in our own kitchens.

ENJOY EGGS
Egg yolks have been mostly acquitted of the charges against them, although nutrition policy still says to restrict them. While egg yolks are high in cholesterol, eating them causes only slight increases in blood cholesterol.[5] Your body has to have cholesterol. Cholesterol plays an essential part in the makeup of the walls of all the cells in the body and is a major component of brain and nerve tissue. Your body uses cholesterol to manufacture essential hormones like estrogen, testosterone, and adrenal hormones. If you don't eat cholesterol, your body makes its own. If you eat less cholesterol, your body makes more; if you eat more cholesterol, your body makes less. As a consequence, varying the amount of cholesterol you eat has little impact on your blood cholesterol.

That is wonderful news for all of us eaters. Eggs are a versatile, convenient, nutritious, and inexpensive food that can be prepared in so many appealing ways! Children like eggs and generally eat them well. For feeding a family, they simply can't be beat you should excuse the pun. Eggs are an important source of protein, vitamins E and A, and even the elusive

vitamin D, which has only three common food sources. Milk and fatty fish are the other two.

I do have a caveat about dietary cholesterol. About 15 to 20 percent of people are "cholesterol responders." Their bodies make the same amount of cholesterol no matter how much they get in their diet, so their blood cholesterol does fall modestly if they cut down on dietary cholesterol. For that reason, a low-cholesterol diet could be helpful for cholesterol responders. If you have high blood cholesterol, try lowering your intake of cholesterol to see if you are a cholesterol responder. If you aren't, go ahead and eat eggs. In my view, we don't all have to go without eggs just because some people are cholesterol responders.

ENJOY POULTRY AND FISH
In defending the inclusion of meat and eggs in your menus, I do not mean to slight poultry and fish. They, too, provide protein, vitamins, minerals, and some meat factor. Eat poultry the way you like it—baked, sautéed, fried, stewed. It isn't necessary to be slavish about removing the skin. True, most of the fat is in or just under the skin. True, you get rid of that fat if you strip the skin away. True, even if you add a marinade, it doesn't equal the amount of fat in the skin. *But*, if you like the skin and enjoy eating it, why deprive yourself? If you check figure 12.1, "Fat in Meat, Poultry, and Fish," on page 194, you will see that leaving the skin on poultry changes it from a lean meat to a not-quite-so-lean meat. Is the added pleasure worth it to you? Only you can decide.

ENJOY DRY BEANS AND NUTS
Cooked dried beans are on the meat list as well. Beans offer fiber, minerals, and B vitamins, and they are filling, economical, and delicious. A benefit of meat skepticism is that people have discovered an assortment of wonderful beans. Tofu is making its way onto our tables, we like hummus and falafel, and we are beginning to use seeds and nuts as a source of protein. All that is well and good. However, you do not have to forsake meat to embrace beans and nuts. Include them all, and your diet will be the better for it. The greater the variety, the better your diet. Have beans as a main dish that includes a little meat as a condiment (see the recipe for **Savory Black Beans** on page 130), or combine beans with meat (see the recipe for **Minestrone Soup** on pages 128), or have beans as a side

dish, as in hot dogs and beans. For ideas about using seeds and nuts in main dishes, see figure 11.2, "Complementary Plant Proteins," on page 178. Do keep in mind, however, that whole nuts are a choking risk for young children. Wait to give them to your child until he is about 3 years old and able to chew and swallow well.

PEANUT BUTTER

This mainstay of children's diets has raised concern recently because some people experience life-threatening reactions to it. Children most likely to be seriously allergic to peanuts are those with a strong family history of allergies. Whether from food or from environmental agents such as house dust, pollen, or animal dander, allergies make themselves apparent through skin rashes, breathing problems, stomachaches, or intestinal upsets. If someone in your family has allergic reactions, keep your child away from peanuts and peanut butter until he is 2 or even 3 years old. Peanuts and peanut butter, however, are not such a concern for children without a family history of allergies. Your 1-year-old can have peanut butter on bread or toast if you spread it thinly to minimize the risk of choking. By age 12 months, his immune system will have matured and his intestine will be less likely to take in the whole protein molecules that cause allergic reactions.

VEGETARIAN DIETS

Given a few precautions, lacto-ovo vegetarian diets—those that include dairy and eggs—allow children to grow and do well. Figure 13.6 outlines those precautions.

Plant proteins, in contrast to animal proteins, are incomplete: They don't have all the components (amino acids) needed to build and repair muscle and other body tissue. Since plants vary in their amino acid contribution—and limitation—a plant from one food group can combine with a plant from another food group to make a complete protein. See figure 11.2, "Complementary Plant Proteins," on page 178, for a guide to combining plant proteins. To address iron, see appendix K, "Iron in Your Child's Diet."

I haven't attempted to give guidelines for a vegan diet—a diet that avoids eggs and dairy products as well as meat—because maintaining nutritional adequacy on such diets is so challenging, especially for children. If you are considering a vegan diet, consult a registered dietitian or a *certified* nutritionist. Make sure the

nutritionist is certified; anybody can appropriate the title "nutritionist," and uncertified nutritionists may or may not know what they are doing.

FIGURE 13.6 VEGETARIAN MEAL PLANNING
Follow the Mother Principle for meal planning.

- Plan meals around high-quality protein. Include some animal protein, such as milk, eggs, or cheese, or combine incomplete vegetable protein sources such as legumes, seeds, and grains to provide more complete protein.

- Attend to iron nutrition. Cutting out meat, poultry, and fish with their well-assimilated heme iron and meat factor makes it more difficult to get enough iron. Choose enriched or whole-grain cereal products as well as fruits and vegetables that contribute iron.

- Include a good vitamin C source at the same meal you offer the iron-rich food; vitamin C increases the absorption of iron.

- Use whole grain no more than half the time—the fiber and phytate in whole grain cuts down on iron, copper, and zinc absorption.

- Because grains and legumes are low in fat, be sure to include fat in your vegetarian recipes—about 2 teaspoons fat per serving. Recipes in vegetarian cookbooks are often too low in fat. Put butter, margarine, dressings, and sauces on the table and let your child eat as much or as little fat as he wants.

Enjoy Milk, Yogurt, and Cheese

Milk contributes high-quality protein, calcium, and vitamin D. All are desperately important for building strong teeth and bones. If you make milk your mealtime beverage and you and your family regularly drink milk, why not skip this section? If you and your family do not regularly drink milk, it could be the most important section in this chapter.

I am belaboring the issue of calcium and vitamin D because those nutrients are in increasingly short supply in our diets. In 1999–2000, only 30 percent of the population age 2 and over met the dietary requirement for milk and other

high-calcium foods.[2] Today's children and adolescents have a higher frequency of bone fractures than in the past.[6] Women with low milk
intake during childhood and adolescence have
less bone mass in adulthood and greater risk of
fracture.[7] While you can get protein from the
meat group, milk is our most reliable dietary
source of calcium and vitamin D. Calcium alone
won't build bones and teeth—you must have
milk's vitamin D to absorb and utilize the calcium. To reliably get as much dietary calcium
and vitamin D as you need, you almost have to
consume milk or a milk substitute that has been
fortified to the level of calcium and vitamin D
in milk.

A few people are allergic to milk or lack the
intestinal enzyme, lactase, that digests milk
sugar, lactose. If you are lactase-insufficient,
you are likely to be able to manage milk if you
drink only a few ounces at a time. Using milk
with fat in it helps, as it slows down the emptying time of the stomach and keeps the lactose
from reaching the intestine all at the same time.
You can also use lactase-treated milk or take
lactase tablets to help digest the sugar in milk.

A study of 10-year-old girls indicates that it is
the *perception* of difficulty digesting milk that
creates the barrier to milk consumption and
calcium nutrition, not the difficulty itself. Girls
who actually *are* lactose-insufficient drink milk
and have adequate spinal bone mineral content.
On the other hand, girls who *perceive* themselves as being lactase-insufficient, whether or
not they really are, have lower calcium intakes
and lower spinal bone mineral content.[8]

Ironically, part of the reason our vitamin D
intake has become critical is that we have
become sensible about being out in the sun.
Your skin makes adequate vitamin D when it is
exposed to 10 or 15 minutes of ultraviolet rays
from sunlight per day. However, sunblock
interferes with vitamin D production. Because
today's parents are keeping their children out
of the sun and covering them with sunblock,
rickets—a serious disease characterized by
poor mineralization of bones—is on the
upswing. Breastmilk does not contain vitamin
D. The American Academy of Pediatrics recommends that breastfed infants be supplemented
with 200 international units (IU) of vitamin D
per day.

While enough vitamin D is good, too much
is bad—very bad—and the margin between

enough and too much is narrow. Too much
vitamin D can cause nausea, vomiting, poor
appetite, and constipation. Too much vitamin D
makes your bones break down and raises your
blood calcium levels. Too-high blood calcium
levels can make your heart beat irregularly,
make your muscles weak, and even make you
confused. I could go on. The point is, don't take
too much vitamin D. Nutritional supplements
and cod liver oil are potential culprits. For
infants, the toxic level of vitamin D is 1,000 IU
per day; for everyone else, it is 2,000 IU.

You can get calcium and vitamin D from milk
and milk substitutes, from some brands of fortified orange juice, and from vitamin-mineral
supplements. To help you get enough but not
too much, figure 13.7 gives calcium and vitamin
D requirements for people at different ages.[1]

FIGURE 13.7 CALCIUM AND VITAMIN D REQUIREMENTS AT DIFFERENT AGES

	Calcium	Vitamin D
Child, birth to 12 months	210 mg	200 IU
Child, 12 months to 8 years	500 mg	200 IU
Adolescent, 9 to 18 years	1,300 mg	200 IU
Young adult, 19 to 30 years	1,000 mg	400 IU
Older adult, 31 years and over	1,200 mg	600 IU
mg = milligram; 40 IU = 1 microgram		

Bones are built during childhood and adolescence. After that, it is all downhill, as bones
gradually demineralize throughout adult life.
The best bet is to lay down a good store of calcium during the early years, although if you are
faithful during your adult years about getting
your calcium and vitamin D and doing weight-
bearing activity—which also helps strengthen
bones—you are likely to be able to keep your
bones stronger, longer. The increased requirement of calcium and vitamin D for older adults
is to compensate for age-related limitations in
absorption and metabolism.

Figure 13.8 tells you the where and how
much of getting calcium and vitamin D in your
diet. Eggs naturally contain small amounts of
vitamin D, and fatty fish and fish oil contain

quite a lot. Milk is fortified with vitamin D. Dairy products such as cheese and yogurt are generally made from nonfortified milk, so they do not contain vitamin D, but check the label—this seems to be changing. To substitute adequately for milk, soy or rice beverages must provide 300 milligrams of calcium and 130 IU of vitamin D per 8 ounces. Generally, this will be stated on the Nutrition Facts label as a percentage of daily value: calcium, 30 percent and vitamin D, 25 percent. Calcium-enriched orange and grapefruit juice may or may not contain vitamin D.

FIGURE 13.8 SOURCES OF CALCIUM AND VITAMIN D

Food	Amount	Calcium (mg)	Vitamin D (IU)
Dairy products			
Milk, fluid	1 cup	300	100
Milk, powdered	1 Tbsp	60	16
Soy milk, rice milk	1 cup	Read label	Read label
Cheese, natural or processed	1 oz	200	0
Cottage cheese	1/4 cup	40	0
Yogurt	1 cup	300	0, but read the label
Ice cream	1/2 cup	110	0
Cream cheese	1 Tbsp	10	0
Meat and other protein sources			
Meat, poultry	3 oz	10–20	0
Fatty fish	3 oz	20	80–200
Canned salmon with bones	3 oz	250	600
Cod liver oil	1 tsp	0	500
Eggs	1	30	25
Cooked dried beans	1/2 cup	45	0
Nuts and seeds	2 Tbsp	20–40	0
Peanut butter	2 Tbsp	20	0
Tofu made using calcium lactate	4 oz	50–250	0, but read label
Bread, cereal, pasta			
Bread	1 slice	25	0
Biscuits, rolls	1	25	0
Corn tortillas	1	60	0
Cooked and dry cereals, unfortified	1 serving	15	0
Noodles, macaroni, rice	1/2 cup	15	0
Vegetables and fruits			
Vegetables, average	1/2 cup	20–40	0
Green leafy vegetables, average	1/2 cup	100	0
Fruits, average	1/2 cup	20–40	0
Calcium-fortified juice: orange, grapefruit, others	1/2 cup	150	0–45

THE HOW OF MILK

The rumors (and even press conferences by supposed authorities) ballyhooed every so often that milk is bad for people in general and for children in particular are simply wrong. Such ideas are based on flimsy evidence put forth by people on crusades. Charges against milk do not hold up to careful examination. Pasteurized milk sold in regular grocery stores is safe and wholesome for your child. It is subject to strict regulation. Unpasteurized milk is not.

Give your baby breastmilk or iron-fortified formula until he is at least a year old and is eating a variety of other food. Then, if he is growing well and doing well nutritionally, switch to pasteurized whole milk. By that time, the other foods your baby eats make up for the nutrients lacking in milk, such as iron and vitamin C. In addition, his other food will mix with milk in his stomach to make milk easier to digest. Don't feed your child unpasteurized milk of any type at any age.

Why whole milk? Because fat is an important source of energy. Younger children, especially, depend on milk to provide them with fat. After age 2, whole milk is still okay. So is 2 percent, 1 percent, or skim milk, *if* your child likes it and drinks it well (many children don't) and *if* he has other good sources of fat in his diet. *But be careful!* Pennsylvania State researchers found that it is all too easy to overdo fat restriction, especially for toddlers. Computer modeling led to the conclusion that the use of more than one fat-reduction strategy can cause dietary deficiency for 4- to 5-year-olds, and the use of even one strategy can impair dietary quality for 2- to 3-year-olds.[9] Do *not* use low-fat milk if you use mostly lean meats *or* use low-fat food preparation techniques. Even if your child drinks whole or 2 percent milk, make butter, salad dressings, and other fatty food available at meals and do not limit the amount your child uses at the table. If you are in doubt about whether your child is eating enough fat, give him whole milk.

Make milk the mealtime beverage. If you can, drink it yourself. Offer only water as an alternative. For a while after your child is weaned from the breast or bottle, he is likely to not drink much milk. Just make milk available and wait—before long he will begin drinking milk from the cup. Don't push him to drink his milk or you will turn it into something he wants to avoid. Do not, whatever you do, reintroduce the bottle as a way of getting your child to drink

milk. It will bring a whole other set of nutritional problems.

I realize that many cultural traditions don't support milk as a mealtime beverage. Such cultures have other food traditions that ensure they get enough calcium and vitamin D.

It is okay to occasionally put flavorings in milk, but be careful of your attitude. If you are so invested in getting your child to drink milk that you are willing to go to a lot of trouble to make it happen, your child will know that. He will make drinking milk your thing, not his, and he will use it to manipulate you. Even the child who drinks milk will go through periods when he doesn't drink much milk. Don't make a fuss about it; don't try to push milk. Just wait. And drink *your* milk. He will go back to drinking milk when he's ready. After all, if you drink it, it must be the thing to do.

Enjoy Fats and Oils

While advice about fat consumption has lightened up, the damage is done. People in general feel that fat is bad for them and get into a food-is-dangerous trap when they consider fat. In a 2003 Food Marketing Institute survey, the primary nutritional concern of 40 percent of respondents was dietary fat avoidance, with concern about the nutritional value of food at 12 percent and a "desire to be healthy and eat what's good for us" assigned priority by so few that numbers were not statistically significant.[10] That's backwards. Being attuned to the nutritional value of food and eating what is good for us is far more important than avoiding fat.

While many consumers avoid fat in the name of weight control, the nutrition community does it in the name of degenerative disease avoidance. Of course, even nutrition professionals think that restricting fat will help manage weight. My reading[11] and experience tell me that restricting fat achieves neither weight management nor disease management. As I told you before, adults with high eating competence have low risk factors for heart disease.[12] Unless you have a strong family history of heart disease, you can safely relax about your own fat consumption and that of your child. By *relax* I mean strive for a middle-of-the-road approach between avoiding fat altogether and eating it in great quantities. I use this middle-of-the-road approach with my recipes. I have defined moderate fat levels in recipes as roughly 1 to

2 teaspoons of fat per serving, and I have ensured that the recipes call for a variety of dietary fats. If you want to know why you don't have to be so scared about diet and disease and so restrictive with fat, see appendix L, "Diet and Degenerative Disease: It's Not as Bad as You Think."

Ironically, the livable middle-of-the-road approach I describe will allow you to put together a pattern of fat consumption that closely approximates that recommended by nutrition policy makers. It's all in the spin. I advise you to lighten up on fat restriction and hedge your bets. The Dietary Guidelines say to limit fat consumption to 35 percent of calories or less (which is moderate), and saturated fat consumption to 10 percent or less, (which is restrictive), and keep trans fat consumption as low as possible (which is easy to achieve). I will get to trans fat later. Which approach carries the specter of food-is-dangerous? It seems to me that it is the one with the percentages. To keep yourself out of the food-is-dangerous mind-set, be practical rather than prescriptive, provide rather than deprive, and seek food rather than avoid it.

LIGHTEN UP ON FAT RESTRICTION
You must have fat. Fat provides essential fatty acids and carries fat-soluble vitamins. Fat conveys flavor in food, tastes good on its own, and gives food appealing color, texture, and moistness. Fat gives food staying power because eating fat with a meal retards the emptying time of the stomach and makes energy available to your body more slowly and for a longer time. Fat in the intestine stimulates the release of cholecystokin, a hormone that acts as a hunger suppressant.[13] Eating fat will not overwhelm your ability to regulate food intake. While you will eat and enjoy some high-fat foods, a steady diet of them is not pleasant. Internal mechanisms that seek variety provide guidance with low- and high-fat food, as well as with other foods. If you pay attention, you will observe that you will get enough of even luscious fried food and look around for alternatives.

Eating fat doesn't make you fat, unless you get into the restraint/disinhibition cycle. Do use butter on vegetables or sauces on foods, if you enjoy them. At the table, let your child use as much or as little butter or salad dressing as he wants, even if he eats it all by itself. Use fat in food preparation. The 1 or 2 teaspoons of fat per serving I use in my recipes still allows those

recipes to be moderate in fat. Using a tasty sauce or some butter in food preparation will make your food more rewarding.

Butter's wonderful taste adds greatly to good food flavor, and because it tastes so good, you may end up using less than if you settle for margarine. Butter and lard brown beautifully. For some dishes, like authentic, south-of-the-border refried beans, lard is an essential ingredient.

HEDGE YOUR BETS
To hedge your bets against heart disease, use a variety of fats. It can't hurt to take this simple action, and it might help. Emphasize liquid monounsaturated fats—like olive, canola, and peanut oils—in your cooking, frying, and salad dressings. To get essential fatty acids, include liquid polyunsaturated fats as well—like corn, sunflower, and soybean oils. If you use margarine, make sure the first ingredient is a liquid form of one of the unsaturated fats.

Butter and lard are not all saturated fat and actually contribute a fair amount of monounsaturated and polyunsaturated fat. Both have gotten an undeserved bad name by being put on oversimplified "bad" lists. Recent research on trans fats, in fact, indicates that butter and lard are better choices than partially hydrogenated vegetable shortenings.

For more detail about fat composition, see appendix N, "A Primer on Dietary Fat."

TRANS FATS
Currently, the most vilified fat is trans fat. For the most part, trans fats are industrially created partially hydrogenated fatty acids that have the hydrogen fixed in a particular pattern on the carbon chain. This chemical configuration is formed when vegetable oils are converted into the semisolid fats used in solid vegetable shortenings, margarines, commercial cooking, and food manufacturing. We eat industrially produced trans fats mostly in deep-fried fast foods, store-bought bakery products, packaged snack foods, margarine, and crackers. We eat small amounts of natural trans fats in meats and dairy products from cows, sheep, and other ruminants.

There is a small statistical correlation between the consumption of trans fats and heart disease.[14] It can't hurt to avoid industrially created trans fats, and it might help. Avoiding them is getting easier all the time because manufacturers are developing other processes for producing semisolid fat. Trans fat avoidance is now a selling point in manufactured and restaurant foods, and consumers look for foods that don't contain trans fats. Nutrition labels must declare trans fat content, and ingredients labels must declare the type of fat. The food component to avoid is *partially hydrogenated fat*.

Unfortunately, food hysteria waits always in the wings, as evidenced by the reactions of New York restaurateurs to the New York Department of Health and Mental Hygiene request to eliminate industrially produced trans-fatty acids and partially hydrogenated oils. That's *industrially produced* trans-fatty acids, a distinction that escaped the chefs who discovered that butter contains small amounts of trans fat and set about eliminating butter from their ingredients lists.

What is the bottom line? Read nutrition labels and choose baked products that are low in trans fats; read ingredients lists and avoid products with partially hydrogenated fats. If you eat out a lot, patronize restaurants that do not use industrially produced trans fats and partially hydrogenated fats. Use butter, lard, and vegetable oils and read the labels on margarines and hardened vegetable shortenings to determine whether they are free of trans fats and partially hydrogenated oils.

TREAT LOW-FAT FOOD WITH RESPECT

Research shows that over the last few years, as the percentage of fat in our diets has gone down, our weight has gone up. What does this mean? The nutrition enthusiasts say that we have to be more disciplined about watching our portion sizes, even for low-fat food. But that is a *control* message. The *trust* message is that your body knows how much to eat and that adhering to a low-fat diet could undermine that ability to regulate.

Why would that be? Because for most people, eating a low-fat diet involves restriction. People tire of restriction, so they take a vacation from it and overeat. In fact, periodic overeating is built into the restrictive low-fat lifestyle through the erroneous idea that "if it is low-fat, I can eat a lot of it." Low-fat food gives an escape from restriction and is used as license for disinhibition. In a Penn State study, when given yogurt of consistent fat content, healthy women who did *not* identify themselves as dieters or restrained eaters ate far more yogurt when it was labeled low fat. Not only that, but even though the yogurts were the same in fat and calories, they ate more at the meal following the low-fat-labeled yogurt

snack than after the unlabeled yogurt snack.[15] Presumably they tuned in on internal controls when they ate the unlabeled yogurt and ignored them when they ate what they thought was low-fat yogurt.

Those people are typical. Why is it necessary for us to overeat on low-fat foods? Why don't we just eat until we are satisfied? Because low-fat foods don't taste as good. In desserts as in other food, fat carries flavor and contributes a smooth and creamy texture. We also overeat because we feel deprived.

The irony is that low-fat desserts have about the same number of calories as the higher-fat alternatives. Removing fat impairs taste and texture, and sugar is added to compensate.

RELAX ABOUT CHILDREN AND DIETARY FAT

You may think my advice is too wildly liberal, and you may choose to be more restrictive with your fat intake. Keep in mind, however, that if you are going without and then making up for lost satisfaction, you are not being consistent. If you can be cautious and *consistent*, then carry on. It is not wise, however, to be restrictive with your child. Children depend on fat to get the calories they need, and they depend on fat to make food appealing to them. Children's energy needs are high, and their stomachs are small. Fat is generally hooked onto high-nutrient foods such as main dishes and vegetables. A low-fat diet is so bulky that a young child can't eat enough to get the calories he needs. Often, a child on a low-fat diet seeks sweets to get the high-energy food he needs and, unlike fat, sugar is less likely to be associated with high-nutrient food. To find out *what* I recommend for children and fat, keep reading. To find out *why*, see appendix M, "Children, Dietary Fat, and Heart Disease: You Don't Have to Panic."

Your child's energy needs vary a lot from meal to meal and from day to day. To support that variation, choose foods for meals and snacks that vary in fat and calories. Include some foods that are high in fat, some that are moderate, and some that are low. The main dishes and vegetables in this book are moderate in fat. Salads, fruits, and yeast breads are low in fat. Butter, margarine, salad dressing, quick breads (such as muffins and biscuits) and sauces are high in fat. Offer and use a variety of fats and fat sources, including monounsaturated, polyunsaturated, and saturated fats from both animal and vegetable sources. Then let your child choose and eat what he will. When he is hungry because he is active or growing fast, he will likely eat more high-fat, high-calorie foods. When he is less hungry, he will eat fewer high-fat, high-calorie foods.

Let your child pick and choose from what is on the table. Sometimes he will eat a lot of fat; other times, not so much. I ask my parent audiences, "Has anyone lived with a toddler who eats butter as if it were cheese?" There are a lot of chuckles and many raised hands. Recently weaned toddlers eat a lot of fat, probably because the fat content of their food drops so abruptly. Half or more of the calories in breast-milk or formula are from fat. Table food has, at best, 30 or 35 percent of the calories in the form of fat, and a lot of toddlers have to get by on diets that have 20 percent of their calories, or less, as fat. That's bad. Toddlers absolutely have to have more fat than that. The toddler who eats butter is intuitively compensating for the sudden drop-off in dietary fat content. When the toddler gets to the point where he is comfortable and capable eating table food, he will go cold turkey on the butter. Unless you and your child struggle about butter, he eats a lot of butter because he needs the calories.

One mother worried when her 5-year-old daughter Julie piled on the butter. She doubted me when I warned her not to put on the brakes and predicted that Julie would find her own moderation. "You were right," she announced recently. "The other night we had cornbread and Julie put on a lot of butter. Then she said, 'You know, I put on so much butter I can't taste my cornbread.' " When parents restrict foods, children want them all the more, and they don't have the opportunity to discover, like Julie did, that some is good but too much isn't.

Enjoy Sweets

Although people generally think of sugar as bad and sugary foods as forbidden, children benefit from eating some sugar. Their energy needs are high, their stomachs are small, and sugar gives them concentrated energy. But, to state the obvious, it's not a good idea for either you or your child to fill up on sweets.

Sugar doesn't have to be a nutritional no-no. Some of the calories in your fudge factor—the margin between the calories that have to go for nutritious food and your total energy requirement—can go for sugary foods. You can also use sugar to help make nutritious foods more interesting, like the spoonful of sugar we put in the **Herbed Peas** (recipe on page 157) to make them taste fresher, or the brown sugar we put in **Microwave Chunky Applesauce** (recipe on page 163) to make it chunkier. Sugar can carry a variety of nutrients if you make most sweets nutritious, like pudding or oatmeal cookies. Candy and Kool-Aid are okay, but offer them only occasionally, and include them in meals or sit-down snacks rather than giving them as food handouts. Kool-Aid has added vitamin C but lacks the variety of nutrients in fruit juice or milk. Supplemented candy may have vitamins and even minerals, but it lacks the variety of nutrients in flour- or milk-based sweets such as cookies and puddings.

The only disease caused by sugar is tooth decay. Sugar of all kinds nourishes the acid-producing bacteria in the mouth. Mouth bacteria can learn to live not only on the sugar in candy and soda (sucrose), but also on the sugar in milk (lactose) and fruit (fructose) as well as on sugar broken down from starch (glucose). The primary considerations with food and tooth decay are frequency and duration—how often bacteria-supporting nutrients are in the mouth and for how long. Munching all day on raisins can decay your child's teeth as surely as chewing on caramels; both are sticky and sugary and stay in contact with teeth. Drinking fruit juice all the time can cause tooth decay as surely as drinking Kool-Aid. For up-to-date information about nutrition and oral health, talk with your dentist. Dental professionals care about nutrition and go to some trouble to support their patients' nutritional health.

There is no reliable evidence that eating sugar causes children to have behavior problems. However, *hungry* children have behavior problems. Eating sweets instead of something more substantial can soon leave a child empty—and cranky. To keep your child from having that post-sugar emptiness and crankiness, reserve the sweets for meal and snack times and offer other foods that contribute protein and fat at the same time. The other food will stay with him longer and keep him comfortable until the next feeding time.

Currently, the food rumor mill indicts high-fructose corn syrup consumption for multiple health problems, and particularly for increased levels of obesity. The accusation is based on epidemiological coincidence: High-fructose corn syrup became the sweetener of choice for food and beverage manufacturers at about the same time that Americans started gaining more weight. Like any other hypothesis based on population studies, it is equally likely that some or many of the other cultural changes that were made about the same time caused increasing rates of obesity. The erosion of family meals and the increased prevalence of dieting are just a couple of examples. To disrupt the body's ability to regulate food intake, high-fructose corn syrup would have to outwit or overwhelm food regulation capabilities. Researchers in the Netherlands found no such disruption. Experimental subjects who drink soda sweetened with high-fructose corn syrup before mealtime compensate by eating less at mealtime to exactly the same extent as subjects who drink milk or drink soda sweetened with regular table sugar.[16] What about the other accusation, that high-fructose corn syrup causes multiple health problems? Not likely. Our health is getting better and better, and the incidence of chronic diseases continues to decrease.

MAKE A CHOICE ABOUT SODA

But what about the impact of chronic soda-drinking on eating behavior and nutrition? In chapter 4, "Eat as Much as You Want," I warned you that sipping calorie-containing beverages between meals can take the edge off your hunger and appetite and make it more difficult for you to detect your internal regulatory cues. Artificially sweetened soda can undermine regulation as well—it keeps the always-have-to-be-eating-or-drinking-something habit going. Soda is not a nutritional problem if you consider it as part of your fudge factor. It *is* a nutritional problem if it replaces nutritious foods in your diet. For many of today's adults and children, soda represents a nutritional problem. They drink way too much soda and way too little milk.

If you are hooked on soda, consider limiting the damages. In the best of all worlds, you would kick the soda habit, but how realistic is that? Rather than sipping along throughout the day, deliberately include soda at mealtime or coffee break. Consider it dessert, then have milk for your mealtime beverage. Consider whether you are drinking soda on the mistaken conviction that it will keep you from eating so much. I have been encouraging you to feed yourself regularly and reliably and to reassure yourself that you will get enough to eat. If you do that, you won't be saddled with such a constant

sense of going without that you have to shore yourself up with soda.

Despite the fact that "everybody" drinks a lot of soda, you do not have to provide your child with unlimited soda. Consider the mother I overheard in the grocery store, complaining to her preadolescent daughter. "You drink way too much soda," she said, as she loaded a 12-pack into the shopping cart. Her daughter looked pained, but smug. She knew her mother wasn't capable of nixing soda. Treat soda as a controlled substance—buy it occasionally, have it at picnics, have it once in a while as part of a sit-down snack that also provides protein and fat, then put it away. If you simply can't live without regular infusions of soda, maintain a double standard. You get to drink it; your child doesn't. Drink soda at work and after your child goes to bed. Be honest if you drink it in front of him—he will be on to you if you try to hide it in an opaque cup. Tell him, "This is for grown-ups." It is. Grown-ups get to choose whether to ruin their teeth by sipping on soda and weaken their bones by not drinking their milk. Your child depends on you to preserve his health.

Provided you have treated soda as a controlled substance, your child may drink a lot of soda when he gets out on his own, but he will get over it. Eventually, he will return to the habits you gave him.

Enjoy Salt

If you want to know what I recommend for your salt use, read on. If you want to know why I recommend it, see appendix O, "Sodium in Your Diet." It is more important to eat—and enjoy—a variety of nutritious food than it is to restrict salt—or anything else, for that matter. Use the salt you need to make your food taste good. Don't drive yourself to eating out so you can let someone else do the salting. As with the rest of your eating, find the moderate middle ground. Getting enough salt is important, particularly during pregnancy and when doing hard physical labor. It is not necessary to be enslaved by salt or afraid to use it, nor is it a good idea to eat an unrelieved diet of high-salt foods.

I stay in the middle ground with my cooking strategies. I use moderate amounts of salt in cooking, include canned vegetables, sauces, mixes, and even soups, and I occasionally use bacon and other high-salt foods. Cooking—and eating—in that way gives you about 3,000 to

4,000 milligrams of sodium per day—a reasonable and moderate amount. More important, it allows you to be *consistent* in your sodium intake.

With sodium, as with the rest of your eating, think about sustainability. Find a way of eating that you can maintain without the extremes of restraint and disinhibition. If you want to restrict salt and can be consistent about it, you have my blessing, unless you are pregnant, sweat a lot, or take certain medications. Be aware, however, that if you, like most people, can't consistently maintain that level of restriction, you'd better lighten up. If you restrain and disinhibit with salt, you will lead your body's sodium-processing system on a merry chase, and it won't be good for you.

Food Safety

Earlier I alluded to the notion that our food is dangerous. Such notions lead to labeling certain foods "bad" and others "good." The idea is that it is more healthful to eat vegetables than animals, and that "health," "natural," or "organic" foods are most healthful of all. As I have said before, both animal and vegetable foods make important contributions to the diet. You run a nutritional risk when you avoid entire food groups.

To keep your family safe from food-related illness, you have to be clean, but you don't have to become a vegetarian or buy organic or natural food. Food scientists agree that the biggest danger associated with food is bacterial contamination. To be safe for consumption, all food needs to be handled appropriately. It must be properly stored: Hot food has to be kept hot, cold food cold. All washable food must be carefully washed to get rid of bacteria, pesticides, or fertilizers. This is simply part of safe food-handling practice. In chapter 11, "Planning to Get You Cooking," and in the cooking chapters, I go into detail about sanitation.

People purchase organic foods for a variety of reasons: based on the debatable notion that it is more nutritious, to avoid the traces of pesticides and artificial fertilizers that may ride along on nonorganic foods, or to support farming methods that preserve and restore the land. Both ordinary food from the ordinary grocery store and organic food are nourishing. Ordinary food is a lot less expensive. You can address your personal pesticide and fertilizer issues by washing food well before you eat it

and by eating a variety. To protect yourself with anything you consume, consider dose and frequency. If you eat the same food all the time, even if it's nutritious food, you run the risk of overdosing. Did you know that if you eat a lot of raw cabbage, kale, broccoli, or cauliflower, it can interfere with your thyroid gland function? That raw soybeans can interfere with protein metabolism? As I told you earlier, too much vitamin D, even natural vitamin D, can be toxic.

In my view, the major value of organic foods is ecological—they are grown using methods intended to preserve and restore the land they are grown on. Such considerations lead naturally into the whole issue of being a *conscious consumer*—of behaving in ways that show respect for the social as well as the physical environment. Ideally, organic foods are grown locally so the transportation costs are low. But that isn't guaranteed: Currently, a significant portion of name-brand organic food is grown on factory farms and transported long distances to our supermarkets. However, workers on those organic factory farms are not exposed to the high levels of pesticides and herbicides that characterize conventional agriculture (nor, of course, are the family farmers involved in small-scale organic agriculture). Maybe what it comes down to, as Michael Pollan observes in *The Omnivore's Dilemma*, is this: If you care about the issues and can afford to subsidize sustainable agriculture by purchasing expensive organic or sustainably grown food, then do it. If you can't afford it, don't apologize. Remember that the priority is seeing to it that you and your family are well nourished. Do that first, then concern yourself with social and environmental activism.

Don't Be Enslaved by Portion Sizes

A serving is how much you put on your plate. A portion is a nutritional unit of measurement. It's up to you how much you serve yourself. To determine how you are doing nutritionally, convert your servings into standard portion sizes. If you drink 12 ounces of milk, you get credit for one and a half of your two to three portions; if you eat a cup of watermelon, it counts as two portions. Estimate a child-sized serving as a tablespoon per year of age or a fraction of the adult serving, starting with 1/4, then 1/2, and so on. For instance, toddler servings would be 1 tablespoon of peas, 1/4 slice of bread, 1/2 ounce of meat, and so on. To keep from overwhelming your child with a lot of food, give small servings and then make seconds, thirds, and fourths readily available. Keep in mind that a child might eat more or fewer servings, larger or smaller servings; the recommendations are just a place to start. Remember, the serving size doesn't dictate the amount that you—or your child—need to eat.

Beyond that, I don't worry about portion sizes. I assume that if you eat enough of a food to count it, you are eating enough to make it carry its nutritional weight. It goes back to the principles of eating competence. If you have positive and trusting attitudes about eating and if you regularly have structured meals and snacks, you will satisfy your nutritional requirements. You will regularly provide yourself with a variety of food to choose from, you will eat what you are hungry for and what tastes good on any given day, and over time you will get what you need.

Be forewarned, however, that many nutrition professionals are keen to teach portion sizes. Control-model thinkers depend on portion sizes to tell you how much to eat. Portion sizes go with MyPyramid and other diets that emphasize eating from your head and by the numbers. People who care deeply about portion sizes are convinced by research hypothesizing that children and adults who are offered small helpings eat less than those offered large helpings. I am not. Those studies are short in duration and don't give experimental subjects time to do what comes naturally: Compensate over time for small portion sizes by eating more or large portion sizes by eating less.

You get to decide how much to put on your plate. Perhaps you take reassurance from a crowded plate with big helpings; perhaps such a plate turns you off. Take smaller helpings if you want to. Just be sure there are plenty of those helpings in the serving bowl and that you and your child have as many helpings as it takes to get filled up.

Make Practical Use of Nutrition Facts Labels

Nutrition Facts labels, such as the one for macaroni and cheese in figure 13.9, are created by nutrition enthusiasts to encourage you to

achieve the goals of the Dietary Guidelines: eating a lot of fruits, vegetables, and whole grains and limiting fat, salt, and sugar. If you use the Nutrition Facts label as it is intended, it gives you detailed guidance for your planning, cooking, and shopping. You will also use the portion-size and calorie-content information to determine how much to eat.[17] In my view, that is too much detail too be useful. In fact, being competent with eating is undermined by that much detail.

FIGURE 13.9 NUTRITION FACTS LABEL FOR BOXED MACARONI AND CHEESE

Nutrition Facts
Serving Size 2.5 oz
(70g/about 1/3 Box)
(Makes about 1 cup)
Servings Per Container   about 3

Amount Per Serving	In Box	Prep
Calories	260	380
Calories from Fat	25	140

	% Daily Value*	
Total Fat 2.5g	4%	23%
Saturated Fat	5%	20%
Trans Fat 0g		
Cholesterol 10mg	3%	3%
Sodium 580mg	24%	31%
Total Carbohydrate 49g	16%	17%
Dietary Fiber 1g	4%	4%
Sugars 7g		
Protein 9g		
Vitamin A	0%	15%
Vitamin C	0%	0%
Calcium	20%	25%
Iron	10%	10%

* Percent Daily Values are based on a 2,000 calorie diet. Your daily values may be higher or lower depending on your calorie needs:

	Calories:	2,000	2,500
Total Fat	Less than	65g	80g
Sat Fat	Less than	20g	25g
Cholest	Less than	300mg	300mg
Sodium	Less than	2,400mg	2,400mg
Total Carb		300g	375g
Dietary Fiber		25g	30g

Note that there are two sets of figures: the composition as it comes from the box, before you prepare it, and the composition after you prepare it according to package directions.

However, the food composition and nutrition information on Nutrition Facts labels can be a useful adjunct to meal planning. As always in our discussion about nutrition principles, the task is to make use of the detail without getting caught in the rules. Let me give you some examples. Reading the Nutrition Facts label can tell you whether a commercial PPM (you know, Prepared Meal) makes a nutritional contribution. If a PPM claims to give vegetables, look for at least some vitamin A and vitamin C on the Nutrition Facts label. To substitute for a home-prepared main dish, a purchased soup or stew should have 7 or more grams of protein per 1-cup serving. The macaroni and cheese from figure 13.9 has 9 grams of protein, which makes it an adequate main-dish substitute.

Here are some other examples of how you can make use of nutrition labeling. On page 218, I encouraged you to read the Nutrition Facts label to determine whether a soy or rice beverage contributes enough calcium and vitamin D to make it an adequate substitute for milk. On the label, that contribution would be expressed as a percentage of daily value: calcium, 30 percent and vitamin D, 25 percent. (Daily value is the estimated requirement for an adult who eats 2,000 calories per day.) I told you the percentages to look for, but you can figure them out for yourself by comparing the label on the soy or rice beverage with the milk label. In figure 8.4, "Ground Beef," on page 99, I suggest using ground chuck. At times, ground chuck is labeled as 80/20 ground beef. That means that 20 percent of the *weight* of the meat is made up by fat. Those two weights are declared on the label. In 100 grams of raw hamburger, about 3 ounces, you would have 80 grams of lean and 20 grams of fat. The 80/20 figure is confusing because we generally think of fat percentage as meaning the percentage of *calories* that are contributed by fat. When we are told to have diets with 35 percent fat, that means that 35 percent of the calories in the total diet should come from fat.

Protect Yourself Against the News

Almost every day some new bit of research about what we eat scares us or sends us off on another wild-goose chase in search of a magic potion to keep us healthy. Advertisers for food companies, weight loss businesses, and health care establishments promote the message, "Eat right or you will die, and so will your children." That's bad. It's bad because it is so pessimistic and alarming. It's also bad because it takes away self-trust and makes us controlling with our eating. The media feature scary messages about nutrition and health because such messages sell, and they sell because we are concerned and want to do the right thing.

Because health and nutrition are such popular topics, many issues that used to be argued only in professional meetings and publications are now being argued in the media. In the past, scientists would test each other's ideas and experiments. Eventually, most of the ideas would be discarded, the few ideas that stood up to scrutiny would emerge, and we would hear about them. Now we hear about somebody's ideas before they have been scrutinized: They are, at best, *preliminary results.* A lot of the "findings" we hear about in the media are *preliminary results.* To keep yourself steady with eating, take these media releases, as they say, with a grain of salt. Appendix P, "Interpreting the News," tells you how to protect yourself from wild-goose chases precipitated by alarming headlines.

We have covered a lot of information in this chapter, and it is pretty detailed. Here is the bottom line:
• Focus on meal planning.
• Seek variety.
As Grandpa Eddie says: "A little of everything will keep you alive. Too much of anything will kill you." You don't know Grandpa Eddie, but like other sages, he makes a good point. Maybe you can think of him the next time you read one of the news releases about a new miracle food that will ward off disease, or when you hear one of those alarming statements that tell us we are killing ourselves with our forks and knives.

Hedge your bets by eating a variety. Variety increases your chances of eating the right thing and decreases the risks associated with eating the wrong thing. Striving for variety allows you to be positive in exploring food and keeps you in touch with the joy of eating. It lets you expose your child to the wonderful world of food and helps him grow up with the joy of good eating. Every food has something to offer. You can help your family be comfortable in the world of food and hedge their bets against disease by helping them learn to enjoy a *variety.*

References

1. Food and Nutrition Board. Dietary reference intakes table [Web page]. Institute of Medicine Web site. http://www.iom.edu/CMS/3788/4574.aspx. Accessed December 12, 2007.

2. Briefel RR, Johnson CL. Secular trends in dietary intake in the United States. *Annu Rev Nutr.* 2004;24:401-431.

3. Subar AF, Krebs-Smith SM, Cook A, Kahle LL. Dietary sources of nutrients among U.S. adults, 1989 to 1991. *J Am Diet Assoc.* 1998;98:537-547.

4. Thijssen MA, Mensink RP. Small differences in the effects of stearic acid, oleic acid, and linoleic acid on the serum lipoprotein profile of humans. *Am J Clin Nutr.* 2005;82:510-516.

5. Fernandez ML. Dietary cholesterol provided by eggs and plasma lipoproteins in healthy populations. *Curr Opin Clin Nutr Metab Care.* 2006;9:8-12.

6. Khosla S, Melton LJ 3rd, Dekutoski MB, Achenbach SJ, Oberg AL, Riggs BL. Incidence of childhood distal forearm fractures over 30 years: a population-based study. *JAMA.* 2003;290:1479-1485.

7. Kalkwarf HJ, Khoury JC, Lanphear BP. Milk intake during childhood and adolescence, adult bone density, and osteoporotic fractures in US women. *Am J Clin Nutr.* 2003;77:257-265.

8. Matlik L, Savaiano D, McCabe G, VanLoan M, Blue CL, Boushey CJ. Perceived milk intolerance is related to bone mineral content in 10- to 13-year-old female adolescents. *Pediatrics.* 2007;120:e669-e677.

9. Sigman-Grant M, Zimmerman S, Kris-Etherton PM. Dietary approaches for reducing fat intake of preschool-aged children. *Pediatrics.* 1993;91:955-960.

10. FMI Research Department; Trends in the United States. Consumer Attitudes and the Supermarket. Washington, DC: Food Marketing Institute; 2003:72.

11. Howard BV, Manson JE, Stefanick ML, et al. Low-fat dietary pattern and weight change over 7 years: the Women's Health Initiative dietary modification trial. *JAMA.* 2006;295:39-49.

12. Psota T, Lohse B, West S. Associations between eating competence and cardio-vascular disease biomarkers . *J Nutr Educ Behav .* 2007;39 (suppl):S171-S178.

13. Little TJ, Horowitz M, Feinle-Bisset C. Modulation by high-fat diets of gastro-intestinal function and hormones associated with the regulation of energy intake: implications for the pathophysiology of obesity. *Am J Clin Nutr.* 2007;86:531-541.

14. Mozaffarian D, Katan MB, Ascherio A, Stampfer MJ, Willett WC. Trans fatty acids and cardiovascular disease. *N Engl J Med.* 2006;354:1601-1613.

15. Shide DJ, Rolls BJ. Information about the fat content of preloads influences energy intake in healthy women. *J Am Diet Assoc.* 1995;95:993-998.

16. Soenen S, Westerterp-Plantenga MS. No differences in satiety or energy intake after high-fructose corn syrup, sucrose, or milk preloads. *Am J Clin Nutr.* 2007;86:1586-1594.

17. U.S. Food and Drug Administration. How to understand and use the nutrition facts label. [Web page]. http://www.cfsan.fda.gov/~dms/foodlab.html. Accessed December 12, 2007.

Part
III

EPILOGUE

Having worked our way through Section III, "How to Cook," I expect that you have developed enough of a repertory of food-management strategies to support your meal habit. Whatever your approach to providing meals, stop to think about what you have achieved, and consider yourself successful. Cultivate a positive attitude about your ability to manage food. Give yourself full marks for getting a meal on the table whether it is cooked from scratch, thawed in the microwave, delivered to your door, ordered at a fast-food restaurant, or pulled out of a brown paper bag. The bottom line is reassuring yourself and your family that you will be fed.

In chapter 1, "The Secret in a Nutshell," I encouraged you to address the three sections of *Secrets* in any order that you wished, and reassured you that gaining mastery in any of the three areas—how to eat, how to raise good eaters and how to cook—would stimulate your energy and curiosity and introduce you to the possibilities of the other two. As you may have discovered by now, mastery in any of the three areas increases your mastery in the other two. Consider the impact of your being able to manage and prepare food for your family. In our research, we found that people who cook have higher eating competence.[1] They also pass eating competence on to their children.[2] Adults who have regular meals show many indicators of having superior nutritional status.[1] Regular meals are essential to doing a good job of parenting with food. As I have observed in many places but most persuasively in Appendix B,

"What the Research Says about Meals," children and adolescents who have family meals do better in all ways—nutritionally, socially and emotionally. Young adults who had family meals as adolescents tend to cook for themselves when they get out on their own.[2]

In turn, our research shows that people with high eating competence tend to plan meals, to cook, and to feel successful with cooking. Most indicate that they like to cook and that they cook every day. Each day, few invest less than 15 minutes or more than 45 minutes in cooking, meaning that they tend toward the types of homestyle or speed scratch cooking that I have discussed in this *How to Cook* section. They tend not to choose cooking methods that require ether very little time—frozen, convenience meals—or very much time—so-called gourmet cooking.[1] However, I would doubt that they were slavish in their food-preparation standards. Since the survey respondents were asked to check all their food-preparation methods, we can assume that the homestyle method predominated for the eating competent but that they used the other methods as well. In other words, they were flexible with respect to the approach they used to cooking. With cooking as in any other human endeavor, flexibility is an extremely useful trait.

If you have worked your way through the "How to Eat" and "How to Cook" sections, you will have discovered that they add up. You will have discovered for yourself that mealtime structure and your eating capabilities interact in the way I told you about in the section I epilogue: Your structured meals plus your internal regulation skills guide you in knowing how much to eat; Your structured meals plus your food acceptance skills guide you in determining what to eat. As you have discovered that you can eat enough of even enjoyable food without going out of control, your attitudes about eating will have become more positive. Your overall eating competence will continue to improve as you demonstrate to yourself over and over again that for you to cook and to eat the amount and type of food that you need, your meals must be rewarding to plan, prepare, provide and eat. You will put time and energy into food preparation because eating that meal is enjoyable, and it leaves you feeling comfortable and satisfied.

If you have worked your way through the "How to Raise Good Eaters" section, you will have discovered how much your child can teach you about what competent eating is all about. Your maintaining a division of responsibility will have preserved your child's curiosity about food and willingness to push herself along in learning to eat the food you eat. She will intuitively know how much to eat because that is natural for her and because you have done nothing to interfere with her natural ability. You will have also discovered that developing your trust in your own internal regulators supports you in trusting those of your child. Finally, you will have discovered that for your child to be competent with eating, you simply must maintain the structure of reliable meals and sit-down snacks.

References

1. Lohse B, Satter E, Horacek T, Gebreselassie T, Oakland MJ. Measuring Eating Competence: psychometric properties and validity of the ecSatter Inventory. *J Nutr Educ Behav* . 2007;39 (suppl):S154-S166.
2. Larson NI, Neumark-Sztainer D, Hannan PJ, Story M. Family meals during adolescence are associated with higher diet quality and healthful meal patterns during young adulthood. *J Am Diet Assoc.* 2007;107:1502-1510.

Appendixes

A

Interpreting and Using the ecSatter Inventory (ecSI)

The ecSatter Inventory (ecSI) tests the degree to which adults show evidence of eating competence, as defined by the Satter Eating Competence Model, ecSatter. According to ecSatter, competent eaters 1) have positive attitudes about eating and about food, 2) have food acceptance skills that support eating an ever-increasing variety of the available food, 3) have internal regulation skills that allow intuitively consuming enough food to give energy and stamina and to support stable body weight, and 4) have skills and resources for managing the food context and orchestrating family meals.[1]

ecSI is a valid tool for measuring ecSatter in a population of healthy adults,[2] for evaluation and followup,[3] and for identifying educational needs and assessing outcomes.[2] Further testing will be needed to examine ecSI usefulness with other populations.

Research under the direction of the Barbara Lohse, PhD, RD, Pennsylvania State University, indicates that adults who score high on ecSI have indicators of better diets: They like a greater variety of food, are likely to eat meals and plan those meals to include all the food groups, and are likely to be in the post-action stage of change with respect to fruit and vegetable consumption. Adults who score high on ecSI have weights that tend toward the average—neither unusually high or unusually low. They are more satisfied with their weights, are less likely to cycle between dieting and not-dieting, and are less likely to have an unhealthy drive for thinness and tendency toward bulimia.[2] Adults who score high on ecSI show better health indicators: They have higher HDL, lower blood pressure, total cholesterol, LDL and triglycerides, and show fewer of the components of "sticky plaque," today's high-tech approach to predicting the tendency to cardiovascular disease.[4] Finally, adults who score high on ecSI appear to do better socially and emotionally. They feel more effective, are more self-aware and are more trusting and comfortable both with themselves and with other people.[2]

Categories and Questions

Each component of eating competence is essential in making up the whole. Questions relating to each component include:

> **Eating attitudes**: "I am relaxed about eating;" "I feel it okay to eat foods that I like."
> **Food acceptance skills**: "I experiment with new food and learn to like it."
> **Internal regulation skills**: "I eat as much as I am hungry for."
> **Contextual skills**: "I tune in to food and pay attention to myself when I eat;" I make time to eat."

Using ecSI

ecSI is a copyrighted instrument. Usage is available on a limited basis to projects that contribute toward developing and examining the instrument and furthering the study of the eating competence construct. It available by permission from the Ellyn Satter Foundation after an application process that includes an access fee. Gaining permission *for each intended usage* requires filling out a short application, available at **www.EllynSatterFoundation.org**, and agreeing to participate in the *ecSI Registry*. Registry information will be used to generate a picture of the usage of ecSatter and ecSI. While investigations thus far are highly encouraging, ecSI continues to be studied, clarified, and refined. ecSI Registry members are part of an experience and evaluation community.

References

1. Satter EM. Eating Competence: definition and evidence for the Satter Eating Competence Model. *J Nutr Educ Behav.* 2007;39 (suppl):S142-S153.
2. Lohse B, Satter E, Horacek T, Gebreselassie T, Oakland MJ. Measuring Eating Competence: psychometric properties and validity of the ecSatter Inventory. *J Nutr Educ Behav.* 2007;39 (suppl):S154-S166.
3. Stotts JL, Lohse B. Reliability of the ecSatter Inventory as a tool to measure eating competence. *J Nutr Educ Behav.* 2007;39 (suppl):S167-S170.
4. Psota T, Lohse B, West S. Associations between eating competence and cardiovascular disease biomarkers. *J Nutr Educ Behav.* 2007;39 (suppl):S171-S178.

Appendix
B
What the Research Says about Meals

Surveys show that structured and deliberate opportunities to eat are on the wane. Snacking and grazing—frequent, small food-intake occasions at irregular or unstructured times, often in association with other activities—now account for a significant proportion of daily calories.[1,2] A survey of almost 16,000 adults shows that about half have breakfast, lunch, and dinner, another 13 percent skip lunch, and still another 8 percent skip breakfast.[3] In a 2005 *Parade* survey, half of adults say they eat fewer than three meals a day. The majority describe as "homemade" a meal that combines fresh fare (such as steak) with convenience foods (bagged salads and frozen vegetables).[4] On any given day, about 60 percent of adults have a meal away from home, mostly at fast-food places. Those meals contribute about 25 percent of calories.[2]

Ninety-two percent of mothers of preschoolers surveyed by telephone by Central Michigan University Public Broadcasting report having family meals, 58 percent without the television.[5] Data from the Better Homes and Gardens Food Marketing Institute survey indicate that most families eat dinner together 4 or 5 days a week with about 10 percent eating together 2 or fewer days per week.[6] The Nurses' Health Study shows that among the offspring of subjects, more than half of 9-year-olds but fewer than one-third of 14-year-olds eat a family dinner every day.[7] A survey of almost 5,000 11- to 18-year-old middle school and high school students from ethnically and socioeconomically diverse communities in metropolitan Minneapolis/St Paul, Minnesota,

found the numbers to break down roughly by thirds: A scant third report having seven or more meals per week, a generous third report three to six, and a solid third have two or less. Fourteen percent of children report never having family meals.[8]

For households with children, the incidence of family meals decreases as children enter and move through the teen years. A 2007 survey conducted by Columbia University's National Center on Addiction and Substance Abuse found that while 50 percent of 12-year-olds said they had family dinner seven times per week, by age 17 only 27 percent reported that frequency of family dinners.[9]

Meals Support Nutritional Status

National Health and Nutrition Examination Survey (NHANES) respondents reporting three meals per day plus one or two snacks show superior dietary quality compared with breakfast skippers, who report two meals and one or two snacks.[3] For adults, a pattern of regular meals and snacks appears to be more metabolically desirable than today's increasingly common grazing pattern. Subjects who follow a regular meal pattern of six eating occasions per day compared with a random pattern of three to nine eating occasions have lower energy intake, greater post-prandial thermogenesis, and lower fasting total and LDL cholesterol. Peak insulin concentrations and the area under the curve of insulin responses to the test meal are lower after the regular meal pattern than after the irregular meal pattern.[10] Pregnant women who eat three meals and one or more snacks per day show a lower frequency of pre-term births compared with women who miss meals, snacks, or both.[11]

For middle and high school students, frequency of family meals is positively associated with intake of fruits, vegetables, grains, and calcium-rich foods and negatively associated with soft-drink consumption. Positive associations are also seen between frequency of family meals and energy, protein (percentage of total calories), calcium, iron, folate, fiber, and vitamins A, C, E, and B6.[12] The Nurse's Health Study cited earlier found similar positive associations between family meals and adolescents' nutritional status and further found that children and teens who eat dinner with their families consume less fat, soda, and fried foods.[7]

The benefit of family meals extends beyond adolescents' leaving home. Young adults who had family meals during adolescence assign importance to mealtime structure. They are likely to provide regular meals for themselves and to arrange for social eating occasions. They are also likely to have diets of high nutritional quality.[13] Social eating occasions attest to the importance placed on structured meals.

Meals Support Adolescent Social and Emotional Well-Being

Both adolescents and parents regard family meals as important. While they agree that it is difficult to find time for a family meal, they value family meals as a way of bringing family members together in an enjoyable way and providing a time for talking and listening.[14]

There is considerable evidence that children who have regular family meals do better socially and emotionally. A University of Michigan study of how 3- to 13-year-old children spend their time found that more meal time at home is the single strongest predictor of better achievement scores and fewer behavioral problems. Relative to children's positive outcome, meal time is far more powerful than time spent in school, studying, church, playing sports, and doing art activities. These results hold true regardless of the child's age, sex, race

and ethnicity, and regardless of the age and education of the head of the family, the family structure (two-parent, one-parent, multi-enerational), employment, income, and family size.[15]

The Minneapolis/St. Paul study found that as family meals and family connectedness go up, grade point average and self-esteem go up.[8] The Adolescent Health Study, a large, federally funded study of adolescence, found a strong association between regular family meals (five or more dinners per week with a parent) and academic success and psychological adjustment. Results hold for both one-parent and two-parent families and after controlling for social class.[16]

Children who have regular family meals show fewer negative indicators, as well. Five- to six-year-olds who have a higher meal frequency show a lower incidence of overweight.[17] The prevalence of overweight is reduced by 15 percent among 9- to 14-year-olds who eat a family dinner on "most days" or "every day" compared with those who eat a family dinner "never or some days."[18] As the regularity of family meals increases, rates of depression go down, as do suicidal ideation and attempts, cigarette and alcohol use, illegal drug use, and early sexual behavior.[8,16] The younger the adolescent, the stronger the relationship between lack of family dinners and substance abuse. Compared with 12-year-olds who have frequent family dinners, 12-year-olds who have infrequent family dinners are 6 times as likely to try marijuana, 4 1/2 times as likely to smoke cigarettes, and 1 1/2 times as likely to drink alcohol.[9]

Adolescents who report more frequent family meals, high priority for family meals, a positive atmosphere at family meals, and a more structured family meal environment are less likely to engage in disordered eating. Another Minneapolis/St. Paul study found that 18 percent of girls who report one to two family meals per week engage in extreme weight control behaviors compared with 9 percent of girls who report three to four family meals per week. Making family meals a priority in spite of scheduling difficulties emerges as the most consistent protective factor for disordered eating. Associations between family meal patterns and disordered eating behaviors tend to be stronger among girls than among boys.[19] Youngsters with mental health complaints eat less frequently with both parents than the youngsters in the comparison group do. They also share fewer activities and practice fewer family rituals than the families of the youngsters in the comparison group, and they show a lower level of satisfaction with the way their family functions.[20]

The evidence is compelling. As I told you in chapter 7, "Stuff to Know to Have Family Meals," the day-to-day routine of structured, sit-down family meals and snacks reassures children that they are loved and that they will be provided for—nutritionally and in all other ways.

References

1. Zizza C, Siega-Riz AM, Popkin BM. Significant increase in young adults' snacking between 1977-1978 and 1994-1996 represents a cause for concern! *Prev Med.* 2001;32:303-310.
2. Briefel RR, Johnson CL. Secular trends in dietary intake in the United States. *Annu Rev Nutr.* 2004;24:401-431.
3. Kerver JM, Yang EJ, Obayashi S, Bianchi L, Song WO. Meal and snack patterns are associated with dietary intake of energy and nutrients in US adults. *J Am Diet Assoc.* 2006;106:46-53.
4. Hales D. What America really eats. Mark Clements Research; Parade November 11, 2005.
5. Central Michigan University Public Broadcasting , Michigan Nutrition Network. *Telephone Interviews With the Low-Income Parents of Preschoolers: Pretest Evaluation of the "Healthy Lifestyles in Preschool Children" Project.* 2005.
6. Food Marketing Institute and Better Homes and Gardens. *MealWatch Survey.* Washington, D.C.: Research Department of FMI; 1995.
7. Gillman MW, Rifas-Shiman SL, Frazier AL, et al. Family dinner and diet quality among older children and adolescents. *Arch Fam Med.* 2000;9:235-240.
8. Eisenberg ME, Olson RE, Neumark-Sztainer D, Story M, Bearinger LH. Correlations between family meals and psychosocial well-being among adolescents. *Arch Pediatr Adolesc Med.* 2004;158:792-796.
9. National Center on Addiction and Substance Abuse at Columbia University (CASA). [Web site] *The Importance of Family Dinners IV.* New York, NY; September 2007. http//www.casacolumbia.org/ViewProduct.aspx?PRODUCTID={296A5E1E-B68F-44fa-A64D-95ABC1FB6CA0} Accessed April 25, 2008.
10. Farshchi HR, Taylor MA, Macdonald IA. Beneficial metabolic effects of regular meal frequency on dietary thermogenesis, insulin sensitivity, and fasting lipid profiles in healthy obese women. *Am J Clin Nutr.* 2005;81:16-24.
11. Siega-Riz AM , Herrmann T, Savitz DA, Thorp J. The frequency of eating during pregnancy and its effect on preterm delivery. *Am J Epidemiol.* 2001;153:647-652.
12. Neumark-Sztainer D, Hannan PJ, Story M, Croll J, Perry C. Family meal patterns: associations with sociodemographic characteristics and improved dietary intake among adolescents. *J Am Diet Assoc.* 2003;103:317-22.
13. Larson NI, Neumark-Sztainer D, Hannan PJ, Story M. Family meals during adolescence are associated with higher diet quality and healthful meal patterns during young adulthood. *J Am Diet Assoc.* 2007;107:1502-1510.
14. Fulkerson JA , Neumark-Sztainer D, Story M. Adolescent and parent views of family meals. *J Am Diet Assoc.* 2006;106:526-532.
15. Hofferth SL. How American children spend their time. *Journal of Marriage and the Family.* 2001;63:295-308.
16. Council of Economic Advisers to the President (CEAC) . *Teens and Their Parents in the 21st Century: An Examination of Trends in Teen Behavior and the Role of Parental Involvement.* 2000.
17. Toschke AM, Ruckinger S, Bohler E, Von Kries R. Adjusted population attributable fractions and preventable potential of risk factors for childhood obesity. *Public Health Nutr.* 2007;10:902-906.
18. Taveras EM, Rifas-Shiman SL, Berkey CS, et al. Family dinner and adolescent overweight. *Obes Res .* 2005;13:900-906.
19. Neumark-Sztainer D, Wall M, Story M, Fulkerson JA. Are family meal patterns associated with disordered eating behaviors among adolescents? *J Adolesc Health.* 2004;35:350-359.
20. Compan E, Moreno J, Ruiz MT, Pascual E. Doing things together: adolescent health and family rituals. *J Epidemiol Community Health.* 2002;56:89-94.

Appendix
C
What Surveys Say about Our Eating

Despite decades of emphasis on "healthy" food selection and lowered body weight in the Dietary Guidelines[1] and their operationalization by the Food Guide Pyramid (now MyPyramid),[2] only a third of today's consumers score an average of 70 or above on the 100-point Healthy Eating Index (HEI)[*] and only 20 percent get their 5-a-day of fruits and vegetables.[3] Adherence appears not to make us healthier. The Women's Health Initiative, which followed almost 50,000 women for 7 years, showed that women who follow a low-fat diet high in fruits and vegetables are no thinner and have no fewer health problems than those who don't.[4] Body weights have continued to increase[5] despite the fact that currently 60–80 percent of adults[6] and over 65 percent of adolescents[7] are restricting food intake to lose or maintain body weight.

While eating attitudes are not addressed in either the Dietary Guidelines[1] or MyPyramid,[2] it appears that current nutrition policy is having unintended negative consequences with respect to eating attitudes. As early as 15 years ago, the American public expressed considerable ambivalence about adhering to nutrition standards. Over half of respondents in an ADA-commissioned Gallup poll said that eating a healthy diet took too much work. While consumers report enjoying eating, 36 percent say factoring in health takes the fun out of it and that they feel guilty about eating the foods they like.[8] In general, consumers say they don't want to give up the food they like and think a healthy diet takes too much time.[9] Surveys capture the tension created by the expectation of pleasure on the one hand, and guilt about taking pleasure on the other. In the 2005 *Parade* survey, "What America Really Eats," respondents report eating a "healthy mix" of foods, then indulging in snacks and "pleasure foods" as rewards.[**] Fifty-nine percent say they are "familiar with the Food Guide Pyramid" but "do not really follow it."[10]

That discord between the expectation of pleasure from eating and guilt about taking that pleasure is regularly measured by the American Dietetic Association Survey of

---

[*] HEI is a 10-component scale measuring degree of compliance with the Dietary Guidelines and MyPyramid. Five of the components measure adherence to recommended amounts of low-fat grains, vegetables, fruits, milk, and meat. Two of the components directly measure restriction and avoidance of components that contribute flavor: fat and salt. Two measure adherence to recommended amounts of saturated fat, and cholesterol. One measures variety and assigns points based on eating 16 different food items over 3 days in recommended serving amounts.

[**] *Parade* commissioned Mark Clements Research to administer the "What America Really Eats® 2005 Survey" by mail in March 2005. The results are based on a national sample of 2,088 adults, aged 18–65, and selected to conform to the latest U.S. Census data. Findings are projectable to all households nationally, with results accurate to within ±2.2 percent at the 95 percent level of confidence.

Dietary Habits, first done in 1991 and repeated periodically ever since. Survey respondents numerically rank both the importance they *assign* to adhering to nutritional standards and their actual *behavior* in selecting foods that conform to nutritional standards. The respondents break roughly into three groups: "I know I should, but …", "I'm already doing it," and "don't bother me." For the "I know I should, but …" group, which accounts for an increasing percentage of survey respondents, the gap between personal standards and actual behavior is 34 percent. For the "I'm already doing it" group, who see their nutritional behavior as being exemplary, the gap is 15 percent. Not surprisingly, the "don't bother me" group, who profess to assign no value to nutritional standards, report a small gap between internalized standards and actual behavior—only 9 percent.[11]

Interestingly, the "don't bother me" attitudes about food selection are positive; those respondents just don't get worked up about it. When asked to rate the importance of nutrition on a scale of 1 to 7, 62 percent of the "don't bother me" group assign a score of 5 or more. I could settle for that. When asked how careful they are in selecting what they eat to achieve a healthy diet, 89 percent assign a score of 4 or more out of 7. That sounds reasonable to me. Eating is, after all, only one of life's great issues. Conversely, 60 percent of the "already doing it" group check the box that says it is important to check *every* food item for nutritional content. Think of it! Every food item! That makes shopping quite a chore!

We have become more focused on the nutritional and other healthful qualities of our food—or concerned about negatives in the food supply. It need not be so, as evidenced by differences in attitudes among adults and college students from Flemish Belgium, France, the United States, and Japan. Generally, the Americans are most food-health-oriented and least food-pleasure-oriented, the French are the opposite on both counts, and the Japanese are somewhere in the middle. In all four countries, women are most likely to resemble the Americans. Ironically, the Americans, who do the most to alter their diet in the

service of health, are the least likely to classify themselves as healthy eaters.[12]

In spite of the advice that bombards consumers about following the nutrition rules, and in spite of the fact that some consumers have made following rules their nutritional priority, most still seek pleasure and predictability. A national survey based out of the University of Hawaii indicates clearly that for most consumers, taste is still the most important influence on food choices, followed by cost and convenience.[13] The question, of course, is whether consumers feel comfortable making taste the priority. The gaps we just talked about between nutritional goals and actual behavior indicate that no, they do not. Certainly, nutrition professionals do not feel comfortable with that priority, as indicated by the comment in the discussion section of the Hawaiian survey article that, given the importance assigned to taste by consumers, nutrition educators need to "stress the good taste of healthful foods." The assumption, of course, is that there is a contradiction between good nutrition and good taste.

Despite their disagreement on whether the evidence supports making disease prevention an appropriate priority for national nutrition policy, nutrition enthusiasts and moderates do agree that the nutritional bottom line is positive: to sustain life and support vitality. Attitudinally, at least, that nutritional bottom line is being eroded. In a 2003 survey by the Food Marketing Institute on the nature of concerns about nutritional content, the primary concern for 40 percent of respondents was dietary fat avoidance (down from 59 percent in 1998), with concern about nutritional value of food at 12 percent and a "desire to be healthy and eat what's good for us" assigned priority by so few that the numbers were not statistically significant.[14]

While fat restriction originated as a disease-avoidance tactic, in the minds of many professionals and consumers, fat avoidance has become synonymous with weight management. While the effectiveness of fat restriction as a means of weight management continues to be debated, the epidemiological evidence is clear: As the percentage of fat in diets has gone down,[15] body weights have gone up.[5]

References

1. U.S. Department of Health and Human Services and U.S. Department of Agriculture. *Dietary Guidelines for Americans, 2005.* Washington, DC: U.S. Government Printing Office; January 2005. http://www.health.gov/dietaryguidelines/dga2005/document/default.htm. Accessed December 12, 2007.

2. U.S. Department of Agriculture. MyPyramid Plan [Web page]. http://www.mypyramid.gov/mypyramid/index.aspx. Accessed December 12, 2007.

3. Center for Nutrition Policy and Promotion. Healthy Eating Index [Web page]. U.S. Department of Agriculture Web site. http://www.cnpp.usda.gov/HealthyEatingIndex.htm. Accessed December 12, 2007.

4. Howard BV, Manson JE, Stefanick ML, et al. Low-fat dietary pattern and weight change over 7 years: the Women's Health Initiative dietary modification trial. *JAMA.* 2006;295:39-49.

5. Ogden CL, Carroll MD, Curtin LR, McDowell MA, Tabak CJ, Flegal KM. Prevalence of overweight and obesity in the United States, 1999-2004. *JAMA.* 2006;295:1549-1555.

6. Serdula MK, Mokdad AH, Williamson DF, Galuska DA, Mendlein JM, Heath GW. Prevalence of attempting weight loss and strategies for controlling weight. *JAMA.* 1999;282:1353-1358.

7. Neumark-Sztainer D*, Hannan P, Story M, Perry C. Weight-control behaviors among adolescent girls and boys: implications for dietary intake. *J Am Diet Assoc.* 2004;104:913-920.

8. Wellman N. The good and the bad: how Americans are making food choices. *Nutrition News.* 1990;53:1-3.

9. American Dietetic Association. *Survey of American Dietary Habits.* Chicago, IL: The American Dietetic Association; 1997.

10. Hales D. What America really eats. *Parade Magazine.* November 13, 2005:. http://www.parade.com/archive.jsp. Accessed December 12, 2007.

11. American Dietetic Association. *Nutrition Trends 2002: Final Report of Findings.* Chicago, IL: The American Dietetic Association; 2002.

12. Rozin P, Fischler C, Imada S, Sarubin A, Wrzesniewski A. Attitudes to food and the role of food in life in the U.S.A., Japan, Flemish Belgium and France: possible implications for the diet-health debate. *Appetite.* 1999;33:163-180.

13. Glanz K, Basil M, Maibach E, Goldberg J, Snyder D. Why Americans eat what they do: taste, nutrition, cost, convenience, and weight control concerns as influences on food consumption. *J Am Diet Assoc.* 1998;98:1118-1126.

14. FMI Research Department; Trends in the United States. Consumer Attitudes and the Supermarket. Washington, DC: Food Marketing Institute; 2003:72.

15. Briefel RR, Johnson CL. Secular trends in dietary intake in the United States. *Annu Rev Nutr.* 2004;24:401-431.

Appendix

D

BMI, Mortality, Morbidity, and Health: Resolving the Weight Dilemma

Our predicament with weight is that at the same time as we are being told by health policy makers—repeatedly and with a great deal of judgment and urgency—that any degree of overweight is medically dangerous, there is no successful method for reducing and maintaining a lowered body weight. In fact, weight loss tends to have a boomerang effect: Most people regain lost weight and many gain to a higher level with each loss-regain cycle. That pattern of weight instability is likely to be associated with negative health outcomes. But the policy makers say that overweight is so dangerous that it is better to lose and regain than to not lose at all. Those are the same policy makers who set the cutoff point for defining overweight at BMI (Kg/M^2) 24.9, which is essentially the population average. One is reminded of the quandary of Sisyphus, the Greek who was condemned by the gods to an eternity of continually pushing a boulder up a mountain, only to have it roll down again.

To free ourselves from the weight dilemma, we must stop going along with what we are told, and instead make up our own minds about the issues. Because it is so involved to address the issues related to overweight and health, this appendix is long and complex. What *is* normal body weight? What are the true consequences of having an "above-normal" BMI? What are the consequences of trying to force BMI below its biologically preferred level? What are the alternatives—realistic and achievable approaches to addressing the issue of weight and health?

Normal Body Weight

Before you read this next section, prepare to be astonished. The logic about body weight and the lack of logic about weight standards are so obvious that you may wonder how anybody could believe otherwise.

Except for moderate increases related to aging, the natural adult tendency is to achieve and maintain a constitutionally determined BMI. Biological characteristics are distributed in nature according to the bell-shaped curve illustrated in figure D.1.

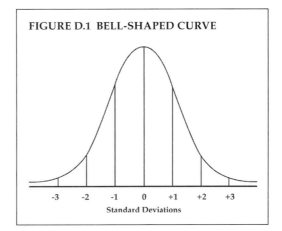

FIGURE D.1 BELL-SHAPED CURVE

Standard Deviations

The principle of the bell-shaped curve applies, for instance, to energy requirement, blood pressure and height, and, with a caveat, to weight. The principle means that the biological value in question simply *is*; there is no right or wrong to it. Being close to the mean is not superior to being far away from it. You simply have more company if your characteristic, whatever it is, puts you close to the mean. To make more sense of this explanation, take a quick look at biology professor Dr. Gregory Pryor's Web site.[1] To demonstrate the principle of the bell curve distribution, Pryor arranged the students in his biology class on the school bleachers in order of height, from shortest to tallest.

The statistical principle of the bell curve is that 68 percent of values are at the mean or within 1 standard deviation (SD) above or below the mean (which on the bell curve is the same as the average), approximately 95 percent are within 2 SD above or below the mean, and 99.9 percent are within 3 SD above or below the mean.[2] For adults, BMI 25 is roughly at the mean with a standard deviation of 4. That small standard deviation means that there isn't a lot of variation above or below the average value. BMI 29 is approximately +1 SD (that is, 1 standard deviation above the mean), BMI 33 is +2 SD, and BMI 37 is +3 SD. Running the figures in the opposite direction, BMI 21 is –1 SD (1 standard deviation below the mean), BMI 17 is –2 SD, and BMI 13 is –3 SD.[3] The last figure is biologically improbable.

What I don't show on figure D.1 is that BMI distribution is somewhat skewed toward the upper end. That is, the tail trails out farther to the right than in the picture because a few people's BMIs are 4, 5, or even 6 SD above the mean. The curve is imbalanced because the tail doesn't trail out to the left in the same way. It couldn't. If your BMI were that low, you would be dead. This is not to say that BMIs in that long upward-trailing tail are the result of a genetically normal distribution. In my experience, people get that heavy because of serious and chronic distortions in feeding and eating that likely exacerbate a genetic tendency to gain excess weight.

The point of this lesson in statistics is that the cutoff points for adult overweight are set so low that half of us are diagnosable as being overweight. In my opinion, this is as illogical as saying half of Dr. Pryor's students are too tall—or too short. In other words, overweight diagnosis is a numbers and semantics construct that pathologizes what is in most cases a normal, genetically determined BMI. Except for moderate increases related to aging, the natural adult tendency is to achieve and maintain a unique and constitutionally determined BMI. Large parents tend to have large babies who grow up to be large children and large adults.[4] Because it is biologically preferred, the body defends this BMI with numerous processes including hunger, appetite, and satiety on the *in* side and metabolic processes that conserve or squander energy on the *out* side. (Appendix E, "Energy Balance and Weight," addresses these processes.) In short, advice to maintain weight at BMI 24.9 or below is literally impossible to follow for a large proportion of the population.

BMI and Mortality

The mortality studies—the ones that correlate death with lifestyle and physical characteristics—clearly indicate that above-average BMIs are not as lethal as we have been led to believe. Among the government agencies that promote the BMI cutoff point of 24.9 is the Centers for Disease Control and Prevention (CDC). Thus, there was a delicious irony in the huge and prestigious study that was done by the CDC's own Katherine Flegal, who led a team of statisticians in analyzing National Health and Nutrition Examination Survey data of hundreds of thousands of people like you and me. Flegal's analysis, which is summarized in figure D.2, clearly indicates that people who have BMIs within 1 or 2 SD above the mean show no greater mortality than those whose BMI is closer to the mean. Compared with the "normal" BMI of 18 to 24.9, BMIs of 25 to <30 correlate with a slight *decrease* in relative risk of mortality in 25-to-59-year-olds, and BMI 30 to <35 correlates with only a slight increase in mortality. For people age 60 and older, and particularly for people above 70 years old, the differences are even more slight.

Mortality risk appears to increase significantly at BMIs above 35,[5] but when BMIs above 35 are further broken down statistically into the 35-to-40 and the 40-plus categories, mortality risk increases most notably at or above BMI 40. In the context of all the worry about overweight and the lack of worry about underweight, it is striking that excess mortality associated with BMIs below 18.5 for people up to age 60 is higher than the excess mortality in the BMI 30 to 35 category. For people age 60 and older, mortality in the under-18.5 BMI category is far higher than that in the BMI 35-plus category.[6]

FIGURE D.2 RELATIVE RISK OF EXCESS DEATHS ASSOCIATED WITH UNDERWEIGHT, OVER-WEIGHT, AND OBESITY

Age	BMI				
	Under 18.5	18.5 to <25	25 to <30	30 to <35	Over 35
25 to 59	1.38	1.00	0.83	1.20	1.83
60 to 69	2.30	1.00	0.95	1.13	1.63
70 and older	1.69	1.00	0.91	1.03	1.17

Source: Flegal KM, Graubard BI, Williamson DF, Gail MH. Excess deaths associated with underweight, overweight, and obesity. JAMA. 2005;293:1861–1867.

The release of Flegal's analysis was greeted with a delightful assortment of reactions. The weight-loss enthusiasts warned that a public freed from fear of the consequences of overeating and weight gain would throw away all constraints with eating. "For those of us who enjoy a full menu of choices and don't like to be hectored about what to eat, things are looking up," chortled the Center for Consumer Freedom, a group financed by the food industry. Then there was the statistical bickering. Critics of the analysis raised arcane issues related to which subjects were kept in or thrown out in the statistical analysis—criticism that was successfully refuted by Flegal and her colleagues.[7] Other critics claimed that higher morbidity with lower BMI was the result of recent weight loss—that people in the lower BMI categories were truly fat people whose weights were temporarily or recently lowered. Flegal and her colleagues pointed out that only 2 percent of those age 65 and older in the BMI 18.5 to 24.9 range had been obese 10 years previously, and 6 percent in the BMI 25 to <30 range had been obese 10 years previously.[8] Ironically, this bit of information gives still more evidence of the body's tenacity with respect to defending its preferred body weight.

Irony on irony—from the howls of protest that greeted the Flegal study, it seemed as if this information was new and unexpected. In reality, since 1992, five other huge and well-conducted studies *that I know of* have reported highly similar results.[6,9-12]

BMI and Morbidity

Despite this convincing data on mortality and body weight, health policy defines overweight and obesity as independent risk factors for heart disease and diabetes or metabolic syndrome and sets the cutoff point for overweight at BMI 24.9. "Independent risk factor" means that high body weight, in and of itself, causes disease. Metabolic syndrome is a combination of symptoms that correlate with increased cardiovascular disease or diabetes: elevated blood sugar or type 2 diabetes, high blood pressure, overweight with fat deposits mainly around the waist, decreased HDL cholesterol, and elevated triglycerides.

This contradiction between evidence and policy arises from the tendency of policy makers to ignore the mortality studies and the secular trends and concentrate instead on *morbidity* studies and epidemiological studies—both of which *correlate* degenerative disease with high body weight.[13] Before we discuss those studies, consider that the process of arriving at health policy with respect to overweight and obesity is very much the same as the process I describe in appendix L, "Diet and Degenerative Disease: It's Not as Bad as You Think." It is a matter of consensus, which means that dissenting points of view and evidence to the contrary are minimized. Also consider that the operative word is *correlate*, meaning that high body weight and disease are linked statistically. It does not mean that a cause-and-effect relationship has been established. The definition of obesity as an independent risk factor for disease originated with the 1985 National Institutes of Health (NIH) Consensus Conference on Overweight. There were many thoughtful and responsible scientists and health professionals at the conference who disagreed with the conclusion, among them epidemiologist Elizabeth Barrett-Connor, who understood clearly the limitations of epidemiological studies and wrote a persuasive dissenting paper.[14]

Many thoughtful and responsible people have disagreed ever since. Morbidity studies suffer from the bias of the Pygmalion effect: the self-fulfilling prophecy based on selective perception. If I expect something to happen, I am likely to find evidence to confirm my expectations. Diagnosticians expect a *high body weight = disease* connection, so they look more carefully for illness in people of size.[17] Secular trends in weight and risk factors for disease clearly belie the association between weight and health. As the rate of overweight (BMI greater than 24.9) between 1970 and 2000 went up from 45 to 68 percent, the rate of hypertension decreased from 40 to 29 percent and the incidence of elevated blood cholesterol decreased from 29 to 18 percent.[15]

The morbidity and epidemiological studies supporting health policy suffer from the flaws outlined in appendix P, "Interpreting the News." They are preliminary studies; most of them are epidemiological, show correlations rather than cause and effect, give relative rather than actual numbers, use statistical processes and comparisons that overstate the evidence, and draw conclusions that are not supported by their own data. With the exception of diabetes, the actual numbers in studies that claim impressive correlations between high body weight and disease are low.[16]

Correlations between high BMI and diabetes are relatively strong, but those correlations are frequently reported in relative rather than absolute numbers, which exaggerates the negative effects of overweight. The correlational data is also discussed as if the relationship between high BMI and diabetes is one of cause and effect: that diabetes is *caused* by the high body weight. There is no evidence to support that. It is equally possible that some other factor—one that has not yet been identified and therefore not examined or correlated—causes the metabolic thriftiness that is characteristic of diabetes. It is also possible that high body weight and diabetes are both caused by something altogether different that we don't yet know about. For instance, preliminary studies *correlate* low intakes of vitamin D and calcium from dairy products and a modest increase in the incidence of type 2 diabetes.[15] Since the 1970s, our intake of milk and other high-calcium foods has progressively decreased; currently only 20 percent of us consume enough.[15]

CONSIDER THE INDIVIDUAL
The *high body weight = disease* connection is by no means universal, nor is it as malignant as we have been led to believe. Stanford University

researchers studying 211 subjects in the BMI 30–35 category found insulin resistance—an indication of prediabetes—to vary sixfold. Metabolic indicators—blood pressure, blood glucose, blood triglycerides, and high-density lipoproteins—varied along with insulin resistance, although all metabolic indicators for all BMI categories were within normal ranges. When compared with the most insulin-sensitive third, the most insulin-*in*sensitive (that is, insulin-resistant) third of the population had higher systolic and diastolic blood pressures, more prevalent impaired glucose tolerance (47 percent versus 2 percent), higher triglycerides, and lower high-density lipoproteins.[17] In other words, just because your BMI is above the cutoff point, it doesn't mean that you are unhealthy. I remember fondly two of my over-40-BMI patients—roommates who came to their sessions together—laughing hilariously at the desperation of their lipophobic doctor to find something medically wrong with them. He couldn't.

But, I digress. The nature of scientific inquiry is that it groups experimental subjects and thereby irons out differences. Most studies put everyone of similar weights in the same category rather than distinguishing among individuals within the category. But even such a study by CDC statisticians found that relative to the reference weight category (BMI 18.5 to 24.9), overweight (BMI 25 to 30) was associated with only *modest* increases in the percentage showing risk factors for heart disease: elevated total cholesterol (over 240 mg/dL), high blood pressure (systolic above 140 or diastolic above 70), and diabetes.[18] Even with these modest results, the study design creates misconceptions. Failing to distinguish among individuals in a given category means that those who show distorted values contaminate the whole category. Moreover, researchers failed to distinguish among categories. They lumped everyone into the over-30 BMI category rather than breaking it down into 30–<35, 35–<40, and over 40. People whose BMI is over 40 *do* unquestionably have a higher risk that, when pooled together with everyone else in the over-30 BMI category, contributes statistically to the average risk.

Why the Alarums and Excursions?

In case you don't know the meaning of this useful expression, it means "clamor, excitement, and feverish or disordered activity."[19] In response to the obesity hysteria, we engage in a great deal of desperate and disordered activity to remedy a problem that is nowhere near as bad and dangerous as we think it is. The *high body weight = disease* connection is by no means clear, and even if it were, the mortality data *is* clear that high body weight isn't lethal. We know for sure only that *some* people who have an exceptionally high BMI may have an increased risk of degenerative disease and death, the same as some people whose BMI is closer to the mean.

So what keeps the idea alive that any degree of overweight is unhealthy? Vested interests. The people who cling most tightly to the idea that high body weight is malignant get something out of it, whether it is personal or professional. The personal is easy to define: It feeds bigotry in general and a sense of moral superiority among those who happen to be genetically favored with lower body weights and need to make something of it. It is the concept of "born on third and thinks he hit a triple."

The professional investment is enormous, diverse, and therefore difficult to define—funding, publishing, reporting, weight-loss business, professional recognition. There is a *lot* of grant money available for those who study obesity. Funding agencies and consensus panels are peopled by those who believe the conventional wisdom that *high body weight = disease*. The same conventional-model people show up on the editorial boards of journals, and authors may spin their data to make it seem to support the conventional wisdom. The media has a great appetite for the idea that overweight kills and gives selective attention and placement to stories that support that idea.

Weight reduction is big business, whether you are talking about commercial weight-loss organizations, drug companies, or publishing. Conventional-model obesity researchers, consultants, and policy makers get money from those big businesses. The weight-loss industry held its breath while the NIH-convened National Task Force on the Prevention and Treatment of Obesity was considering the relationships among dieting, weight loss, weight cycling, eating disorders, and psychological functioning in overweight and obese adults. There was a collective sigh of relief in that industry when the task force concluded that, while dieting may be associated with weight cycling, it causes minimal harm with respect to eating attitudes and behaviors as well as

psychological functioning. The task force acknowledged that "nondieting" approaches are associated with improvements in mood and self-esteem but negated those approaches on the grounds that weight loss is generally minimal. Their conclusion: It is better to lose and regain than to not lose at all.[20] In other words, business as usual.

Nature or Nurture?

The discussion about the bell curve tells us the genetic truth: Not everyone is constitutionally endowed with slimness. Many people, through no fault of their own or anyone else, have BMIs that are naturally higher than those deemed acceptable by the policy makers and the fashion industry. But the conventional-model argument countering this discussion about the *nature* of weight is that we, as a nation, are getting fatter. There are clearly environmental factors making us fatter, the argument goes, and those environmental factors must be addressed by getting us to eat less and move more.

To a point, the argument is valid. My clinical work with children as well as adults indicates that many people *are* heavier than nature intended them to be. I write about this in detail in *Your Child's Weight*.[21] Every child is born with a powerful ability to regulate food intake and a strong and resilient tendency to grow in the way that nature intended for him or her. However, distortions in feeding and parenting can overwhelm a child's powerful natural tendencies and distort growth, causing a child's weight to falter or to accelerate.

The biggest culprit in children's weight acceleration is the weight cycling associated with weight-reduction dieting. People of all ages whose food intake is restricted tend to reactively overeat and regain weight, often to a higher level. The policy-based standard of universal slimness leads parents to conclude—often on the instigation of health professionals—that their large but normal infants and children are too fat and to attempt to slim them down. Only the most determined, thick-skinned, and relentless parents can ignore a hungry child's pleas for food and maintain consistent underfeeding. More tuned-in and empathetic parents are incapable of underfeeding and either impose the weight-reduction effort sporadically or give it up altogether. While setting aside weight-reduction efforts minimizes the damage, parents are left feeling ashamed of their own "failure" and mistrusting of their child's normal growth processes. Thus, the child's eating attitudes and behaviors become distorted.

Many adults who are chronic dieters are the product of such early efforts to force weight loss. When they are adolescents or even pre-adolescents, they take up the endeavor for themselves and continue the same cycles of restraint and disinhibition, weight loss and regain. Three-quarters of adolescent boys and girls diet to try to lose weight; their efforts make them fatter, not thinner.[22] The struggle continues into adult life. The 1999 Behavioral Risk Factor Surveillance Survey found 64 percent of men and 78 percent of women are trying to lose or maintain weight.[23] While one could argue that what is *normative* is *normal*, the fact remains that restrained eating is an ineffective approach to regulating food intake and body weight. Not only are attempts to maintain body weight below biologically preferred levels unsuccessful,[24] but such attempts likely contribute to tendencies to overeat and gain weight in the population as a whole. Systems of externally dictated food management, particularly when they mandate negative energy balance, are fundamentally fragile and inconsistent because they activate the body's physiological and psychological defense mechanisms. Among those counter-regulatory mechanisms is gaining excess weight and accumulating excess fat subsequent to food restriction.[25] Repeated weight loss and regain is accompanied by sequentially increasing body weight.[26]

RESTRAINED EATING

Restrained eating is the attempt to eat less food or less-appealing food than desired in the attempt to lose weight or maintain a lowered body weight. The research is clear that restrained eating profoundly disrupts eating attitudes and behaviors as well as destabilizes body weight. Rather than overeating *per se* in response to stressors, restrained eaters *suspend restraint*: They stop undereating. Then, because restraint has been violated, rather than simply eating enough to satisfy hunger, they go on to overeat. Irrespective of weight, restrained eaters consume more when stressed or depressed compared with nonrestrained eaters, who tend to consume less under stress.[27] Restrained eaters consume more food after an identifiably high-calorie preload and when exposed to palatable "forbidden" food.[28] They also consume relatively large amounts in response to stress,[29]

or even when doing exacting intellectual tasks.[29,30] The degree of distortion resulting from restrained eating appears to depend on the degree of restriction. Compared with rigid control, flexible control is associated with lower disinhibition (less frequent and less severe binge-eating episodes), lower overall self-reported energy intake, and lower BMI.[31] That is, eating distortion still exists with flexible control, it just is not as great.

Even people who say they are nonrestrained eaters show signs of having been conditioned to overeat by prior restraint or conditions that mimic restraint. Unreliable availability of food mimics food restriction and creates the tendency to eat greater amounts when food is plentiful. A Continuing Survey of Food Intakes by Individuals of 4,509 women shows that the prevalence of overweight increases as food insecurity increases, from 34 percent of the 3,447 who are food-secure, to 41 percent of the 966 who are mildly food-insecure, to 52 percent of the 86 who are moderately food-insecure.[32] Distinctions among levels of food insecurity have to do with the proportion of time that food is in short supply.

Experimental subjects eat more than usual when they are led to anticipate restraint[33] and after a short-term weight-reduction intervention.[34] Analysis of weekend versus weekday dietary recall data in the Continuing Survey of Food Intakes by Individuals shows that 19- to 50-year-olds eat more on the weekend than on weekdays: an average of 115 calories a day.[35] When given yogurt of consistent fat content, healthy women who do *not* label themselves as dieters or restrained eaters eat more yogurt when it is labeled low-fat. They also consume more during a subsequent lunch meal after eating the yogurt labeled low-fat than they do after they receive the same yogurt either unlabeled or labeled high-fat.[36] Apparently the women respond to the low-fat label by disinhibiting their eating—by taking license to ignore internal regulators and eat larger quantities.

To summarize our nature vs. nurture discussion, from the perspective of the destructive impact of situationally or self-imposed food insufficiency, today's obesity "crisis" is to a great extent an iatrogenic condition: It is physician-induced. In this case, the "physician" is health policy, but the fact remains: We are becoming too fat because we are being told we are too fat and that we must do something about it.

WEIGHT STABILITY

Thus, it appears that in the process of trying to outwit and overwhelm Mother Nature, we are paying the price with respect to being heavier than nature intended us to be. A number of well-conducted studies indicate that we are also paying the price with respect to health and longevity. Below-average-weight boys who become average weight, moderately overweight, or markedly overweight men have twice the incidence of cardiovascular disease of the general population of men, whereas above-average-weight boys who maintain the same relative weight level have only an average risk.[37] Boys whose BMIs accelerate from childhood to adulthood are more likely to show adult metabolic syndrome.[38] Women's Health Initiative participants who report weight cycling have triple the risk of renal cell carcinoma compared with women whose weight is stable. Weight cycling is defined as losing and regaining 10 pounds or more at least 10 times in adult life.[39]

A summary of reports from 11 diverse population studies, 7 from the United States and 4 from Europe, show the lowest mortality rates to be generally associated with modest weight gains of the sort that are normally associated with aging. It is normal to have about a 5 percent increase in BMI for each decade. The highest mortality rates occur in adults who have either lost weight or had pronounced weight gains.[40] In the Iowa Women's Health Study of almost 35,000 women, those who have had a 10 percent or more weight loss or weight fluctuation show the greatest number of risk indicators for cardiovascular disease, diabetes, and cancer. Women who have lost weight and maintained it have a 70 percent higher risk of death from heart disease but not from cancer. Even if they are heavy, the women whose weight is by definition stable—fluctuating less than 5 percent up or down—have fewer overall risk indicators.[41]

Twenty-three-year follow-up data from the prestigious Framingham Study shows that subjects who have highly variable body weights have increased total mortality from coronary heart disease. The researchers concluded that the increase in cardiovascular disease in obese patients can be entirely explained by taking two facts into account. First, obese people are more likely to go up and down in weight than thin people. Second, weight cycling is associated with increased rates of death from cardiovascular disease.[42] Research at the Cooper Institute in Houston followed the death statistics on 10,529

men 35–57 years old who were in the upper 10 to 15 percent of risk for heart disease by virtue of being overweight and having high blood pressure and high cholesterol. The men whose weights had remained stable had a lower likelihood of premature death than those whose weights changed. Men who had lost more than 5 percent of their body weight had a 61–242 percent higher mortality than men whose weights remained within 5 percent of their initial body weight. (That is not a typographical error nor is that figure missing a decimal. It is *242* percent.) In a subgroup of men who were 20 pounds or more above average weight (BMIs between 26 and 29), a 5 percent weight loss correlated with a 195 percent increase in cardiovascular disease mortality compared with men of similar BMIs who did not lose weight.[43]

Define the Problem in a Way That It Can Be Solved

The data on BMI tell us that the range associated with positive outcomes is broader than we have been led to believe. The mortality and morbidity data thoroughly undermine the *high body weight = disease (and death)* assumption. It is weight *instability*, not high weight *per se*, that appears to be the culprit. Thus, we arrive at a conclusion of crashing irony: In trying to force body weight below its biologically preferred level, we are creating the very medical problems we have been told weight loss will address.

What shall we do instead of striving for weight loss? Set aside weight loss as an outcome indicator—it can't be achieved anyway. The modest increases in health risks associated with high BMI can be dealt with on an individual basis and independent of weight loss. Instead of trying for weight loss, focus on improving your health behaviors. Establish goals that *can* be achieved:

- Develop and maintain eating competence.
- Develop sustainable patterns of activity.
- Learn to feel good about yourself, just as you are.

EATING COMPETENCE

Our survey data tell us that people who have higher eating competence have better health indicators—blood lipids, blood glucose, blood pressure.[44] Will improving your eating competence improve your metabolic parameters? Maybe, maybe not. Will improving your eating competence make you live longer? We don't know yet.

People with higher eating competence have higher levels of body satisfaction and lower levels of psychosocial dysfunction.[45] Will improving your eating competence improve your body satisfaction and psychosocial functioning? It is possible. Becoming eating competent implies a degree of self-knowledge and self-acceptance, and that can make you feel better about yourself and allow you to be more effective in the world.

Clinical data give some encouragement of benefits from developing eating competence. People who replace restraint and disinhibition with eating competence stabilize weight, improve eating attitudes and behaviors and physical self-esteem, and decrease blood lipids.[46] Less comprehensive Health at Every Size interventions that suspend restraint, institute internally regulated eating, and obviate weigh loss as an outcome variable still produce weight stability, improve physical self-esteem and self-esteem overall, decrease blood pressure and blood lipids, and decrease eating disorder pathology.[47]

ACTIVITY

The data on activity are clear. Low fitness is an independent predictor of mortality in all BMI groups after adjustment for other mortality predictors. For fit men, all-cause mortality rates are essentially the same across all BMI categories.[48] For men, with respect to all-cause mortality, it is better to be fit and fat than unfit and lean.[49] For women, the relationships are not as clear, primarily because until age 80 years and over, women's heart attack rate is so low that it is difficult to make predictions.[50,51] However, regular activity decreases blood pressure in both men and women.[52]

PHYSICAL SELF-ESTEEM

In my clinical work, I have found that developing eating competence improves physical self-esteem, particularly for people whose self-esteem is not that low to begin with. Getting a sense that you can trust your body and yourself to manage food intake neutralizes a great deal of the demoralization that goes along with having a high BMI and with being caught in a relentless and fruitless struggle to lose weight.

However, physical self-esteem is closely tied up with self-esteem overall. If physical self-esteem is particularly low, it will only yield to psychotherapy or corrective life experience.

What is the bottom line? Question health policy. According to Australian Health Sciences professors Lily O'Hara and Jane Gregg, framing body weight as the source of health problems—the weight-centered health paradigm that currently rules—does harm in the form of body dissatisfaction, weight-reduction dieting, disordered eating, weight discrimination, and even death resulting from extreme demoralization and extreme weight-loss methods.[53] To keep from being caught by this weight dilemma, work *with* your body rather than *against* it. Eat well and joyfully, move your body in a way that you enjoy and can sustain, develop loyalty and respect for your body, and stop postponing living until you get thin. I have seen far too many attractive, talented, charming people go through life feeling handicapped and ashamed of themselves because their weight is high. What a waste! Don't let it happen to you!

References

1. Pryor, G. S. Class photo at Ben Hill Griffin Stadium ("The Swamp" at UF, 2001) [Web page]. Francis Marion University Web site. http://acsweb.fmarion.edu/Pryor/bellcurve.htm. Accessed December 13, 2007.
2. Niles, R. Standard deviation [Web page]. Robert Niles Web site. http://www.robertniles.com/stats/stdev.shtml.
   Accessed December 13, 2007.
3. Najjar MF, Rowland M; BMI for females and males 28-74 years of age: tables 10 and 11. *Vital and Health Statistics, Series 11, No 238, DHHS Pub. No. (PHS) 87-1688.* Washington, D.C.: Public Health Service; 1987:21-22.
4. Stettler N, Zemel BS, Kumanyika S, Stallings VA. Infant weight gain and childhood overweight status in a multicenter, cohort study. *Pediatrics.* 2002;109:194-199.
5. Flegal KM, Graubard BI, Williamson DF, Gail MH. Excess deaths associated with underweight, overweight, and obesity. *JAMA.* 2005;293:1861-1867.
6. Bender R, Trautner C, Spraul M, Berger M. Assessment of excess mortality in obesity. *Am J Epidemiol.* 1998;147:42-48.

7. Flegal KM, Graubard BI, Williamson DF, Gail MH. Impact of smoking and preexisting illness on estimates of the fractions of deaths associated with underweight, overweight, and obesity in the US population. Am J Epidemiol. 2007;166:975-982.

8. Flegal KM, Williamson DF, Pamuk ER. Flegal, et. al. respond. Am J Public Health. 2005;95:932-a, 933.

9. Troiano RP, Frongillo EAJr, Sobal J, Levitsky DA. The relationship between body weight and mortality: a quantitative analysis of combined information from existing studies. *Int J Obes (Lond)*. 1995;20:63-75.

10. Durazo-Arvizu RA, McGee DL, Cooper RS, Liao Y, Luke A. Mortality and optimal body mass index in a sample of the US population. *Am J Epidemiol*. 1998;147:739-749.

11. Seccareccia F, Lanti M, Menotti A, Scanga M. Role of body mass index in the prediction of all cause mortality in over 62,000 men and women: the Italian RIFLE Pooling Project. *J Epidemiol Commun Health*. 1998;52:20-26.

12. Hirdes JP, Forbes WF. The importance of social relationships, socioeconomic status and health prices with respect to mortality among healthy Ontario males. *J Clin Epidemiol*. 1992;45:175-192.

13. Ernsberger P, Koletsky RJ. Biomedical rationale for a wellness approach to obesity: an alternative to a focus on weight loss. *Journal of Social Issues*. 2000;55:221-259.

14. Barrett-Connor EL. Obesity, atherosclerosis and coronary artery disease. *Ann Intern Med*. 1985;103:1010-1019.

15. Briefel RR, Johnson CL. Secular trends in dietary intake in the United States. *Annu Rev Nutr*. 2004;24:401-431.

16. Must A, Spadano J, Coakley EH, Field AE, Colditz G, Dietz WH . The disease burden associated with overweight and obesity. *JAMA*. 1999;282:1523-1529.

17. McLaughlin T, Abbasi F, Lamendola C, Reaven G. Heterogeneity in the prevalence of risk factors for cardiovascular disease and type 2 diabetes mellitus in obese individuals: effect of differences in insulin sensitivity. *Arch Intern Med*. 2007;167:642-648.

18. Gregg EW, Cheng YJ, Cadwell BL, et al. Secular trends in cardiovascular disease risk factors according to body mass index in US adults. *JAMA*. 2005;293:1868-1874.

19. Webster's Third New International Dictionary, Unabridged, 2002 [Web page]. Miriam-Webster Web site. http://unabridged.merriam-webster.com. Accessed December 13, 2007.

20. National Task Force on the Prevention and Treatment of Obesity. Dieting and the development of eating disorders in overweight and obese adults (review). *Arch Intern Med*. 2000;160:2581-2589.

21. Satter EM; Chapter 10, Understand Your Child's Growth. *Your Child's Weight: Helping Without Harming*. Madison, WI: Kelcy Press; 2005:323-380.

22. Neumark-Sztainer D, Wall M, Guo J, Story M, Haines J, Eisenberg M. Obesity, disordered eating, and eating disorders in a longitudinal study of adolescents: how do dieters fare 5 years later? *J Am Diet Assoc*. 2006;106:559-568.

23. Serdula MK, Mokdad AH, Williamson DF, Galuska DA, Mendlein JM, Heath GW. Prevalence of attempting weight loss and strategies for controlling weight. *JAMA*. 1999;282:1353-1358.

24. Jeffery RW, Drewnowski A, Epstein LH, et al. Long-term maintenance of weight loss: current status. *Health Psychol*. 2000;19(1 Suppl):5-16.

25. Keys A, Brozek J, Henschel A, Mickelsen O, Taylor H. *The Biology of Human Starvation*. Minneapolis: University of Minnesota Press; 1950.

26. Wadden TA, Bartlett S, Letizia KA, Foster GD, Stunkard AJ, Conill A. Relationship of dieting history to resting metabolic rate, body composition, eating behavior, and subsequent weight loss. *Am J Clin Nutr*. 1992;56:203S-208S.

27. Herman CP, Polivy J. Anxiety, restraint, and eating behavior. *J Abnorm Psychol*. 1975;84(6):666-672.

28. Stirling LJ, Yeomans MR. Effect of exposure to a forbidden food on eating in restrained and unrestrained women. *Int J Eat Disord*. 2004;35:59-68.

29. Van Strien T, Ouwens MA. Counterregulation in female obese emotional eaters: Schachter, Goldman, and Gordon's (1968) test of psychosomatic theory revisited. *Eat Behav*. 2003;3:329-340.

30. Ward A, Mann T. Don't mind if I do: disinhibited eating under cognitive load. *J Pers Soc Psychol*. 2000;78:753-763.

31. Westenhoefer J, Stunkard AJ, Pudel V. Validation of the flexible and rigid control dimensions of dietary restraint. *Int J Eat Disord.* 1999;26:53-64.

32. Townsend MS, Peerson J, Love B, Achterberg C, Murphy SP. Food insecurity is positively related to overweight in women. *J Nutr.* 2001;131:1738-1745.

33. Urbszat D, Herman CP, Polivy J. Eat, drink, and be merry, for tomorrow we diet: effects of anticipated deprivation on food intake in restrained and unrestrained eaters. *J Abnorm Psychol.* 2002;111:396-401.

34. Lowe MR, Foster GD, Kerzhnerman I, Swain RM, Wadden TA. Restrictive dieting vs. "undieting" effects on eating regulation in obese clinic attenders. *Addict Behav.* 2001;26:253-266.

35. Haines PS, Hama MY, Guilkey DK, Popkin BM. Weekend eating in the United States is linked with greater energy, fat, and alcohol intake. *Obes Res.* 2003;11:945-949.

36. Shide DJ, Rolls BJ. Information about the fat content of preloads influences energy intake in healthy women. *J Am Diet Assoc.* 1995;95:993-998.

37. Abraham S, Collins G, Nordsieck M. Relationships of childhood weight status to morbidity in adults. *HSMHA Health Rep.* 1971;86:273-284.

38. Morrison JA, Friedman LA, Gray-McGuire C. Metabolic syndrome in childhood predicts adult cardiovascular disease 25 years later: the Princeton Lipid Research Clinics Follow-up Study. *Pediatrics.* 2007;120:340-345.

39. Luo J, Margolis KL, Adami H-O, et al. Body size, weight cycling, and risk of renal cell carcinoma among postmenopausal women: the Women's Health Initiative (United States). *Am J Epidemiol.* 2007;166:752-759.

40. Andres R, Muller DC, Sorkin JD. Long-term effects of change in body weight on all-cause mortality. A review. *Ann Intern Med.* 1993;119:737-743.

41. Folsom AR, French SA, Zheng W, Baxter JE, Jeffery RW. Weight variability and mortality: the Iowa Women's Health Study. *Int J Obes (Lond).* 1996;10:704-709.

42. Lissner L, Odell PM, D'Agostino RB, et al. Variability of body weight and health outcomes in the Framingham population. *N Engl J Med.* 1991;324 :1839-1844.

43. Blair SN, Brownell K, Collins G, Lisner L. Body weight change, all-cause mortality and cause-specific mortality in the Multiple Risk Factor Intervention Trial. *Ann Int Med.* 1993;119(749-757).

44. Psota T, Lohse B, West S. Associations between eating competence and cardio-vascular disease biomarkers. *J Nutr Educ Behav.* 2007;39 (suppl):S171-S178.

45. Lohse B, Satter E, Horacek T, Gebreselassie T, Oakland MJ. Measuring Eating Competence: psychometric properties and validity of the ecSatter Inventory. *J Nutr Educ Behav.* 2007;39 (suppl):S154-S166.

46. Hammond-Meyer A. *Stabilizing Eating and Weight Using a Nondieting Treatment As a Means to Improve Biomedical Health Parameters in an Overweight Population of Women: A Health at Any Size Perspective [Dissertation].* Seattle, WA: Seattle Pacific University; 2005.

47. Bacon L, Stern JS, Van Loan MD, Keim NL. Size acceptance and intuitive eating improve health for obese, female chronic dieters. *J Am Diet Assoc.* 2005;105:929-936.

48. Wei M, Kampert JB, Barlow CE, et al. Relationship between low cardiorespiratory fitness and mortality in normal-weight, overweight, and obese men. *JAMA.* 1999;282:1547-1553.

49. Sui X, LaMonte MJ, Laditka JN, et al. Cardiorespiratory fitness and adiposity as mortality predictors in older adults. *JAMA.* 2007;298:2507-2516.

50. National Center for Health Statistics [Web site]. LCWK1 Deaths, percent of total deaths, and death rates for the 15 leading causes of death in 5-year age groups, by race and sex: United States, 1999-2004. [Web page] Centers for Disease Control and Prevention Web site. http://www.cdc.gov/nchs/datawh/statab/unpubd/mort-abs/lcwk1_10.htm. Accessed December 13, 2007.

51. Sui X, LaMonte MJ, Blair SN. Cardio-respiratory fitness as a predictor of nonfatal cardiovascular events in asymptomatic women and men. *Am J Epidemiol.* 2007;165:1413-1423.

52. Barlow CE, LaMonte MJ, FitzGerald SJ, Kampert JB, Perrin JL, Blair SN. Cardio-respiratory fitness is an independent predictor of hypertension incidence among initially normotensive healthy women. *Am J Epidemiol.* 2006;163:142-150.

53. O'Hara L, Gregg J. The war on obesity: a social determinant of health. *Health Promot J Austr.* 2006;17:260-263.

Appendix
E
Energy Balance and Weight

It is impossible to predict how much someone "should" eat. While average daily energy requirements for *groups* of people can be estimated, energy requirements for individuals cannot. If you look past the averages and examine the fine print, energy recommendations cover a range. The National Research Council estimates average energy requirements, plus or minus 20 percent, for individuals of a given age and gender, then goes on to say that those estimates are appropriate for only about 70 percent of people.[1] For the statistically knowledgeable, that 20 percent is the standard deviation (SD) around the mean and the 70 percent refers to the bell-shaped curve. I discuss and illustrate the bell-shaped curve in appendix D, "BMI, Mortality, Morbidity, and Health: Resolving the Weight Dilemma." If you are a 30-year-old woman of average height (64 inches), a rough estimate of your calorie requirement would be 2,000 calories with a 400 calorie variation up or down—between 1,600 and 2,400 calories per day. Energy requirements are better based on height rather than weight because height gives a better estimate of active metabolic tissue.

But that is only if you are one of the 70 percent of people whose requirement falls within that range. What about everyone else? To capture 95 percent of 30-year-old women in our estimate—the ones whose energy requirements are 2 SD above or below the mean—we have to expand the range to 1,200 to 2,800 calories. To capture 99 percent of women whose energy requirements are 3 SD above or below the mean, we have to expand the range to from 800 to 3,200 calories. And even that leaves 1 percent of women unaccounted for.

To run the figures for men, for the 70 percent of 30-year-old men of average height (70 inches), the average calorie requirement would be 2,700 with a range of 2200 to 3,240 calories. To predict for 95 percent of men, the range would be 1620 to 3,780 calories. To predict for 99 percent of men, the range would have to be 1080 to 4,320 calories.

George the Amazing Plumber

The remaining 1 percent leave me awestruck. It was a red-letter day for me when one of the doctors in the clinic where I worked as an outpatient dietitian referred George, a stocky, middle-aged plumber with a modest potbelly, for instruction in an 1,800-calorie diet. By this time, I had learned from my sins of being a diet vending machine and had developed the routine of taking a diet history and then tweaking what the patient told me he usually ate. "Do the least you can to get the results you want" became my mantra as I scouted out small changes that could be made consistently and that carried little attendant sense of deprivation.

George was concerned about his health, committed to change, and totally lacking in either shame or bravado as he reported what he generally ate. For breakfast, George said he had half a dozen fried eggs, 8 or 10 slices of heavily buttered toast, and a quart or two of orange juice.

For lunch, George said his wife used up most of a loaf of store-bought bread in making him peanut butter, meat, and cheese sandwiches. He also had cookies, fruit, and a quart of milk. Dinner was more of the same—a number of steaks, chops, or pieces of chicken or fish, several helpings of potatoes and gravy, a pile or two of vegetables, two or three pieces of pie, and several glasses of milk. My quick calculation told me that George regularly consumed about 10,000 calories a day! Actually, I calculated that George ate 16,000 calories a day, but none of us would believe that!

Finding this nutritional anomaly was a dietitian's fantasy—a *Ripley's Believe It or Not* display right in my own office! But I suspected George of chicanery, so while he set up his next appointment I sidled up to his wife in the waiting room. What did she pack for George's lunch, I asked her. She allowed as how she used up most of a loaf of bread for his sandwiches. "You know," she observed mildly, "George does seem to eat a lot."

I remember what George told me; I don't remember what I told him. I hope I said to cut down a little. I hope against hope that I didn't give him that 1,800-calorie diet! That would have been the most extreme cruelty! I would like to believe that I evaluated his weight history as part of making my recommendations, but I don't think I had gotten that far yet in my own thinking and practice. If I saw George now, I would ask him to describe the pattern of his weight since his mid-20s (men achieve their full growth by then). If his weight had been pretty stable with the usual modest increases as he aged, I would advise him to keep doing what he was doing and not mess with his energy balance. I would explain to both George and his doctor that George's extraordinary energy-in, energy-out system was in equilibrium, and trying to restrict his food intake carried a high risk of destabilizing it and undermining what was working well for him. I doubt if the doctor would have believed George's story. I did, and I don't consider myself to be gullible.

Appetite Adjusts to Requirement

Whether your metabolism is set up to require few calories or a lot, if you are tuned in to your internal cues of hunger, appetite, and satiety, you will be satisfied on the amount your body

needs. George's metabolism was set to need 10,000 calories a day, and he was comfortable when he ate that amount. If he ate 8,000 or 9,000 calories a day, he would be hungry all the time. Unless you have a metabolism like George does, if you try to eat 10,000 calories a day—or even 8,000 or 6,000—you will feel absolutely stuffed. If your body is set up to need 800 or 1,000 calories a day, you will be comfortable on that amount of calories. If I ate that little, I would be starved, tired, and cranky as all get-out. I would also have trouble keeping warm in our Wisconsin winters.

THE BODY DEFENDS ITSELF

Except for moderate increases related to aging, the natural adult tendency is to achieve and maintain a constitutionally determined body weight that is unique for each of us. To maintain this preferred weight level, your body fine-tunes its desire for food and also its way of *using up* the calories you take in. If you don't eat much, it conserves heat, and you feel colder. You get tired more easily, and whether you realize it or not, you fidget less. Have you ever felt tired and dragged out and discovered you were peppier after you ate? If you eat an unusually large amount, your body squanders energy and you feel warmer. Have you ever had trouble sleeping after eating a big meal because you were so warm and revved up?

It's bogus to say, as many weight-loss coaches do, "If you eat 50 calories less a day, you will lose 5 pounds in a year." The math works, if you figure 3,500 calories equals a pound—which it may or may not, depending on how much protein and water are in that pound. But the body's ability to conserve or squander calories and maintain energy balance defeats such calculations.

The body adjusts ingestion of food to maintain bodily homeostasis through processes of short-term regulation, which roughly balance energy intake with expenditure on a day-to-day basis, and long-term regulation of food intake, which corrects the errors of day-to-day regulation.[2] Thus, food intake regulation occurs in weekly, monthly, or even seasonal cycles. The body doesn't forget that it is hungry, and it keeps trying to replenish itself.

Moderate levels of activity support homeostatic energy-regulation processes and therefore stable body weight. In a classic experiment in a Bengalese market, researchers found that above a minimum level of activity, subjects balance activity with energy intake and maintain stable body weights. However, subjects whose activity is very low have higher levels of energy intake and gain weight.[3] Clinical observations show that moderate levels of activity make internal regulation cues more prominent.

If you force your body weight below its preferred level, you will have to consistently eat less than you are hungry for. You will have to live with being chronically hungry, food-preoccupied, and prone to overeat when something happens to undermine your willpower. After years of nationwide advertising, the National Weight Control Registry currently claims only 5,000 people have lost at least 30 pounds and kept it off for a year or more.[4] On the average, registry members report consuming 1,400 kcal/day (24 percent of calories from fat) and expending about 400 kcal/day—about 90 minutes—in physical activity.[5] Even though registry members maintain "normal" or even "above-normal" weights, with rare exceptions their bodies want to eat more and weigh more. As a consequence, they are constantly hungry, running on adrenalin, and investing a great deal of time and creative energy to stay thin.

THE MINNESOTA SEMI-STARVATION STUDY

The body's biological pressures to restore physiologically preferred body weight are simply enormous. This has been demonstrated by every dieter who has regained lost weight. But dieters tend to blame themselves for lack of willpower. It has also been demonstrated by research, and the research is not new. The famous World War II Minnesota Semi-Starvation Study demonstrated, in an irrefutable way, the body's drive to protect itself.[6]

Thirty-two young male volunteers were maintained on an average of 1,570 calories per day for 6 months and lost about 24 percent of their body weight. During this time, the men became absolutely miserable. They were impaired physically, emotionally, and socially. They felt cold and weak and tired easily, had diminished strength and work capacity, and were giddy and had momentary blackouts. They became apathetic, irritable, depressed, and moody and their life interests narrowed to thinking about food and anticipating the next meal.[6]

That 6 months of undereating had a destructive impact that persisted. As one of the volunteers, Jim Graham, put it, "After the experiment was over, I was still hungry for a long time. Even when I could eat all I wanted, I would finish a meal and still feel hungry. My stomach would just not hold any more." Within 6 months, Graham gained 100 pounds, going from a low of 125 pounds to a high of 225. Three years later, he was back to his initial weight of 175 pounds.[7] He was lucky. Others in the study regained weight to a higher level and never lost it. But even those who gained weight and then lost it again as Graham did ended up with bodies that were higher in fatty tissue and lower in muscle and organ tissue than they had been at the beginning of the study.

GENETICS DETERMINES WEIGHT

It is tremendously difficult to maintain lowered body weight because the body defends its preferred weight. Identical-twin studies, which have also been around for a while, indicate that genetics is a primary determinant of body weight. The studies include Albert Stunkard's findings that weights of Scandinavian adult identical twins separated during infancy resemble those of each other far more than they do those of their adoptive families,[8,9] and Thomas Bouchard's Minnesota-twin studies that demonstrated that when they are overfed, identical twins gain weight and fatten—or resist fattening—similarly to each other.[10]

To understand Bouchard's twin-overfeeding studies, consider Ethan Sims's classic weight gain experiment with nine Vermont prisoners.[11] The men volunteered to gain between 20 and 25 percent of their original body weight by eating about twice their usual caloric intake for about 6 months. Most of the men gained the initial few pounds with ease. Then, their weight gain experiences diverged. One prisoner stopped gaining weight even though he ate 10,000 calories per day. It appeared his metabolism shifted into overdrive and he squandered the calories rather than continuing to gain weight. Two others found it relatively easy to gain eating "only" about 5,000 calories per day. Afterwards, each of the prisoners returned to his pre-study weight.

There Are Always Exceptions

My work with children, however, tells me that while genetics are tremendously powerful, constitutional endowment does not tell the whole story of food regulation and unstable body weight. Weight rebound from food restriction and weight loss makes children fatter than nature intended them to be.[12] Weight-reduction dieting makes adults gain and maintain weight above previously well-defended levels.[13] Clinical experience shows that the morbidly obese have histories, throughout their lives, of periods of extraordinary food deprivation alternating with periods of overeating and weight gain.

In appears that for some people—probably for those who are genetically predisposed to be fatter rather than thinner—energy regulation and weight are similar to a ratchet wrench that only goes one way. It goes up but doesn't come back down again. Each time it climbs to a higher level, the body establishes a new set point for energy regulation and weight and that is where it wants to stay.

References

1. National Research Council (NRC). Recommended Dietary Allowances. 10th ed. Washington, DC: National Academy Press; 1989.
2. Mayer J. Some aspects of the problem of regulation of food intake and obesity. *N Engl J Med.* 1966;274:610-616, 662-673, 722-731.
3. Mayer J, Roy P, Mitra KP. Relation between caloric intake, body weight and physical work. *Am J Clin Nutr.* 1956;4(2):169-175.
4. Hill JO, Wing R. NWCR Facts [Web page]. National Weight Control Registry Web site. http://www.nwcr.ws/Research/default.htm. Accessed December 13, 2007.
5. Shick SM, Wing RR, Klem ML, McGuire MT, Hill JO, Seagle H. Persons successful at long-term weight loss and maintenance continue to consume a low-energy, low-fat diet. *J Am Diet Assoc.* 1998;98:408-413.
6. Keys A, Brozek J, Henschel A, Mickelsen O, Taylor H. *The Biology of Human Starvation.* Minneapolis: University of Minnesota Press; 1950.
7. Smith B. Minnesota Semi-Starvation Experiment [videotape]. Fort Collins, CO: Office of Instructional Services, Colorado State University; 1990.
8. Stunkard AJ, Sorenson TIA, Hanis C, et al. An adoption study of human obesity. *N Engl J Med.* 1986;314(4):193-198.
9. Stunkard AJ, Harris JR, Pedersen NL, McClearn GE. The body-mass of twins who have been reared apart. *N Engl J Med.* 1990;322:1483-1487.
10. Bouchard C, Tremblay A, Despres JP, et al. The response to long-term overfeeding in identical twins. *N Engl J Med.* 1990;322:1477-1482.
11. Sims EAH, Horton ES. Endocrine and metabolic adaptation to obesity and starvation. *Am J Clin Nutr.* 1968;21(12):1455-1470.
12. Faith MS, Scanlon KS, Birch LL, Francis LA, Sherry B. Parent-child feeding strategies and their relationships to child eating and weight status. *Obes Res.* 2004;12:1711-1722.
13. Wadden TA, Bartlett S, Letizia KA, Foster GD, Stunkard AJ, Conill A. Relationship of dieting history to resting metabolic rate, body composition, eating behavior, and subsequent weight loss. *Am J Clin Nutr.* 1992;56:203S-208S.

Appendix
F
The Story of Sharon

As Sharon walked into her session, I could tell she was thrilled. She could barely wait for me to close the door before she started talking. "I found it!" she exclaimed. "I actually found my stopping place. And I found it in my favorite down-home restaurant. On my way up north, I had lunch at Lester's. That's Lester's of the Swedish meatballs with mashed potatoes and gravy and the melt-in-your mouth pies.

"Always before, when I went there, I did one of two things, and neither one made me happy. Either I ordered just the vegetable soup and tried to stop after one slice of homemade rye bread, or I would say to heck with it and have the whole meal including pie. One way I felt cheated and hungry; the other way I felt stuffed and miserable. This time, I did what we talked about. I said to myself, 'What looks good to me? What do I really want?'

"What I really wanted was roast pork, stuffing, potatoes and gravy, salad, no dressing, bread, and iced tea. I really like iced tea and salad with no dressing," she hastened to explain. "I wasn't trying to cut calories.

"Then I said to myself, 'That's an awful lot of food. I shouldn't have the pie.' Well, the minute I said that, I could feel myself tightening up. I could hear your voice. 'You've starved yourself for years,' you were saying, 'and it scares you when you feel you'll have to go without. You've got to reassure yourself that you'll be able to eat.' 'Well, what I need to reassure myself,' I thought, 'is a piece of three-berry pie with crumb topping, sitting here waiting for me.'

"So all that food came, and it looked wonderful. There was a lot of it, and I liked that. It felt like there would be enough. You know, come to think of it," she said thoughtfully, "I wasn't even self-conscious about having the waitress put that big plate of food down in front of me. It used to be I'd think they were all looking at me and wondering what that big woman was doing eating all that food. You know how it is: 'No wonder she's so fat.' I'm not sure what's made the difference. Maybe it's because I feel so in control. I know for the first time I can remember, I feel like I'm entitled to eat.

"But, back to my lunch. I was just hungry enough—not famished, but hungry. Now that I can enjoy my meals, I don't want to spoil my appetite with nibbling and snacking like I used to. As I looked at the food, I got excited. But I took a moment and did my centering breath. 'It's all right to eat this,' I said to myself. 'I just have to take it slow and pay attention.'

"I took a bite of roast pork with a bit of potato and gravy on it, and it was *wonderful*. I took a bite of dressing and it was even better. It was so good, I could feel my knees get weak." She laughed a little self-consciously. "It was positively sensual." I made a mental note to go back to the sensual part. People feel ashamed for responding so strongly to eating. Those feelings are natural, but Sharon needed a chance to talk about them.

"I was so excited," she continued, "that I felt like just wolfing the food down. But all those focused eating exercises we did paid off.

'Relax,' I said to myself. 'Easy does it. You can eat as much as you want. You just have to go slow and savor it.' Well, that's the way the meal went. I kept talking to myself through it. I tasted every bite. I would get started going fast, and then I'd say, 'Settle down, Sharon. You can have this.' I would stop a minute and take a deep breath.

"I kept on eating and paying attention, and I could tell when I stopped being hungry. It used to be I would have tried to make myself stop. But I didn't want to stop, so I didn't. It still tasted good. So I kept on eating. I was getting a little scared by this time, because I wondered if I would ever stop. But I just said again, 'Relax, just see what happens.'

"And then I was done! Full! Just no longer interested! I took another bite and then another one to make sure. But I was done. And there sat the pie. I didn't even want it. I tried a bite to make sure. Nothing! Do you have any idea what it feels like to look at a piece of pie and truly not want it? I really was full, I was done, I was not stuffed, I wasn't too full, I was just *finished*. I know when to stop! Oh, sure, it worried me a little that I didn't want the pie, but I just talked to myself. 'Sharon, old girl,' I said, 'you can have pie any time. Besides, that would make a good breakfast. Take it along and have it tomorrow morning with your coffee.'

"And I did. And I didn't even feel guilty. It's what I wanted. You told me it wouldn't kill me to have some meals that are nutritionally worthless—but I'm not sure you meant pie for breakfast. What do you say?"

Sharon sat grinning impishly at me. I know what *I* said, but what would *you* say?

Appendix
G
Select Foods That Help Regulation

A well-selected meal with a good distribution of protein, fat, and carbohydrate can help with regulation of food intake. Each nutrient plays a role in satiety. Interaction among the nutrients influences the staying power of a meal or snack.

Food Composition

Let's start with a lesson in food composition. The three major sources of calories in the diet are protein, fat, and carbohydrate—starch and sugar. The only other source of calories is alcohol. Figure G.1 indicates which foods contribute which major

FIGURE G.1 PROTEIN, FAT, AND CARBOHYDRATE CONTENT OF FOODS				
Food	Protein	Fat	Complex carbohydrate: starch	Simple carbohydrate: sugar
Milk	X	X (if not skim)		X
Vegetables	x		X,x	
Fruit, fruit juice				X
Breads, cereals	x		X	
Meat, fish, poultry, eggs, cheese, peanut butter	X	X (if not fat-free)		
Cooked dried beans	X		X	
Butter, margarine, salad				
dressing, cooking oils		X		
Cookies, chocolates, cakes	x	X	X	X
Jelly candies, soda, fruit drinks				X

nutrients. A big "X" means the food contains a lot; a small "x" means the food contains some. Vegetables have both Xs because some contain a lot of starch, others contain little.

As you can see, you get protein from the meat group as well as from milk and milk products. You also get protein from cooked dried beans and peas and in small amounts from bread and cereal products. Fat is often a separate food such as butter or oil, but it is often also contained *in* foods, where it may not be noticeable. Cookies, cakes, and ice cream have fat in them. Most meats have fat in them, as do many dairy products. Skim milk, fat-free yogurt, and fat-free cottage cheese are exceptions. Fat is often used in food preparation, as in frying or in buttering or creaming vegetables. Fat is also used as a spread or as a dressing on other foods.

Carbohydrate comes in two forms: the *simple,* or sugar form, and the *complex,* or starch form. The basic chemical structure of both forms is sugar; starches are made up of many, many molecules of sugar linked together. The important difference, metabolically, is that starch has to be digested into sugar—the links have to be broken—before it can be made available to the body, whereas sugar can be promptly transported into the bloodstream with little or no digestion. You get starch from the bread and cereal group as well as from starchy vegetables such as potatoes, corn, and lima beans. You get a little starch from vegetables that contain a higher proportion of fiber and water, such as broccoli or spinach. We get most of our sugar from sodas, sweetened fruit-flavored beverages, and processed foods that contain sugar, high-fructose corn syrup, or white grape juice. We take sugar straight in refined sugar, honey, and syrup. We get sugar in fruits and fruit juices as well as in cookies, cakes, and candies.

Satiety from Carbohydrate, Protein, and Fat

The series of figures that follow illustrate how eating food high in sugar, starch, protein, fat, or all four impacts satiety. The *satiety* axis on the left-hand side has no numbers because it is subjective. The *time* axis along the bottom also lacks numbers; it, too, is an approximation.

Both start at zero: You are hungry and ready to eat. How quickly you feel satiety after you eat is affected by your bodily state and your mental state as well as by the food itself. So let's start you out hungry and imagine feeding you a series of test meals to find out what happens to satiety.

SUGAR
Figure G.2 demonstrates what would happen if you consumed only sugar. Finding a sugar-only food to consume would be a trick, but on to the experiment. Notice the fast and sharp increase in satiety. That probably comes from an increase in blood glucose, one of many biochemical signs to the body that it has been fed. But the curve drops off just as fast as it went up; the sugar doesn't have much staying power.

FIGURE G.2 SATIETY FROM CONSUMING SUGAR

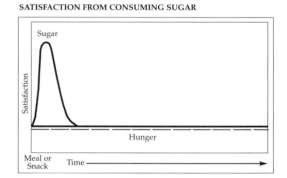

SATISFACTION FROM CONSUMING SUGAR

STARCH
Figure G.3 demonstrates that the addition of starch helps extend satiety. The starch has to be digested before it can be absorbed, and it can't be digested all at one time, so the nutrients get into the bloodstream more slowly and over a more extended time. The nutrient that enters the blood is still glucose, because when starch is digested it is absorbed and carried in the bloodstream as glucose.

Breads and other starchy foods add other components of satiety to the meal: bulk, chewing, and pleasure. Bread's solidness and bulk give the stomach a sense of being filled. Depending on the kind of bread, it will require a greater or lesser amount of chewing. Some people depend heavily on chewing to let them feel that they have had enough to eat, so eating chewy bread such as toast or bagels will help with satiety. Finally, bread adds pleasure. People generally like bread, and we all depend on pleasure to feel satisfied after a meal.

FIGURE G.3 SATIETY FROM CONSUMING SUGAR AND STARCH

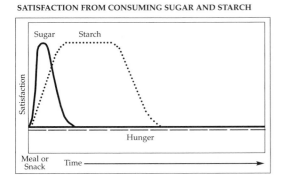

SATISFACTION FROM CONSUMING SUGAR AND STARCH

PROTEIN

As Figure G.4 illustrates, adding protein to the test meal helps quite a lot to make the meal last longer. It takes time for the body to convert protein into amino acids that can be absorbed into the bloodstream. As a result, it takes a while for protein to satisfy, and the satiety lasts longer.

FIGURE G.4 SATIETY FROM CONSUMING SUGAR, STARCH, AND PROTEIN

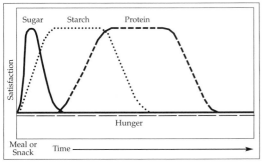

SATISFACTION FROM CONSUMING SUGAR, STARCH AND PROTEIN

The body senses increases in blood amino acids as one of the bits of information supporting a sense of satiety. This is a rather artificial test meal, because most protein sources contribute fat as well. Skim milk is one of the few sources of protein in the diet that doesn't also contain some fat. Egg white is another source of fat-free protein, and some very lean fish, tofu, and fat-free cottage cheese are almost fat-free.

FAT

As illustrated by Figure G.5, adding fat to an otherwise fat-free meal gives quite a different picture of satiety. The curve goes out even farther before it starts to drop. When fat reaches the small intestine, it stimulates the release of cholecystokin, a hormone that signals satiety. Fat is digested and absorbed slowly, so fatty acids continue to be released into the bloodstream for quite a while after sugar and amino acids. In addition, fat with the meal slows the emptying time of the stomach, which slows the digestion and absorption of the whole meal.

FIGURE G.5 SATIETY FROM CONSUMING SUGAR, STARCH, PROTEIN, AND FAT

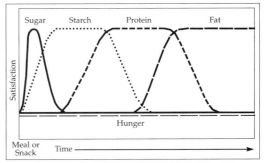

SATISFACTION FROM CONSUMING SUGAR, STARCH, PROTEIN AND FAT

Including fat adds another critical component of satiety: pleasure. Fat carries the flavor in food; the addition of fat allows you to taste the food better and more acutely.

OMITTING SUGAR AND STARCH

As illustrated by Figure G.6, omitting carbohydrate increases the lag time before the meal begins to satisfy. Protein breaks down slowly, and fat more slowly still. When the diet lacks carbohydrate, the body has to manufacture its essential blood glucose from protein. However, the process takes a while, and that slows the blood glucose response. Furthermore, without the bulk of starch, the meal won't feel very filling.

This figure illustrates the metabolic response you would get from eating a very low-carbohydrate meal or diet. While it eventually leaves you feeling full, that fullness comes late in the meal or even after the meal. Such meals may also leave you feeling aesthetically unsatisfied because they lack the pleasure that can be contributed by carbohydrate foods.

FIGURE G.6 SATIETY FROM CONSUMING PROTEIN AND FAT

SATISFACTION FROM CONSUMING PROTEIN AND FAT

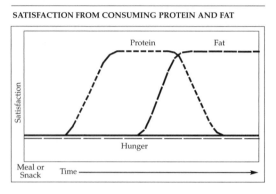

Applications

To support food regulation, plan meals to include carbohydrate, protein, and fat. Consuming these major nutrients together lets them work best nutritionally and makes meals more satisfying and lasting. All of us, but some of us in particular, benefit from such well-selected meals and snacks. The extremely active person benefits from the long-lasting energy. The person with heart disease benefits from avoiding periodically flooding the system with fatty acids. The person with diabetes benefits from sustained release of nutrients without spikes in blood sugar to balance out available insulin.

Appendix

H

Nutrition Education in the Schools

Nutrition education at school that is consistent with the principles of fdSatter (the Satter Feeding Dynamics Model) and ecSatter (the Satter Eating Competence Model) maintains children's intuitive eating capabilities and builds their cognitive and behavioral capabilities in a stage-related, developmentally appropriate fashion. Children are born with the ability to eat as much as they need to grow predictably and with the drive to learn to eat the food their grown-ups eat. Adults support children's inborn eating capabilities by providing leadership and giving autonomy: By regularly and reliably providing children with adequate amounts of wholesome food in a positive environment and by letting children decide what and how much to eat of what grown-ups offer. Slowly and over time, children who receive such good parenting with food become competent with eating. They retain their positive eating attitudes and food regulation capabilities as well as develop practical food acceptance attitudes and behaviors. Young children depend on their grown-ups to manage the food context. It is only toward the end of grade school and under adult guidance that they begin to learn to manage the food context by doing some food selection for themselves.

Nutrition education based on feeding dynamics and eating competence principles leads with experience and with the practical. It follows with the theoretical, provided the child is developmentally ready and has mastered the experiential and practical lessons outlined in Figure H.1.

FIGURE H.1 EXPERIENTIAL AND PRACTICAL NUTRITION EDUCATION
The young child learns eating capability concretely—with her body and through her feelings and attitudes. Here are examples of concrete ways that children learn about food and about eating.
- Having experience with food and with eating situations.
- Being with adults who enjoy a variety of food.
- Being allowed to explore and approach unfamiliar food at her own pace: to look, touch, feel, taste, and watch others eat.
- Being allowed to eat as little or as much as she needs.
- Being supported in feeling good about her body.
- Being with adults who accept diversity with respect to body size and shape.

A child raised by parents who practice positive feeding dynamics has received *intuitive* nutrition education. With her *body* and with her whole *being* she has learned positive attitudes about food and eating, has developed food acceptance skills and retains her ability to regulate food intake. As a result, such a child has the basic capabilities with eating outlined in Figure H.2.

> **FIGURE H.2 INTUITIVE CAPABILITIES WITH EATING**
>
> The child who has been appropriately parented with food and eating preserves her food regulation capabilities and her positive feelings and behaviors with respect to food and her body.
> - She has the meal habit; she is secure in her expectation that her grown-ups will regularly and reliably provide for her.
> - She enjoys eating and is confident and unselfconscious about eating.
> - She has good food acceptance skills. She knows how to behave around food whether at home, in the school cafeteria, or in social eating situations.
> - She assumes she will get enough to eat.
> - She intuitively depends on her internal regulators to let her eat as much or as little as she wants.
> - She feels good about her eating and her body.

The best nutrition education at school reinforces a child's trust in the intuitive capabilities she has gained at home and, when she is older, adds an understanding of those capabilities. Building on a child's capabilities is respectful of her family. After an extensive review of such programs, university specialists found that the few programs that were successful in increasing children's food acceptance were programs that took significant time with nutrition education, that let children *eat or work with food*, and that involved families, schools, and communities.[1] After a thorough review of environmental influences on children's eating, other nutrition educators reminded readers that basic respect for the family unit was the essential means of ensuring children's health and well-being.[2]

Nutrition education in schools can be delivered in the regular classroom or in physical education, consumer science, health, social studies, history, chemistry, or biology class.

Don't Teach Children Adults' Jobs

For the most part, conventional nutrition education units teach children jobs that belong to adults. In the very early grades, children are given concrete experiences with food. Beyond those early grades, curricula tend to become more abstract; they teach nutrition and expect children to apply nutritional principles to food selection. Such expectations are unrealistic. In Minneapolis, researchers found that students in kindergarten through sixth grade have difficulty using the Food Guide Pyramid (current at the time of the study) and other standard nutrition guidelines to evaluate the acceptability of foods. Younger children freely use terms such as "low-fat" and "low-sugar," but they have trouble naming foods in those categories. Children in the third through sixth grades still have difficulty understanding concepts like "avoid high-fat food," "eat a variety of food," and "maintain a healthy weight."[3]

Why would children want to learn these rules? Provided they are being offered regular and nutritious meals and snacks in a positive environment, children have within them far more sophisticated mechanisms for achieving nutritional adequacy, regulating food intake, and maintaining healthy weight. For a young child, learning how to choose food and how to regulate food intake is like learning how to breathe. It doesn't arise. The food is there; you eat it or don't eat it, and you eat as much or as little as you want.

Rule- and avoidance-based nutrition lessons are particularly problematic. Children naturally explore, learn, and grow. Warnings about food impede their exploration. To cope, they become rigid and try to live by rules that are to them illogical, ignore them completely, or give up and become rebellious.

Instead of teaching children adults' jobs, support children in doing *their* jobs. Children's jobs with eating are to learn to eat the foods their grown-ups eat, to eat the amount of food they need to be healthy and energetic, and to grow in accordance with their genetic endowment. Children can do their jobs with eating if adults provide leadership and give autonomy.

Address Food Acceptance

Support children in accumulating positive food acceptance attitudes and behaviors and in restoring those capabilities if they have been impaired:
- Being relaxed and comfortable at mealtime.
- Knowing how to behave in situations where food is available.

- Being calm around food, even when it is unfamiliar or disliked.
- Being able to choose from available foods.
- Being polite and matter-of-fact about saying "yes, please" and "no, thank you."
- Being inclined to experiment with unfamiliar food by examining it, watching others eat it, and eventually tasting it.

PROVIDE FOOD EXPOSURE

Children learn food acceptance from experience. Developing comfort with unfamiliar food and learning to like it takes 10 to 20 neutral exposures or more.[4] To increase exposure, team up with the school lunchroom and arrange to have foods appear both in the classroom and on the lunch menu. Neutral exposure is matter-of-factly presenting the food without outside pressure of any kind and, in fact, reassuring children they do not have to eat, taste, or even *lick* the food. Outside pressure can *appear* to be positive, as when a child is encouraged, enticed, persuaded, applauded, or rewarded for eating or even tasting the food. However, children can't be fooled. They sense they are being pressured and react by slowing or stopping their acceptance of new food.

Neutral exposure means not only avoiding coercing children in any way to eat, but also not modeling or teaching value judgments about food beyond the value judgments that are inherent in choosing food to bring into the classroom or to include in the school nutrition program. Keep messages about food neutral. Avoid reminders that foods are healthful, and don't tell children how many servings of food they "should" eat. Do not say or imply that some food is healthier or better than other food, or that children should or should not eat this or that. Teach children to avoid making negative remarks about food. Every food is somebody else's favorite and sneering at it scorns their family and culture. The respectful study of food and food traditions offers children a vivid understanding of other people, cultures, and eras. In fact, invite parents to visit the classroom and talk about or bring samples of their family food.

- In the early grades, give children concrete experience with food by letting them touch, smell, prepare, taste, and sort into basic food categories.

- In the upper grades, combine food-exposure lessons with lessons that put food in context. Broaden exposure to food by studying food-related issues, such as cultural differences, production, transportation, food in history, and the politics of food. Encourage children to talk about foods that they eat at home, and find out what people in other homes and cultures eat. Reinforce earlier learning about basic food categories by planning and preparing after-school snacks. (See figure 6.2, "Planning a Good-Tasting and Satisfying Snack" on page 62.)
- In high school, explore novel foods and reinforce earlier learning about food acceptance. Capitalize on adolescents' capabilities with abstract thinking by considering the nutritional qualities of foods, the nutritional ingenuity of diets from other cultures, and the chemistry and biology of food.

TEACH FOOD ACCEPTANCE SKILLS

Children learn food acceptance skills experientially—by being shown how to behave in the presence of food. Food acceptance attitudes and skills are more important for a child than what she eats on any one day. Even if she doesn't sample new food in the nutrition education setting, a child who has positive food acceptance skills is prepared for a lifetime of experimenting with new food and learning to like it. To teach food acceptance skills, establish ground rules and give reassurance that children don't have to eat or even taste the food. Children will be braver about tasting new food if you show them how to get food out of their mouth without making a fuss. While they don't have to taste, children are expected to participate in food lessons—to look, touch, prepare, and discuss. They are expected to follow rules about cleanliness. They have to be polite about accepting and refusing food.

Some children in particular benefit from learning food acceptance skills and from being reassured that they don't have to eat if they doesn't want to. A child who is *really* cautious or reacts especially negatively to new food may be forced at home to eat more or different food than she wants, or she may be sheltered from unfamiliar foods by family menus that are limited to foods that she readily accepts. Sometimes the child's lack of experience grows out of family economic pressure. Families who have tight food budgets food acceptance skills, being consistent with both taking leadership and giving autonomy will allow the child to address and correct her own limitations.

- In the early grades, support children's natural inclination to explore by arranging to have a trusted grown-up with them when they eat. At the very least, introduce young children to the school nutrition setting. Help children examine the offerings, show them how to ask for food and coach them in turning it down. Remind children they may accept food and not eat it.
- In the late grades, reinforce children's natural inclination to learn and master by teaching them the principles of learning to like new food and the practicalities of being comfortable with a variety of food. Depend on children's varying food traditions to introduce unfamiliar food.
- In high school, reinforce children's natural inclination to challenge and establish their individuality by introducing the possibility of broadening their food repertory rather than simply breaking the nutritional rules of their elders. Consider food selection behaviors from the personal perspective of assessing risk. For instance, is it an acceptable risk to bone health to shun milk in favor of soda?

Address Regulation of Food Intake

With respect to preserving her ability to eat the right amount of food, a child needs to be offered adequate amounts of enjoyable food at predictable times, and she needs to be allowed to eat as much or as little of those foods as she wants. Beyond providing them with adequate amounts of food at predictable times, support children in preserving their natural regulatory ability and in restoring that ability if it has been impaired:

- Remaining calm in the presence of food.
- Waiting to be served.
- Asking for more if she wants it.
- Being relaxed about eating.
- Being confident and unworried that she will get enough to eat.
- Stopping voluntarily.
- Forgetting about food between regular eating times.

RESTORE FOOD REGULATION SKILLS

If all has gone well for them, children take it for granted that they can trust their bodies to tell them how much to eat. However, it is likely that some if not many children will enter the classroom with deficits with food regulation. A child may seem turned off to food and uninterested in eating. Another child may seem preoccupied with food, desperate to eat and inclined to eat relatively large amounts of food. The deficit in children's ability to regulate food intake is not innate, but grows out of distortions in feeding dynamics. A child who has been coerced into eating more than she wants is likely to become turned off to food and undereat when she gets the opportunity. A child whose food intake has been restricted with respect to either amount or type of food is likely to become food-preoccupied and overeat when she gets the opportunity.

With such children, do the opposite of what seems right. Reassure the uninterested child that she doesn't have to eat, and address factors in the school food environment that may overwhelm her to the point where she loses interest in food. For instance, does she need to sit with a trusted adult, do adults or other children try to persuade her to eat, or is she expected to put foods on her tray when she doesn't want them? Reassure the food-driven child that mealtime or snack time is coming, that she can have as much as she wants to eat at those times, and address factors in the school environment that make her feel that she will have to go without. Her food preoccupation may arise from food restriction, from economically based food insecurity or from conditions that mimic food restriction, such as erratic and unreliable access to food.

ENHANCE SKILLS WITH SELF-AWARENESS TRAINING AND FACTUAL LESSONS

- Children know how much they need to eat. Self-awareness training and factual lessons help them to know what they know. In the early grades, the message, "Your body knows how much you need to eat" is enough. Make teaching about food regulation concrete and related to the child's experience of herself. "How does it feel inside when you are hungry?" "When you are full?" "Do you like being hungry?" "Do you like being full?"
- In the late grades, food regulation lessons make conscious for children the unconscious

mechanisms of hunger, appetite, and satiety. Teaching food regulation is a consciousness-raising activity, and that's *all*. There are no rules or guidelines attached to how much children *should* eat. Ask questions, such as "What does it feel like when our body needs food?" "What does it feel like when you are ready to stop eating?" Address energy regulation from the perspective of supporting innate regulatory processes: "Do you eat the same amount every day?" "Do other people eat the same amount that you do, even those who are a lot like you?"

- In high school, children can explore mechanisms of food regulation. Given the fact that such a high proportion of adolescents diet to manage their weight, it is critical for them to consider their own food-regulation strategies and to evaluate the utility of those strategies.[5] Consider reading and discussing chapter 4, "Eat as Much as You Want," and Appendix E, "Energy Balance and Weight." Support their exploration by asking the question, "What holds true for you with respect to your eating and weight?"[6] Absolutely avoid prescriptive lessons about regulating food intake or striving for target body weight.

SUPPORT RESPECT FOR DIVERSITY IN BODY SIZE AND SHAPE

An essential component of trusting internal regulation is accepting one's own size and shape and that of others. Both the food acceptance and food regulation units support diversity with the underlying theme that "everybody's different" with respect to food preference and energy requirements. Helping children to trust their eating helps them to trust and accept their bodies and supports physical self-esteem. This unit is more direct in its examination of diversity in body size and shape.

The issue of size and shape diversity teaches facts, but the most important lessons are attitudinal. By reinforcing the notion that "everybody's different" with respect to body size, shape, and physical capability, you can help children avoid developing contemptuous or disdainful attitudes toward themselves and other people. Do not weigh children. Children are comfortable about the differences among themselves as long as adults don't introduce value judgments and negative comparisons. In the context of today's pressure on schools to intervene with children's

weight, adults may label even naturally large children as overweight. Such labeling can have devastating consequences. Children who are labeled overweight feel flawed in every way: not smart, not physically capable, and not good about themselves.[7]

- In the early grades, a child benefits from getting a clear and accurate image of her own size and shape. A young child enjoys having her outline traced on a big piece of paper, measuring to see how tall she is, drawing pictures of herself and her family, and writing stories about her eyes, hair, skin color, size, and shape. All of these observations just *are*: there are no rights or wrongs, goods or bads.

- In the late grades, children become more conscious of ideas and expectations about size and shape and are capable of making positive—or negative—use of those ideas. Because older children are oriented toward doing and achieving, it seems natural to them that body size and shape can be done and achieved like other tasks. They assume they can pick out a particular body and get it through their own efforts. As a consequence, for older children it is important to emphasize that size and shape can't be built to specifications. Then help them to explore concrete themes in diversity, address differences in height and body build. Neutralize the topic of body build by having them look at and feel their hands. Examine the similarities and differences with respect to their parents' and other family members' height and body build. Identify each person's particular physical skills and capabilities. To help preadolescents address their feelings about their bodies, consider using the video and discussion guide, *BodyTalk 2: It's a New Language*.[8] In this video, 9 to 12 year olds share their struggles with body esteem, puberty, trying to fit in, and finding support.

- In high school, students can address size and shape concerns from the perspective of identifying, evaluating, conforming to or resisting messages about size, shape, and attractiveness. They can identify realistic physical role models based on their own bodily characteristics. Consider using the video and discussion guide, *Body Talk 1: Teens Talk about Their Bodies, Eating Disorders and Activism*.[9] In this video, teens discuss the pressure they feel on their weight from media, family and friends, and the effects those pressures have on their physical and emotional self-esteem. Having addressed the personal, adolescents can consider the theoretical, examining genetic differences in size, shape, physical capability, and energy regulation.

Address the Eating Context

Fundamental to eating competence is maintaining the food context:
- Making eating a priority.
- Taking time to eat.
- Providing regular and reliable meals and snacks.
- Choosing food for those meals and snacks.
Throughout the early and late grades and high school, learning about food management is in the context of adults' continuing to take primary responsibility for the *what*, *when*, and *where* of feeding. Children of all ages who are fed regularly and reliably internalize the meal habit.

GRADUALLY SHAPE EATING CONTEXT SKILLS

As they get older, children can gradually begin to understand and master the principles and tasks that grownups use for choosing food and planning and preparing meals and snacks.

- In the early grades, it is not appropriate to assign young children responsibility for managing the food context. As noted previously, it is all right to introduce third- or fourth-graders to the food groups so they can have fun categorizing foods, but they are not capable of applying food-selection guidelines to choosing what to eat.
- In the late grades, many children are cognitively developed enough to begin to think abstractly. In a limited fashion, those children can make practical use of food-group categories along with considerations of food preference for deciding what to eat for a meal at school or a snack after school. They can also apply their developing time management skills to taking time for their after-school snack.
- In high school, adolescents master the food context—structure and food management—so they can provide for themselves after they

leave home. They learn to manage their schedule so they can make time for eating— both with the family and on their own. They learn to keep food safe, to plan, shop for and prepare a few simple meals and to put together a reasonably balanced diet from home-prepared, pre-prepared, and restaurant food.

Address Eating Attitudes

The primary attitudinal goal with ecSatter and fdSatter is to establish and maintain positive and flexible attitudes about eating, which in turn allow being responsively attuned to outer and inner experiences relative to eating.[10] Preserving and cultivating positive attitudes about eating and about food is an outgrowth of the modeling and coursework in this curriculum. Children will have a relaxed self-trust about food and eating and will experience harmony among food desires, food choices and amounts eaten.

- In the early grades, children can be asked how they feel when they are working with food or eating it." "How do you feel about eating this?" "Do you like eating?" "Do you like cooking?" "Do you like this food?" "What is your favorite food?"
- In the late grades, children can begin to consider attitudes and address their own feelings and beliefs. "Do you think eating is important?" "Do you think your parents consider eating to be important?" "Do you enjoy eating?" "Do you think it is all right to enjoy your eating?"
- In high school, adolescents can work to understand the role of attitudes and beliefs in guiding behavior and choices. "What are social attitudes about food?" "About eating?" "What attitudes do your parents have about food and eating?" Do their attitudes reflect your own?" "Are you comfortable with those attitudes, or do you want to change them?"

Address Young Adults' Eating Competence

Young adults who have a high frequency of family meals as adolescents make feeding themselves a priority, plan eating into their schedule, and see to it that they get to eat with other people.[11] Most young adults do not prepare food for themselves, but those who do have diets of higher nutritional quality.[12] Clinical experience shows that young adults present with many deficits in eating competence. They may show extreme food selectivity, use weight reduction dieting as a means of regulating food intake, fail to make feeding themselves a priority, and lack the skills for providing for themselves nutritionally. Such students may register for nutrition classes in hopes of finding out how to feed themselves. College courses that focus on nutrition and food selection have been shown to be ineffective for increasing eating competence. In a study of 334 non-nutrition-major undergraduates, ecSI scores remain low for all students and even decrease in males.[13]

The eating competence approach to nutrition education for this population strives to correct deficits in eating competence by working through part I, "How to Eat," systematically addressing eating attitudes, food acceptance skills, food regulation capabilities, and skills with respect to managing the food context. By way of building competence with managing the food context, the curricula addresses the food management issues in part III, "How to Cook." Students plan simple menus from the suggestions in those chapters. Students learn to do grocery shopping, and even go on field trips to observe grocery store organization and marketing strategies, discover possibilities for feeding themselves, and get help with respect to accessing those possibilities according to the principles outlined in *Secrets of Feeding a Healthy Family*: Provide, don't deprive. Seek food, don't avoid it.

Follow, Don't Lead, with Nutrition Lessons

Following the previous suggestions, high school and young adult students will have learned their food management lessons concretely—they will have developed the meal habit, their food acceptance skills support their seeking variety, and their food regulation skills support their eating the amount they need. Such concrete learning may or may not make them curious about the theoretical study of

nutrition and food composition. If energy for such an exploration emerges, chapter 13, "Choosing Food," is written on a level that is accessible to adolescents. However, use this information strictly to reinforce students' capabilities with respect to managing the food context. Do not use it to motivate or persuade students to eat particular foods or to avoid others.

References

1. Lytle L, Achterberg C. Changing the diet of America's children: what works and why? *J Nutr Educ*. 1995;27:250-260.
2. Crockett SJ, Sims LS. Environmental influences on children's eating. *J Nutr Educ*. 1995;27:235-249.
3. Lytle LA, Eldridge AL, Kotz K, Piper J, Williams S, Kalina B. Children's interpretation of nutrition messages. *J Nutr Educ*. 1997;29:128-136.
4. Birch LL, Fisher JO. Appetite and eating behavior in children. *Pediatr Clin North Am*. 1995;42:931-953.
5. Neumark-Sztainer D, Wall M, Guo J, Story M, Haines J, Eisenberg M. Obesity, disordered eating, and eating disorders in a longitudinal study of adolescents: how do dieters fare 5 years later? *J Am Diet Assoc*. 2006;106:559-568.
6. Satter EM; Chapter 7, *Your Child's Weight: Helping Without Harming*. Madison, WI: Kelcy Press; 2005:251-255.
7. Davison KK, Birch LL. Weight status, parent reaction, and self-concept in five-year-old girls. *Pediatrics*. 2001;107:46-53.
8. Body Positive. *Body Talk 2: It's a New Language (Ages 9 to 12)* [videotape]. Berkeley, CA: Body Positive; 2002.
9. Body Positive. *Body Talk 1: Teens Talk about Their Bodies, Eating Disorders and Activism, (Ages 12 & up)* [videotape]. Berkeley, CA: Body Positive; 1999.
10. Satter EM. Nutrition education with the Satter Eating Competence Model. *J Nutr Educ Behav* . 2007;39 (suppl):S189-S194.
11. Larson NI, Neumark-Sztainer D, Hannan PJ, Story M. Family meals during adolescence are associated with higher diet quality and healthful meal patterns during young adulthood. *J Am Diet Assoc*. 2007;107:1502-1510.

12. Larson NI, Perry CL, Story M, Neumark-
     Sztainer D. Food preparation by young
     adults is associated with better diet quality.
     J Am Diet Assoc. 2006;106:2001-7.
13. Shafer K, McCabe A, Condron E, et al.
     Examining eating competence change in
     a general nutrition course reveals gender
     and food preparation issues. *Society for
     Nutrition Education Annual Conference
     Proceedings.* 2003;36:43.

Appendix
I
Children and Food Regulation: The Research

Children know how much they need to eat and, virtually from birth, they are resilient and resourceful regulators. University of Iowa research shows that when infants over age 6 weeks are fed overly concentrated formula or overly dilute formula, they simply eat less of the concentrated formula or more of the dilute formula and grow consistently. Until age 6 weeks, children compensate for variations in formula concentration, but not completely. After 6 weeks, they compensate completely.[1] From age 1 week to 9 months, Houston anthropologist Linda Adair followed the formula and solid-food intake of a little boy being fed on demand. Although the infant ate three times as much some days as other days, and even though his food intake was lower than 90 percent of other babies, his growth was consistent and his weight was average. When he started eating solid foods, he took less formula and continued to regulate well.[2]

Even premature babies can regulate. A study conducted by newborn intensive care unit nurses shows that medically stable infants who weigh between 1,800 and 2,500 grams at birth are able to give signs to their care providers indicating when they are hungry and when they are full. The demand-fed babies grow better on fewer calories than schedule-fed babies.[3]

The amount children eat varies throughout the day. Children are able to compensate for variations in the amounts they eat at mealtimes and snack times.[4] Children automatically seek out high-calorie foods—those containing sugar and fat—when their calorie needs are particularly high.[5] Colorado Public Health studies that followed children from year to year found that the amounts they eat as well as the composition of their food intake varies considerably. Some years, for instance, they eat far less fat, and other years they eat far more.[6]

You can't predict how much a child needs to eat. As with adults, calorie needs vary widely from child to child. Children of all ages who look alike and act alike may vary from one another in their calorie requirement by as much as 40 percent.[7] This is a result of children's constitutional endowment, not because of poor patterns of food consumption or activity. Any assumptions you make about children's calorie intake based on looking at them are likely to be wrong. Studies of young infants by Harvard nutritionist Jean Mayer show that the fattest babies tend to eat the least and are least active, and the leanest babies eat the most and are most active.[8]

Distortions in Energy Regulation

Children's considerable food regulation capability depends on their being supported with the division of responsibility in feeding throughout their growing-up years. Both over-control of the child's prerogative in eating and under-support of the child's access to food can cause disruptions in food regulation and growth. Children of authoritative parents—those who are parented well—grow appropriately, whereas children of permissive, neglectful, or overly strict parents are at increased risk of overweight.[9] Both mothers and fathers who are concerned about child overweight or have anti-fat attitudes are likely to restrict children's food intake and raise fatter children.[10] Being overcontrolling with feeding—trying to get children to eat more or less than they want—interferes with children's knowing when they are hungry and when they are full and contributes to undereating as well as to overeating.[4]

Sugary and fatty foods are often blamed for making children overeat. But children and other people who have structure and support for eating and whose internal regulators are intact can get full without overeating when they are offered sugary and fatty foods, the same as they do when they are offered other foods. But if sugary and fatty foods are forbidden and purged from the family food supply, children overeat on them when they get a chance and are fatter than children whose parents are more matter-of-fact about including them in meals and snacks.[11] Restricting a child's food intake tells the child that his weight is unsatisfactory. A child who gets idea that he is overweight feels bad in all ways: not smart, not physically capable, and not worthwhile.[12]

Distortions in feeding dynamics can start at birth. An Edinburgh, Scotland study with normal, well-born infants shows that parents of smaller-than-average babies tend to be more active in feeding than parents of average sized babies. The more active the parents, the less well the babies grow. Since it is easier to get pushy with bottle-feeding than with breast-feeding, the tendency to be overactive shows up more with bottle-feeding parents than with those who breastfeed.[13]

A few children suffer from growth problems serious enough to be diagnosed as Nonorganic Failure to Thrive (NOFTT). In many if not most cases, disruptions in the feeding relationship are at the root of the problem. Clinicians in a Buffalo, New York, hospital found that half of infants hospitalized with growth failure had feeding problems.[14] Disruption in the achievement of developmental tasks can undermine a child's ability to eat and grow normally. In her work with infants and toddlers, Washington, DC, Children's Hospital psychiatrist Irene

Chatoor found that disorders of homeostasis, attachment, and separation/individuation can contribute to NOFTT and that toddler NOFTT is related to mother-child interaction.[15]

Clinical observations indicate that letting children graze for food can make them either eat too much and grow too rapidly, or eat too little and grow too slowly. Psychologist Kay Toomey found in her clinical work with poorly eating toddlers that toddlers fed in a structured fashion eat 50 percent more than when they are allowed to graze for food.[16] Texas A&M anthropologist Katherine Dettwyler observed New Guinea toddlers roaming the village in groups and eating only if they happened to be present in a home when food was available. Adults did not, in any systematic way, see to it that toddlers got fed. Growth rates of children in New Guinea were very slow.[17]

Parents' concerns about their own weight as well as their children's contribute to distortions in feeding. Mothers report using more restrictive feeding practices when they are invested in weight and eating issues overall, when they perceive daughters as overweight, when they are concerned about daughters' weight, and when daughters are heavier. Mothers also report using more pressure in child feeding when daughters are thinner, and when mothers perceive daughters as underweight.[18] This interference with feeding has been demonstrated to be counterproductive.[4,19]

Children whose food intake is restricted tend to become food-preoccupied and overeat when they get a chance. Children who are urged and coerced to eat more than they want frequently become resistant to eating and undereat when they get a chance. However, whether a child eats too much or too little in response to parental pressure with feeding depends on who gets the upper hand with feeding. The submissive child of a controlling parent may be underfed or overfed in accordance with the parent's wishes. On the other hand, a more aggressive child may resist the parent's feeding efforts and eat in the very way that the parent is trying to prevent.

The tactics parents use to control their own food intake rub off on children, for good or ill. Parents who overcontrol their own eating, with either amount or type of food, tend to throw away all controls from time to time and be fatter than if they ate consistently. In the Framingham children's study, parents who display high levels of disinhibited eating, especially when coupled with high dietary restraint, appear to foster excess weight gain in their children.[20] Children of parents who restrain and disinhibit also tend to disinhibit and are relatively fat.[19] Associations between parents' restrictiveness with respect to their own eating behavior and adolescent eating attitudes and behaviors have not been examined. However, parental attitudes and behaviors undoubtedly play a role in precipitating adolescent characteristics that do correlate with eating disorders: high incidence of dieting behavior, pressure to be thin, modeling of eating disturbances, appearance overvaluation, and body dissatisfaction.[21]

On the other hand, adolescents who report parental meal management behaviors that involve taking leadership and giving autonomy are less likely to engage in disordered eating. Adolescents do better with eating when parents assign a high priority to family meals, provide family meals more frequently, and maintain a positive atmosphere at mealtimes.[22] Regardless of their weight to begin with, 13- to 16-year-olds using both healthful and unhealthful weight-control behaviors are four or five times more likely to have gained too much weight 5 years later than adolescents not using any weight-control behaviors. "Healthful" behaviors include exercising more and eating more fruits and vegetables and less fat and sweets. Unhealthful behaviors include fasting or eating very little food; using a food substitute such as a powder or a special drink; skipping meals; using diuretics, laxatives, or diet pills; and vomiting. Teenagers who don't diet don't gain too much weight.[23]

The point? Children know how much they need to eat, but they need help from adults if they are to act on and retain that capability. Children need to be able to tune in on what goes on inside of them and be aware of how hungry or how full they are. If adults give them insufficient support—if they don't offer food regularly or if they fail to offer appropriate situational and emotional support at feeding times—children can have trouble knowing how hungry or how full they are and can eat too little or too much. If adults are too active and controlling in feeding and interfere with the children's prerogatives of whether and how much they eat of what parents provide, children experience so much static and interference from the outside that they can't tune in on their sensations of hunger, appetite, and satiety. Sometimes children go along with pressure from the outside and eat more or less than they really want. Sometimes they fight against that pressure, and, again, eat more or less than they really want. Either way, they lose sight of how much they need and make errors in regulation. They eat too much or too little, and they get too fat or too thin.

References

1. Fomon SJ, Filer LJJr., Thomas LN, Anderson TA, Nelson SE. Influence of formula concentration on caloric intake and growth of normal infants. *Acta Paediatrica Scandanavica.* 1975;64:172-181.
2. Adair LS. The infant's ability to self-regulate caloric intake: a case study. *J Ame Diet Assoc.* 1984;84:543-546.
3. Collinge JM, Bradley K, Perks C, Rezny A, Topping P. Demand vs. scheduled feedings for premature infants. *JOGN Nurs.* 1982;11:362-367.
4. Birch LL, Davison KK. Family environmental factors influencing the developing behavioral controls of food intake and childhood overweight. *Pediatr Clin North Am.* 2001;48:893-907.
5. Kern DL, McPhee L, Fisher JO, Johnson S, Birch LL. The postingestive consequences of fat condition preferences for flavors associated with high dietary fat. *Physiol Behav.* 1993;54:71-76.
6. Beal VA. Dietary intake of individuals followed through infancy and childhood. *Am J Public Health.* 1961;51(8):1107-1117.
7. National Research Council (NRC). *Recommended Dietary Allowances, 10th Ed.* Washington, DC: National Academy Press; 1989.
8. Rose HE, Mayer J. Activity, calorie intake, fat storage, and the energy balance of infants. *Pediatrics.* 1968;41:18-29.
9. Rhee KE, Lumeng JC, Appugliese DP, Kaciroti N, Bradley RH. Parenting styles and overweight status in first grade. *Pediatrics.* 2006;117:2047-2054.

10. Musher-Eizenman DR, Holub SC, Hauser JC, Young KM . The relationship between parents' anti-fat attitudes and restrictive feeding. *Obesity (Silver Spring)*. 2007;15:2095-2102.

11. Fisher JO, Birch LL. Eating in the absence of hunger and overweight in girls from 5 to 7 y of age. *Am J Clin Nutr*. 2002;76:226-231.

12. Davison KK, Birch LL. Weight status, parent reaction, and self-concept in five-year-old girls. *Pediatrics*. 2001;107:46-53.

13. Crow RA, Fawcett JN, Wright P. Maternal behavior during breast- and bottle-feeding. *J Behav Med*. 1980;3(3):259-277.

14. Sills RH. Failure to thrive: the role of clinical and laboratory evaluation. *Am J Dis Child*. 1978;132:967-969.

15. Chatoor I, Surles J, Ganiban J, Beker L, Paez LM, Kerzner B. Failure to thrive and cognitive development in toddlers with infantile anorexia. *Pediatrics*. 2004;113:e440-e447.

16. Toomey KA. Caloric intake of todders fed structured meals and snacks versus on demand. *Verbal Communication*. 1994.

17. Dettwyler KA. Styles of infant feeding: parental/caretaker control of food consumption in young children. *American Anthropologist*. 1989;91:696-703.

18. Francis LA, Hofer SM, Birch LL. Predictors of maternal child-feeding style: maternal and child characteristics. *Appetite*. 2001;37:231-243.

19. Savage JS, Fisher JO, Birch LL. Parental influence on eating behavior: conception to adolescence. *J Law Med Ethics*. 2007;35:22-34.

20. Hood MY, Moore LL, Sundarajan-Ramamurti A, Singer M, Cupples LA, Ellison RC. Parental eating attitudes and the development of obesity in children. The Framingham Children's Study. *Int J Obes (Lond)*. 2000;24:1319-1325.

21. Stice E, Presnell K, Spangler D. Risk factors for binge eating onset in adolescent girls: a 2-year prospective investigation. *Health Psychol*. 2002;21:131-138.

22. Neumark-Sztainer D, Wall M, Story M, Fulkerson JA. Are family meal patterns associated with disordered eating behaviors among adolescents? *J Adolesc Health*. 2004;35:350-359.

23. Neumark-Sztainer D, Wall M, Guo J, Story M, Haines J, Eisenberg M. Obesity, disordered eating, and eating disorders in a longitudinal study of adolescents: how do dieters fare 5 years later? *J Am Diet Assoc*. 2006;106:559-568.

Appendix
J
Children and Food Acceptance: The Research

Children learn to eat the foods their parents eat, and they will automatically eat a variety. However, typical childhood eating behaviors and poor information about feeding lead parents to feed in ways that hinder, rather than foster, food acceptance. What do we know about children's ability to learn to like and eat a variety of food? What do we know about productive and counterproductive approaches to feeding?

Some of the earliest research was reported in 1928 by Clara Davis, a New York Mt. Sinai Hospital physician. At the time, pediatricians dictated precisely the food amounts, types, and feeding frequencies for children from 7 months to 3 years of age. The rigid feeding advice was based on the convictions that the transition from breastfeeding to adult food should take 3 or 4 years and that infants didn't know how much they needed to eat. Davis questioned these convictions, and she tested them in experiments with three boys ages 8, 9, and 10 months. For 6 to 12 months, she and her team offered the infants trays with a variety of natural, healthy food. At first the babies sampled everything— the dishes and the doilies as well as the food. They soon learned to discriminate between food and non-food, and between what they wanted to eat and what they didn't. It was impossible to predict what a child would eat at a given meal. An infant might eat from one to seven eggs a day or one to four bananas. Milk consumption ranged from 11 to 48 ounces. The infants even ate salt occasionally, crying and spluttering but not spitting it out, then going back for more. At the time he was enrolled in

the study, one infant had rickets caused by vitamin D deficiency. To correct the deficiency, he was offered cod liver oil in one of his little dishes. Over the first several months of the experiment, he voluntarily consumed almost 9 ounces of the strong-tasting oil. His rickets healed and his tests showed that his vitamin D status was corrected. Then he stopped consuming it, even though it was still on his tray.[1]

Davis's study demonstrated that infants could be healthy and grow well on self-selected diets. Essentially, the researchers maintained the division of responsibility in feeding. They chose a variety of simple, single-ingredient, healthful food for the infants and then let them pick and choose from what was available. Unfortunately, Davis's study is often misquoted and used to rationalize letting children freely graze for self-selected food.

Pennsylvania State researcher Barbara Rolls freshened up the Davis research and gave it a new name. Rolls found that through a process she calls *sensory specific satiety*, children and other people tire of even favorite food and choose otherwise.[2]

As with Clara Davis's babies, children's variations in appetite lead them over time to eat a variety of food and, provided grownups take responsibility for feeding them and maintain a nutritionally adequate diet. Observational studies conducted at the University of Illinois preschool illustrate that children are particularly equipped to make use of these internal cues. These studies found that children are tuned in to food and are far more likely than adults to eat in response to whether the food appeals to them at any given time, and that what they eat one time, they don't another.[3] Children like what is familiar. Nutritionist Jean Skinner found in her surveys that Tennessee mothers complain of their year-old infants' marked increase in food likes and dislikes and their tendency to lose interest in a food after one bite.[4] This highly typical food skepticism doesn't stop children from learning to like new food. Illinois researchers found that children taste new food, and the more often they taste it, the more they like it. Children might take 10, 15, or 20 tastes in as many meals before they learn to like a new food. Infants as young 4 to 6 months who are first introduced to solid foods are skeptical about new foods. The solution for children of all ages is the same: repeated *neutral* exposure. Breastfed infants, presumably because they are accustomed to flavors conveyed in their mother's milk, are more receptive on first introduction to foods compared with formula-fed infants.[3]

To move successfully and willingly through the transition period from nipple-feeding to semisolid food to table food, an infant has to have oral-motor readiness. Colorado public health nutritionist Virginia Beal found that babies under 4 months old resist taking solid foods and get into feeding struggles with their mothers. Babies first cheerfully accept solid foods at around age 4 months.[5] Many parents offer solid foods far too early and apparently engage in struggles with their infants similar to those Beal observed. A 1998 survey done by the Beech-Nut baby food company found that spoon-feeding is a least favorite activity of up to 40 percent of surveyed parents, second in undesirability only to changing diapers.[6] It is unclear what long-term impact these early feeding struggles have on food acceptance.

The critical element in children's food acceptance is *repeated neutral exposure*. To learn to like new food, children must be allowed to try the food repeatedly as well as on their own initiative. Pressure of any sort, even persuasion, praise, or reward, slows down or stops their learning. Preschoolers offered a new juice and allowed to experiment with it on their own are more likely to try the juice again than children who are rewarded for tasting it on their first exposure. Eating with a friend who likes the new food increases food acceptance. So does eating with a trusted adult who is simply being companionable, friendly, and supportive, and who doesn't talk about the food.[3] Nebraska nutrition professor Kaye Stanek found that preschoolers do better with food acceptance when they eat with their parents and/or siblings, when they are given enough time to eat, when they are allowed to help prepare foods or set the table, and when they are allowed to take small portions of new foods.[7]

Problems with Food Acceptance

Children learn to eat—or not eat—from the way they are fed. Feeding problems are common, as are negative feeding behaviors. A 2003 review of the literature indicates that 25 to 45 percent of typically developing children and up to 80 percent of developmentally disabled children have feeding problems. These problems include bizarre food habits, mealtime tantrums, delays in self-feeding, difficulty in accepting various food textures, and multiple food dislikes, as well as feeding disorders such as infant rumination, childhood obesity, and infant anorexia nervosa.[8] Stanek found that typical negative food-related behaviors of parents with 2- to 5-year-old children include bargaining, bribing, and forcing; promising a special food, such as dessert, for eating a meal; withholding food as punishment; rewarding "good" behavior with food; persuading children to eat; playing a game to get children to eat; taking over and feeding children who refuse to eat; threatening punishment for not eating; and making children clean their plates.[7]

Parents engrossed in feeding struggles with their children have difficulty perceiving their own contribution to the problem. Children have trouble learning to like new food if they have either too few opportunities to learn or too much pressure. Children eat poorly when parents limit menus to food that children readily accept, fail to provide regular and reliable opportunities to eat, or encourage, persuade, or insist that they eat. Skinner's Tennessee studies show that adults try food only three times before it disappears from the table[9] and that almost three-quarters of mothers of 16-month-olds offer alternatives when their toddlers don't eat "enough." More than 10 percent acknowledge using force or bribery to get children to eat.[4] Pelchat and Pliner found that Toronto children who are reluctant to try new food have mothers who short-order cook or offer only foods that children readily accept. The Toronto mothers prod, reward, and punish to get children to eat. Those alternatively overindulgent and pushy mothers are seemingly unaware of their own counterproductive feeding behaviors and instead complain that their children are finicky, unwilling to try new foods, avoid whole classes of foods such as vegetables, eat too little, prefer junk food, or are simply not interested in food and eating.[10]

Like the Toronto mothers, Pennsylvania parents appear to be both overindulgent and pushy. Parents in focus groups said that they want to provide good nutrition with not too many sweets and processed foods. At the same time, they short-order cook for their children, use bribes and rewards to get their children to eat, believe their children are being untruthful when they say they are full, and encourage children to eat more when they say they are full.[11] Children are tuned in to their grown-ups and know when they are being pressured, even when that pressure wears a seemingly pleasant disguise. Nonetheless, 85 percent of San Francisco parents of kindergarteners observed during feeding include reasoning, praise, and rewards among their repertoire to get children to eat more than they do voluntarily.[12] Studies in Pennsylvania State preschool laboratories indicate that children who are pressured to eat consume less food and make more negative comments about the food than children who are not pressured.[13] Parents have been repeatedly reminded that fruits and vegetables are important and try to get their children to eat them, even if the parents themselves don't like and don't eat them. Texas researcher Jennifer Fisher observed that under such circumstances, children do not eat their vegetables. On the other hand, parents who like and eat fruits and vegetables have children who do the same.[14]

Nature or Nurture?

Research by Lucy Cooke indicating that there is a genetic basis for food selectivity[15] raised the hopes of beleaguered parents that their child's food rejection wasn't, as one mother put it, "my fault." Are children selective with food because of inborn predisposition, or because of their upbringing? With respect to nature, of course there are differences in children. Some children are exquisitely sensitive to tastes and textures, have a strong gag reflex, and throw up easily. Some children are diagnosed as having sensory integration disorders, meaning they react

against pronounced or unusual tastes and textures. Some children are super-tasters—they can detect the bitter taste in foods including cabbage-family vegetables[16] and they may be more tuned into sweet and other flavors as well. Some children are temperamentally negative with respect to new experiences—including food experiences.[17]

However, children do not have to be handicapped by their predilections, and that brings us to nurture. Even children who have temperamental or neurological barriers can learn to cope with their own limitations. The same as all other children, they set out to learn to eat the food their parents eat and they learn to like a variety of food. They do, that is, provided they have regular and unpressured opportunities to learn. That means the food matter-of-factly shows up again and again on the family table and parents eat and enjoy it. It also means that parents do not pressure children in any way to eat: they do not remind, badger, reward, applaud, or withhold dessert until the child eats her vegetables.

What conclusion can we reach from this research? Children are capable of learning to eat the foods their parents and other trusted adults eat. However, they need help from adults if they are to act on and retain that capability. Children observe what foods their parents eat and assume, even if they don't eat them, that "someday I will eat that." Their assumption and their desire to grow up can be squashed by adults' behaving at either, or both, of two extremes: by imposing too much pressure or by providing too little support. Children need adults to be supportive and companionable, to show them what it means to grow up with respect to food, and to give them opportunities to experiment and master. They don't need to be coerced, controlled, or even motivated. Being motivated to learn and grow comes with being a child.

References

1. Davis CM. Self selection of diet by newly weaned infants: an experimental study. *Am J Dis Child*. 1928;36:651-679.
2. Rolls BJ. Sensory specific satiety. *Nutr Rev*. 1986;44:93-101.
3. Birch LL, Fisher JO. Appetite and eating behavior in children. *Pediatr Clin North Am*. 1995;42:931-953.

4. Skinner JD, Carruth BR, Houck K, et al. Mealtime communication patterns of infants from 2 to 24 months of age. *J Nutr Educ*. 1998;30:8-16.

5. Beal VA. On the acceptance of solid foods and other food patterns of infants and children. *Pediatrics*. 1957;20:448-456.

6. Public Relations Department. *Beech-Nut Baby Survey*. St. Louis, MO: Beech-Nut Nutrition Corporation; 1998.

7. Stanek K, Abbott D, Cramer S. Diet quality and the eating environment of preschool children. *J Am Diet Assoc*. 1990;90:1582-1584.

8. Linscheid TR, Budd KS, Rasnake LK; Pediatric feeding problems. M. C. Roberts. *Handbook of Pediatric Psychology (3rd Ed)*. New York, New York: Guilford; 2003:481-498.

9. Carruth BR, Skinner JD. Revisiting the picky eater phenomenon: neophobic behaviors of young children. *J Am Coll Nutr*. 2000;19:771-780.

10. Pelchat ML, Pliner P. Antecedents and correlates of feeding problems in young children. *J Nutr Educ*. 1986;18(1):23-28.

11. Sherry B, McDivitt J, Birch L, et al. Attitudes, practices, and concerns about child feeding and child weight status among socioeconomically diverse white, Hispanic, and African-American mothers. *J Am Diet Assoc*. 2004;104:215-221.

12. Orrell-Valente JK, Hill LG, Brechwald WA, Dodge KA, Pettit GS, Bates JE. "Just three more bites": an observational analysis of parents' socialization of children's eating at mealtime. *Appetite*. 2007; 48:37-45.

13. Galloway AT, Fiorito LM, Francis LA, Birch LL. 'Finish your soup': counterproductive effects of pressuring children to eat on intake and affect. *Appetite*. 2006;46:318-323.

14. Fisher JO, Mitchell DC, Smiciklas-Wright H, Birch LL. Parental influences on young girls' fruit and vegetable, micronutrient, and fat intakes. *J Am Diet Assoc*. 2002;102:58-64.

15. Cooke LJ, Haworth CM, Wardle J. Genetic and environmental influences on children's food neophobia. *Am J Clin Nutr*. 2007;86:428-433.

16. Drewnowski A , Henderson SA, Cockroft JE. Genetic sensitivity to 6-n-propylthiouracil has no influence on dietary patterns, body mass indexes, or plasma lipid profiles of women. *J Am Diet Assoc*. 2007;107:1340-1348.

17. Pliner P, Loewen ER. Temperament and food neophobia in children and their mothers. *Appetite*. 1997;28 :239-254.

Appendix
K
Iron in Your Child's Diet[*]

Iron in red blood cells carries oxygen to all parts of the body. When children don't get enough iron, they may look pale, act cranky, and not have much energy. Iron-deficiency anemia is one of the most common nutritional problems in children. You can, however, prevent anemia without much trouble by doing the following:

- Breastfeeding or using iron-fortified formula.
- Starting your baby by age 6 months on iron-fortified infant cereal. By 6 months, the natural supply of iron your baby had at birth is being depleted.
- Teaching your child to eat solid foods so she doesn't get stuck on milk.
- Having regular meals and taking some moderate care in menu planning.
- Serving nutritious food at snack time. Snacks shouldn't be just "treat" foods, because those have mostly calories and few other nutrients.

Strategies for Improving Iron Nutrition

When you think about your child's iron nutrition, you have to think not only about the amount of iron in his food, but also about how much iron he can absorb from the food into his body. For both adults and children, only a small percentage of iron in food is absorbed. Your child will absorb iron much better from meat, poultry, and fish than from vegetables or grains. But he'll absorb the iron in vegetables or grains better when he eats them at the same time he eats meat, poultry, or fish.

Vitamin C helps with iron absorption, too. Eating a food that is a good vitamin C source along with a meal improves iron absorption from the whole meal. Vitamin C is in many vegetables and fruits, such as oranges, strawberries, spinach, and broccoli. If your child gets meat, poultry, or fish and vitamin C at the same meal, he'll absorb even more iron from all the food in the meal. Examples of these combination meals (with meat, vitamin C, grain, and vegetable sources of iron) include hamburgers and coleslaw, spaghetti with meat-tomato sauce, hot dogs and orange wedges, and chicken with broccoli.

EGGS, MILK, AND LIVER
Although an egg yolk contains 1 milligram of iron, that iron is poorly absorbed. In fact, unless your child gets vitamin C at the same time, egg yolk actually cuts down on the iron he absorbs from other foods. Milk is low in iron; anemic children used to be called "milk babies."

Liver is an excellent source of iron, but eating a lot of liver gives too much vitamin A. If you serve liver, keep it down to twice a month.

Helping Your Child to Eat Iron-Rich Foods

Have regular meals and snacks, keep control of the menu, offer a variety of nourishing food, make eating times pleasant, and then wait. If you try to *force* your child to eat nutritious food he doesn't like, he probably won't eat it.

Typically, iron-rich foods are challenging for children. Green leafy vegetables, for example, have a strong flavor. Eat and enjoy them yourself, and after a while your child will try them and maybe even learn to like them. Meat may be hard for him to chew and swallow, so make it moist and tender. Remember that even eating a *little* meat, fish, or poultry helps his body absorb more iron from all the food in his meal.

IRON CONTENT OF SELECTED FOODS
Children need 6 to 10 milligrams of iron per day and adults need 8 milligrams. The foods listed in figure K.1 provide significant amounts of iron.

FIGURE K.1 FOODS HIGH IN IRON		
Food	Amount	Iron (in milligrams)
Beef, pork, lamb	1 ounce	1.0
Poultry	1 ounce	0.5
Beef or chicken liver	1 ounce	3.0
Calf liver	1 ounce	5.0
Pork liver	1 ounce	8.0
Clams	1 ounce	2.0
Oysters	1 ounce	4.0
Other fish, shellfish	1 ounce	0.5
Nuts, average	2 Tbsp	1.0

Appendix

L

Diet and Degenerative Disease: It's Not as Bad as You Think

The goal of prevention is to tell those of us who are otherwise in fine health how to remain healthy longer. But this advice comes with the expectation that any prescription given—whether diet or drug or change in lifestyle—will indeed prevent disease rather than becoming the agent of our disability or untimely death.[1] As indicated by appendix C, "What Surveys Say about our Eating," considerable distortion in eating attitudes and behaviors is associated with attempts to adhere to current nutrition policy. Is that distortion a necessary evil in order to achieve the greater good of disease prevention, or is the cost greater than the benefit?

Degenerative Disease

Degenerative diseases include the two leading killers, cancer and heart disease, as well as chronic obstructive pulmonary disease (emphysema), stroke, and diabetes. Heart disease is considered to be the biggest diet-related killer, with more speculation than evidence relating diet and cancer. If diet kills by causing heart disease, it must take a long time. Data from the National Center for Health Statistics indicate that for both sexes taken together for all ages as well as for men and women considered individually, about 27 percent of deaths are caused by cardiovascular disease and 23 percent are caused by cancer. However, until ages 45 to 49 years, the leading cause of death for both sexes is accidents. Between 45 and 80 years, the leading cause of death for both

sexes together and for men and women individually is cancer, and the second leading cause is heart disease, accounting for roughly 50 percent of deaths overall. But keep in mind that the death rate in younger-age categories is relatively low. It is only in the over-80 age categories that heart disease becomes the leading killer. At that point, the high overall death rates shift the statistics upward for all age groups to make heart disease appear to be the big killer. In reality, it is the big killer for the *old*, but not for the *young*.[2] These data are all online, and if you wish, you can peruse all 162 pages, just like I did!

Such data call into question a release from the National Heart, Lung, and Blood Institute (NHLBI) of the National Institutes of Health claiming that newly analyzed data show that the number of women who die from heart disease "has shifted from 1 in 3 women to 1 in 4—a decrease of nearly 17,000 deaths from 2003 to 2004."[3] These annual statistics are alarming but meaningless. Surely 1 and 4 women don't die! You *could* say that of the women *who die*, one in four die of heart disease. Only 0.4 percent of women between the ages of 50 and 54 die each year, 17% of heart disease, which means that 0.06 percent of women in any one year die of heart disease. Again, it is only after age 80 that death rates become high. At that age, a lot of women die, and of those who die, about three in five die of heart disease. But are those numbers really so alarming? Keep in mind that we all have to die of *something*.

Dietary Fat and Heart Disease

There is enough disagreement about the correlation between diet and disease to make prevention only a *hope*, not a *guarantee*. Despite the extent to which health professionals, scientists, and educators back the restrictions and modifications of the Dietary Guidelines, the strength of the link between diet and degenerative disease is debatable. The debate goes way back and is complicated.

The *diet = disease* connection began with the University of Minnesota's Ancel Keys (he of the Minnesota Semi-Starvation Study) and his 1953 seven-country epidemiological survey, in which he found an association between dietary saturated fat and heart disease mortality.[4] In the late 1960s, the seemingly alarming increase in death rates from heart disease stimulated clinical observations testing Keys's hypothesis about the link between dietary saturated fat and heart disease. Carrying the research one step further, three major clinical intervention trials in the 1970s claimed to demonstrate that reductions in dietary fat reduced mortality from heart disease: the Framingham Study,[5] the Multiple Risk Factor Intervention Trial (MRFIT),[6] and the Lipid Research Clinics Coronary Primary Prevention Trial (CPPT).[7] Reports from all three studies indicated that middle-aged men with high blood cholesterol were roughly twice as likely to die of heart attacks than those with low blood cholesterol, and that dietary intervention halved the death rate.

These are the studies, and the numbers, that form the foundation for our current nutrition policy: the Dietary Guidelines and MyPyramid. It is in the *interpretation* of the numbers that dietary enthusiasts and dietary moderates diverge. The enthusiasts, who are currently directing nutrition policy, insist that the results are significant enough to warrant putting us all on modified-fat, low-cholesterol diets. The moderates, who are heard only if you happen to read one of their dissenting articles, look at the same research and disagree.[8-10]

Moderates point out that the "alarming increase" in death rates from heart disease was a *false* alarm. More careful examination of the data some years later showed that age-adjusted mortality from heart disease actually declined between 1940 and 1960.[11] The source of the error? Categories for causes of death had changed, and more deaths were attributed to coronary heart disease and fewer to other diseases than before. Moderates also protest that Keys was selective in the seven countries he chose for his epidemiological survey. Repeating his epidemiological research with all 21 countries for which data were available showed a far weaker association between diet and heart disease mortality.[12] Not only that, but a look at the actual numbers in that "halving of the death rate" in those original Framingham, MRFIT, and CPPT studies revealed the results to be far less impressive than reported by their supporters. The death rate among men who lowered their cholesterol was reduced to 0.7 from 1.4 deaths per 1,000 men per year. That is a small difference—so small, in fact, that given the low death rates in both treated and untreated subjects, it was hard to distinguish between deaths associated with high blood cholesterol and those resulting from mere chance.

There are other reasons to doubt whether the original studies warranted putting us all on modified-fat, low-cholesterol diets. The MRFIT and CPPT studies weren't done with a cross-section of the population, but only with high-risk men between the ages of 35 and 59. The studies went beyond dietary changes and also attempted to increase activity and decrease smoking. Not only that, but the CPPT administered a cholesterol-lowering drug. In spite of stacking the deck so thoroughly in favor of a positive impact from "dietary change," the interventions showed slight results with respect to lowering both blood lipids and death rates. However, despite the weakness of the evidence, and despite the fact that the MRFIT and CPPT research was done on high-risk middle-aged men, researchers declared their trials a success, asserting that they provided proof that a high intake of saturated fat is a cause of heart disease.

I realize my little exposé about the diet–heart disease connection may seem astonishing and unbelievable. Others say the same thing. In his book, Gary Taubes sums up his review of the same history by writing, "From the inception of the diet-heart hypothesis in the early 1950s, those who argued that dietary fat caused heart disease accumulated the evidential equivalent of a mythology to support their belief. These myths are still passed on faithfully to the present day."[13] In his book, *The Cholesterol Myths*, Danish Uffe Ravnskov's reaches the same conclusion.[14] Briefer sources of astonishment include Taubes's *Science* article, "The Soft Science of Dietary Fat,"[15] or Thomas Moore's 1989 *Atlantic Monthly* article, "The Cholesterol Myth."[16] If you read Taubes's book, keep in mind that his assertions about the evils of carbohydrate are contradicted by solid research.

Current Research

Research today broadens the *diet = disease* connection to include not only high dietary fat and high saturated fat, but also low fruit, vegetable, and fiber consumption. Two major studies, the Women's Health Initiative and the Nurse's Health Study, raise questions about the connection. Except for "ever-smokers," the Nurse's Health Study found no overall association between "prudent" and "Western" dietary patterns and the risk of breast cancer.[17] The prudent pattern is characterized by high intakes of fruits and vegetables, poultry, and fish; the Western pattern is characterized by high intakes of meat, fat, and refined grains.

The $415 million Women's Health Initiative study tracked for 8 years nearly 49,000 women aged 50 to 79 who were randomly assigned to either to a control group or to follow a diet of 20 percent fat, high fruit and vegetable, and high fiber. The study found that the diet did *not* make a significant difference in the development of breast cancer, colorectal cancer, and heart disease. Both the control group and the intervention group started out eating 39 percent of calories as dietary fat. Despite intensive counseling, the lowest the dieting women could get their fat intake, on average, was 24 percent in the first year, and 29 percent later. Meanwhile, the control women dropped their fat intake from 39 percent to 38 percent of total calories. At the same time, the intervention women increased their fruit and vegetable intake by one serving per day more than the controls (1.5 versus a 0.5 serving increase) and ate fewer grains than before.[18] The 20,000 intervention women had essentially the same incidence of breast cancer, colorectal cancer, heart disease, and stroke as the 29,000 women who followed their normal eating patterns,[19,18,20] and BMIs in the two groups of women were essentially the same.[21]

Dietary enthusiasts maintain that the Women's Health Initiative's emphasis on reducing total fat rather than saturated fat renders it meaningless, and that 8 years isn't long enough to see differences in the development of degenerative diseases.[22] Despite a consistent lack of evidence, dietary enthusiasts continue to maintain that, "together with regular physical activity, avoidance of smoking, and maintenance of a healthy body weight," three major dietary strategies may prevent the majority of cardiovascular disease in Western populations: (1) Substitute nonhydrogenated unsaturated fats for saturated and trans fats; (2) Increase consumption of omega-3 fatty acids from fish, fish oil supplements, or plant sources; and (3) Consume a diet high in fruits, vegetables, nuts, and whole grains and low in refined grain products.[23] The current thrust toward establishing a *diet = disease* connection appears to be directed toward the Mediterranean diet,[24] which is essentially other researchers acknowledge that a prudent diet with olive oil. However, other researchers acknowledge that a Mediterranean diet is not enough for health.[25]

Relative to other degenerative diseases, Harvard researchers found a slight decrease in emphysema for men and women who consume a Prudent diet versus a Western diet.[26,27] In a multisite clinical study, the colon cancer survival rate is slightly higher for men who follow a prudent dietary pattern compared with a Western pattern.[28]

Restricting Fat Is Difficult

Whatever the fine-tuning of the dietary fat recommendations, applying them and getting convincing results has been extraordinarily difficult. The Women's Health Initiative demonstrated yet again that even patients with careful follow-up and support have trouble restricting dietary fat. Clinical research involves intensive education and follow-up throughout the course of the intervention. Community or work-site interventions are much less intensive. People participating in these interventions have not changed their eating behaviors, although they have become more aware and concerned about the connection between diet and disease.[29,30]

People on carefully supervised clinical studies have considerable trouble adhering to a modified-fat, low-cholesterol diet, and when they do, they have a modest and variable response: on the average, a decrease in cholesterol of 3 to 4 percent[31] with a presumed decrease in the incidence of heart disease of 13 percent for each 10 percent blood cholesterol is reduced.[32] Some people respond well to dietary changes; others respond poorly.[33] Do the changes help? Again, it is a matter of interpretation. In reporting their results, researchers tend to describe small changes like a 3 or 4 percent decrease in cholesterol by using phrases like "a sharp decrease." When *you* interpret these numbers, remember that changes from any intervention are likely to be small and that the word "sharp" was used to describe the "50 percent decrease" in relative mortality found in the original studies, the studies in which deaths were reduced in absolute numbers from 1.4 to 0.7 per 1,000 individuals per year.

The conclusion from this literature review is that deaths from heart disease, the major target of dietary modification, are not as high as we fear, particularly at younger ages. Moreover, even successful dietary modification has little impact on blood lipids and mortality. Dietary modification is extraordinarily difficult and carries with it a high risk of distortion in eating attitudes and behaviors.

A Moderate Approach to Wellness

Where does this leave us? With putting the emphasis on *seeking* food, not *avoiding* it. There is no doubt that eating an adequate diet is essential to maintaining health and well-being and to preventing diseases of nutritional inadequacy. There is doubt that diet can prevent degenerative disease. In other words, be as healthy as you can be. Be conscientious about feeding yourself, eat a varied and wholesome diet made up of foods you enjoy, hedge your bets by using a variety of dietary fats, and pat yourself on the back for behaving responsibly. I am, of course, describing being competent with eating. Based on our research and clinical experience, we have good reason to believe that developing eating competence is a good way of hedging your bets against disease. People with high eating competence have lower blood cholesterol, higher HDL, and lower blood pressure, and they show evidence of doing well nutritionally.[34]

If you have a *particular* risk of heart disease, get individual guidance. See a dietitian, have your eating patterns respectfully evaluated, and do the least you can to get the results you want. Remember that eating is more important than avoidance. Start by developing your eating competence. Stabilizing your eating patterns and increasing the variety in your diet may be

all the change you need. Don't forget about activity as a way of increasing HDL. To take it a step further, be systematic about varying the types of fat you eat within the context of being a competent eater. You may respond to diet and exercise, or you may not. As you make changes, have your blood lipids tested to see if you are getting results. Only become formulaic about your food selection as a last resort, and if it spoils your eating, stop doing it. In the long run, you will be worse off. If your doctor recommends medication, read *all* the fine print. Remember that those expensive drugs are tested by enthusiasts funded by drug companies that make money on them, and they often have negative side effects.

More research will be ballyhooed, and much of it will be contradictory to what we presently think we know. You can't run around purging and refilling your pantry shelves every time you hear about a new study. Well, I guess you can. It depends on how you want to spend your time. What to do instead? Put your emphasis on eating competence. Be honest about what you love and don't want to give up. And prepare to be surprised. The mystery of degenerative disease is a long way from being solved.

References

1. Taubes G. Do we really know what makes us healthy? *N Y Times Magazine.* 2007;156:52-80.
2. National Center for Health Statistics [Web site]. LCWK1 Deaths, percent of total deaths, and death rates for the 15 leading causes of death in 5-year age groups, by race and sex: United States, 1999-2004. [Web page] Centers for Disease Control and Prevention Web site. http://www.cdc.gov/nchs/datawh/statab/ unpubd/mortabs/lcwk1_10.htm. Accessed December 13, 2007.
3. Nabel, E.G. Heart disease deaths in American women decline. *FDA Consum.* 2007;41:8.
4. Keys A. Atherosclerosis: a problem in newer public health. *Journal of the Mount Sinai Hospital.* 1953;20:118-139.
5. Kannel WB, Castelli WP, Gordon T, McNamara PM. Serum cholesterol, lipoproteins and risk for coronary heart disease: the Framingham Study. *Ann Intern Med.* 1971;74:1-12.
6. Martin MJ, Hulley SB, Browner WS, Kuller LH, Wentworth D. Serum cholesterol, blood pressure and mortality: implications from a cohort of 361,662 men. *Lancet.* 1986;2:933-936.

7. Lipid Research Clinics Program. The Lipid Research Clinics Coronary Primary Prevention Trial results II: the relationship of reduction in incidence of coronary heart disease to cholesterol lowering. *JAMA*. 1984;251:365-374.

8. Harper AE. Dietary guidelines in perspective. *J Nutr* . 1996;126 (suppl):1042S-1048S.

9. Howell WH, McNamara DJ, Tosca MA, Smith BT, Gaines JA. Plasma lipid and lipoprotein responses to dietary fat and cholesterol: a meta-analysis. *Am J Clin Nutr*. 1997;65:1747-1764.

10. Muldoon MF, Manuck SB, Matthews KA. Lowering cholesterol concentrations and mortality: a quantitative review of primary prevention trials. *Br Med J*. 1990;301:309-314.

11. Kwiterovich POJ. The effect of dietary fat, antioxidants and pro-oxidants on blood lipids, lipoproteins and atherosclerosis. *J Am Diet Assoc*. 1997;97:S31-S41.

12. Yerushalmy JHHE. Fat in the diet and mortality from heart disease: a methodological note. *N Y State J Med*. 1957;2343-2354.

13. Taubes G. *Good Calories, Bad Calories: Challenging the Conventional Wisdom on Diet, Weight Control, and Disease*. New York, NY: Alfred A. Knopf; 2007.

14. Ravnskov U. *The Cholesterol Myths: Exposing the Fallacy That Saturated Fat and Cholesterol Cause Heart Disease*. Washington, DC: New Trends Publishing, Inc.; 2000.

15. Taubes G. The soft science of dietary fat. *Science*. 2001;291:2536-2545.

16. Moore TJ. The cholesterol myth. *Atlantic Monthly*. September 1989: 37-70.

17. Adebamowo CA , Hu FB, Cho E, Spiegelman D, Holmes MD, Willett WC. Dietary patterns and the risk of breast cancer. *Ann Epidemiol*. 2005;15:789-795.

18. Howard BV, Van Horn L, Hsia J, et al. Low-fat dietary pattern and risk of cardiovascular disease: the Women's Health Initiative randomized controlled dietary modification trial. *JAMA*. 2006;295:655-666.

19. Prentice RL, Caan B, Chlebowski RT, et al. Low-fat dietary pattern and risk of invasive breast cancer: the Women's Health Initiative randomized controlled dietary modification trial. *JAMA*. 2006;295:629-642.

20. Beresford SAA, Johnson KC, Ritenbaugh C, et al. Low-fat dietary pattern and risk of colorectal cancer: the Women's Health Initiative randomized controlled dietary modification trial. *JAMA*. 2006;295:643-654.

21. Howard BV, Manson JE, Stefanick ML, et al. Low-fat dietary pattern and weight change over 7 years: the Women's Health Initiative dietary modification trial. *JAMA*. 2006;295:39-49.

22. Stein K. After the media feeding frenzy: whither the Women's Health Initiative dietary modification trial? *J Am Diet Assoc*. 2006;106:794-800.

23. Hu FB, Willett WC. Optimal diets for prevention of coronary heart disease. *JAMA*. 2002;288:2569-2578.

24. Panagiotakos DB, Pitsavos C, Arvaniti F, Stefanadis C. Adherence to the Mediterranean food pattern predicts the prevalence of hypertension, hypercholesterolemia, diabetes and obesity, among healthy adults; the accuracy of the MedDietScore. *Prev Med*. 2007; 44:335-340.

25. Castillo-Garzon MJ, Ruiz JR, Ortega FB, Gutierrez-Sainz A. A Mediterranean diet is not enough for health: physical fitness is an important additional contributor to health for the adults of tomorrow. *World Rev Nutr Diet*. 2007;97:114-138.

26. Varraso R, Fung TT, Hu FB, Willett W, Camargo CA Jr. Prospective study of dietary patterns and chronic obstructive pulmonary disease among US men. *Thorax*. 2007;62:786-791.

27. Varraso R, Fung TT, Barr RG, Hu FB, Willett W, Camargo CAJ. Prospective study of dietary patterns and chronic obstructive pulmonary disease among US women. *Am J Clin Nutr*. 2007;86:488-495.

28. Meyerhardt JA, Niedzwiecki D, Hollis D, et al. Association of dietary patterns with cancer recurrence and survival in patients with stage III colon cancer. *JAMA*. 2007;298:754-764.

29. Frank JW, Reed DM, Grove JS, Benfante R. Will lowering population levels of serum cholesterol affect total mortality? *J Clin Epidemiol*. 1992;45:333-346.

30. Luepker RV, Jacobs DR, Folsom AR, et al. Cardiovascular risk factor change 1973-74 vs 1980-82: the Minnesota Heart Survey. *J Clin Epidemiol*. 1988;41:825-833.

31. Brunner E, White I, Thorogood M, Bristow A, Curle D, Marmot MG. Can dietary interventions in the population change diet and cardiovascular risk factors? An assessment of effectiveness utilising a meta-analysis of randomised controlled trials. *Am J Public Health.* 1997;87:1415-1422.

32. Gould AL, Rossouw JE, Santanello NC, Heyse JF, Furberg CD. Cholesterol reduction yields clinical benefit: a new look at old data. *Circulation.* 1995;91:2274-2282.

33. Krauss RM. Understanding the basis for variation in response to cholesterol-lowering diets. *Am J Clin Nutr.* 1997;65:885-886.

34. Psota T, Lohse B, West S. Associations between eating competence and cardio-vascular disease biomarkers . *J Nutr Educ Behav.* 2007;39 (suppl):S171-S178.

Appendix

M

Children, Dietary Fat, and Heart Disease: You Don't Have to Panic

Concern about children and heart disease, which was taking second place to hysteria about children and overweight, has again been activated by an American Academy of Pediatrics (AAP) position statement, "Lipid screening and cardiovascular disease in childhood."[1] The AAP recommends that 1) All children over age 2 years should follow a diet based on the Dietary Guidelines, including use of low-fat diary products; 2) Children as young as 2 years who have risk factors for heart disease or whose family medical history is not known should be screened for high total cholesterol, LDL ("bad," cholesterol), HDL ("good" cholesterol), and triglycerides; 3) Children whose lipid levels are above the 75th percentile for age should be referred for nutrition counseling in a diet that is, essentially, the Dietary Guidelines; and 4) The very few children 8 or older with very high concentrations of LDL—*way* above the 95th percentile—be considered for statin treatment to drive levels below 160 or even much lower.[1]

The statin recommendation has provoked furious debate among pediatricians. Critics complain that there is no evidence that giving statins to children will prevent heart attacks later in life and that there is no data on the potential side effects of taking the drugs for decades. These recommendations and the subsequent debate have put me in the surprising position of supporting the policy-makers. Target children have LDLs of 190 milligrams per deciliter or higher. Those children have inherited a tendency to errors in fat metabolism, called familial hyperlipidemia, and have a high

risk of premature cardiovascular disease. The someone-we-know who died of a heart attack at age 30 was probably a victim of familial hyperlipidemia. It is a scary process, and if I were asked to make preventive-care recommendations for those children, I genuinely don't know what I would say.

Fortunately, only a very few children are in that very-high-risk category. For the rest, my objection to the AAP statement is the naiveté that attends laying out arbitrary guidelines for what and how much a child should eat. No child ever ate according to a formula, and parents who try to impose a formula condemn themselves and their child to chaos and conflict. The justification given by the new AAP statement for imposing dietary rigidity on young children is that fat modification is effective in preventing heart disease in adults and that it will be even more effective if it is begun at age 2. The flaw in the reasoning, as I pointed out in appendix L, "Diet and Degenerative Disease: It's Not as Bad as You Think," is that dietary changes have only a marginal impact—except for the negative impact on eating attitudes and behaviors.

The atherosclerotic process begins in childhood, warn the enthusiasts, the most recent of which is the AAP, depending heavily on the American Heart Association and the National Cholesterol Education Program. Well, yes and no. Young children who have high blood cholesterol are not likely to be at risk because most children who have high blood cholesterol grow out of it.[2] Almost all children, regardless of national origin, diet, and sex, do develop fatty streaks in their major arteries.[3] Since children everywhere, on every kind of diet, develop fatty streaks, it is unclear what can be done about it. These fatty streaks are reversible and do not necessarily progress to the hardening and plaque formation characteristic of heart disease. It is only after puberty that the hardening process continues, and then only for some people; only after age 30 does the process become significant.[4]

If the hardening of the arteries starts in childhood, it must be a slow process. Heart disease, for the most part, is a disease of aging. As I told you in appendix L, the alarming and often-repeated figures on the risks of heart disease tend to imply that heart disease presents a great risk of *premature* death. That is definitely not the case. Eighty percent of deaths from heart disease occur after age 65.[5]

The safety of attempting to restrict children's fat intake continues to be a major point of disagreement among nutrition and health professionals. The moderates say that it is dangerous and unnecessary to try to restrict children's fat intake and show clinical evidence of poor growth in many children put on such regimens by parents trying to do the "right" thing.[6] The enthusiasts say that it is only overzealous parents who cause such problems and that, if the diet is intelligently applied, children will grow just fine. As evidence, enthusiasts point to intensively supervised clinical interventions in which parents and children were provided with laborious instruction and follow-up.[7,8] Such ambitious clinical interventions show modest changes in children's food intake and slight decreases in children's blood lipids.[9]

The truth of the matter is that applying the Dietary Guidelines with all the complicated fat instructions is complex, difficult to do, and easy to screw up. If you screw up, your efforts don't do any good, and they may even do harm. Restricting children's fat intake without interfering with their intake of energy or other nutrients involves a significant increase in precision, attention to detail, and risk of error. Pennsylvania State researchers doing computer modeling of children's diets found that using more than one fat-lowering strategy produced deficient diets, particularly for children under age 2. Strategies included using low-fat meat and milk, doing low-fat cooking, and avoiding added fats at the table.[10] If your child has a particularly high risk of heart disease, and if you and your doctor have determined that he needs a special diet, I agree with the AAP that you get careful and informed dietary guidance from a registered dietitian to avoid nutritional deficiencies and poor growth.

Most people, however, are not in the high-risk category. Most of us are simply trying to be responsible and practical in feeding our children. From the perspective of eating competence and feeding dynamics, the practical and realistic path is the one most likely to help without harming. Don't try to force your child's fat intake down to 30 percent or below. Instead, follow the division of responsibility in feeding and have regular and reliable family meals with choices from the five food groups. Vary fat concentrations in the meals by offering some foods that are low in fat, some moderate, and some high. Vary fat sources by choosing monounsaturated, polyunsaturated, and saturated fats. Encourage your child to eat what and how much he wants from what you put before him. Enjoy your own food. Given such meal-management strategies, both you and your child are likely to automatically consume a balanced, moderate-fat, low-saturated-fat diet. Finally, avoid dietary hassles. Your child's positive eating attitudes and behaviors will do more for him in the long run than trying to impose a formula on his eating.

References

1. Daniels SR, Greer FR, and the Committee on Nutrition. Lipid Screening and Cardiovascular Health in Childhood. *Pediatrics.* 2008;122:198-208.
2. Lauer RM, Clarke WR. Use of cholesterol measurements in childhood for the prediction of adult hypercholesterolemia: the Muscatine study. *JAMA.* 1990;264:3034-3038.
3. Tejada CJ, Strong JP, Montenegro MR, Restrepo C, Solberg LA. Distribution of coronary and aortic atherosclerosis by geographic location, race and sex. *Lab Invest.* 1968;18:509-526.
4. Pathobiological Determinants of Atherosclerosis in Youth (PDAY) Research Group. Relationship of atherosclerosis in young men to serum lipoprotein cholesterol concentrations and smoking: a preliminary report. *JAMA.* 1990;264:3018-3024.

5. National Center for Health Statistics [Web site]. LCWK1 Deaths, percent of total deaths, and death rates for the 15 leading causes of death in 5-year age groups, by race and sex: United States, 1999-2004. [Web page] Centers for Disease Control and Prevention Web site. http://www.cdc.gov/nchs/datawh/statab/unpubd/mortabs/lcwk1_10.htm. Accessed July 10, 2008.

6. Lifshitz F, Tarim O. Nutrition dwarfing. *Curr Probl Pediatr.* 1993;23:322-336.

7. Van Horn L, Obarzanek E, Friedman LA, Gernhofer N, Barton B. Children's adaptations to a fat-reduced diet: the Dietary Intervention Study in Children (DISC). *Pediatrics.* 2005;115:1723-1733.

8. Salo P, Viikari J, Hamalainen M, et al. Serum cholesterol ester fatty acids in 7- and 13-month-old children in a prospective randomized trial of a low-saturated fat, low-cholesterol diet: the STRIP baby project. Special Turku coronary Risk factor Intervention Project for children. *Acta Paediatr.* 1999;88:505-512.

9. Obarzanek E, Kimm SYS, Barton BA, et al. Long-term safety and efficacy of a cholesterol-lowering diet in children with elevated low-density lipoprotein cholesterol: seven-year results of the Dietary Intervention Study in Children (DISC). *Pediatrics.* 2001;107(2):256-264.

10. Sigman-Grant M, Zimmerman S, Kris-Etherton PM. Dietary approaches for reducing fat intake of preschool-aged children. *Pediatrics.* 1993;91:955-960.

Appendix
N
A Primer on Dietary Fat

This lesson in fat chemistry goes beyond what you really need to know. I include it because you may be curious and because I think understanding the technical terms could help you be more relaxed about eating fat. What do the terms *saturated*, *monounsaturated*, and *polyunsaturated* fat really mean? It has to do with fat chemistry. Fat is made up of fatty acids, which are chains of carbon atoms with hydrogens hooked on. Some carbons in fats have as many hydrogens hooked onto them as they possibly can: They are saturated with hydrogen atoms, thus they are called *saturated* fats. Some fatty acids have double bonds between the carbon atoms with fewer hydrogens hooked on. They are *not* saturated with hydrogen. Fatty acids with one double bond are called *mono*unsaturated fatty acids; those with several double bonds are the *poly*unsaturated fats.

The fat and heart disease theory says that saturated fats raise blood cholesterol more than unsaturated fats, and that high blood cholesterol is correlated with cardiovascular disease. The Dietary Guidelines and MyPyramid have relented about dietary fat percentage; they now say to keep total fat intake between 20 and 35 percent of calories (up by 5 percent), to keep saturated fat down to 10 percent, and to keep trans fat consumption as low as possible. They still say to emphasize polyunsaturated fats, although in other quarters, the Mediterranean diet, which is high in monounsaturates, has gained favor. Recent work in Holland, however, indicates that in terms of their impact on blood cholesterol, HDL, and LDL, the saturated stearic acid, the monounsaturated oleic acid and the polyunsaturated linoleic acid are comparable.[1]

Health policy still gives the general directive to cut down on animal fat and emphasize plant oils, presumably because the former are saturated and the latter unsaturated. The research from Holland calls this into question: Stearic acid comes from animals, yet its impact on HDL and LDL is the same as that of the linoleic and oleic acids that come from plants. To examine the generalization that animal fat is bad and plant fat is good, let's consider the details with the help of a software program called Food Processor, which calculates food composition. Figure N.1 summarizes the percentage of calories from saturated, monounsaturated, and polyunsaturated fats.

Are animal fats all bad? Not really. Our favorite animal fats, butter and cream, do have most of their fat in the form of saturated fat—but not all. The fats in butter and cream are about 30 percent monounsaturated and 4 percent polyunsaturated. And what about the universally deplored lard, a fat whose very name implies sloth? The fat in lard is a desirable 42 percent monounsaturated and 14 percent polyunsaturated. Most people who use chicken and goose fat fear it is entirely reprehensible, but these poultry fats have such a respectable fat profile that I have included them on the monounsaturated fat list as well as the animal fat list. Furthermore, about 25 percent of the saturated fat in red meat and poultry and 10 percent of the saturated fat in butter and cream is stearic acid. The generalization that plant oil is good doesn't hold with nut oils. Coconut oil is particularly saturated. Palm oil isn't as saturated and has some monounsaturated and polyunsaturated fats. The generalization also doesn't hold with plant oils like those in solid shortenings and stick margarines that have been hydrogenated. *Hydrogenated* means partially saturated or saturated. To make them solid, the fatty acids are changed chemically by "saturating" them with hydrogen atoms, which makes them behave in much the same way as naturally saturated fatty acids. Partially hydrogenated fat that is in the *trans* form as opposed to the *cis* form can increase total cholesterol and LDL. *Cis* and *trans* have to do with the arrangement of the carbon chain—if it rotates one way, it is cis, and if it rotates the other way, it is trans. According to recent evidence, there is a small statistical correlation between the consumption of trans fats and heart disease.[2]

It can't hurt to avoid industrially created trans fats, and it might help. Avoiding them is getting easier all the time because manufacturers are developing other processes for producing semisolid fat. Being trans-fat-free is now a selling point in manufactured and restaurant foods, and consumers look for foods that don't contain trans fats. Nutrition labels must declare trans fat content, and ingredient labels must declare the type of fat. The food component to avoid is *partially hydrogenated fat*.

FIGURE N.1 PERCENTAGE OF CALORIES FROM SATURATED, MONOUNSATURATED, AND POLYUNSATURATED FATS IN COMMON PLANT AND ANIMAL FATS

	Saturated	Monounsaturated	Polyunsaturated
High monounsaturated fats			
Olive oil	14	74	8
Canola oil	7	62	27
Goose fat	28	57	11
Peanut oil	17	52	26
Chicken fat	30	45	21
High polyunsaturated fats			
Safflower oil	9	12	74
Sunflower oil	12	16	67
Walnut oil	9	23	63
Corn oil	14	24	59
Cottonseed oil	25	15	59
Soybean oil	14	23	58
Sesame oil	14	40	42
Animal fats			
Butter	62	30	4
Lard	40	42	14
Tallow (suet)	50	42	4
Chicken fat	30	45	21
Goose fat	28	57	11
Nut oils			
Coconut oil	88	6	2
Palm oil	49	37	9

As if the story weren't complicated enough, recent research indicates that not all unsaturated fats work the same. Monounsaturated fat raises HDL. Polyunsaturated fat at three times the level of saturated fat raises HDL,[3] but animal studies indicate that polyunsaturated fat can contribute to lipid peroxidation, a cellular sign of aging.[4] Omega-3 fatty acids lower triglycerides.[3]

Do you see why I encourage you to emphasize variety? Based on constant fluctuations in research, I would encourage you to hedge your bets. Choose your primary fat based on taste or other qualities that you prize, then make an effort to diversify with other fats and oils.

If you have a high blood cholesterol level that needs to be treated by diet, get professional help. Don't settle for having your whole eating life turned upside down by a general chart of "good" or "bad" foods. Make sure your dietitian is up to date on the research and on fat chemistry.

So, are you going to march right down to the grocery store and buy some lard? Or are you, like a shopper I overheard the other day, going to smirk and say, "I guess it's been a long time since we ate *that*!" It depends on how daring you are. There is a certain political correctness about grease. At a recent holiday party, I got into a discussion about fat, of all things. One of my companions smugly announced that he was looking for the perfect olive oil. Refusing to pander to his superior attitude, I announced that lard was my favorite fat. (Actually, that isn't really true, but I was provoked. Butter is my favorite fat.) To my surprise, my other companion put his bid in for suet—beef tallow. He had grown up in Britain and said there is nothing like shaved suet for making flaky pie crust. In his honor, I have included suet in figure N.1. Yvonne Bushland, food scientist and reviewer, topped my story by telling of a Norwegian friend's meatball recipe calling for whale blubber. Sorry, the Food Processor software doesn't show it.

References

1. Thijssen MA, Mensink RP. Small differences in the effects of stearic acid, oleic acid, and linoleic acid on the serum lipoprotein profile of humans. *Am J Clin Nutr.* 2005;82:510-516.
2. Mozaffarian D , Katan MB, Ascherio A, Stampfer MJ, Willett WC. Trans fatty acids and cardiovascular disease. *N Engl J Med.* 2006;354:1601-1613.
3. Denke MA. Dietary fats, fatty acids, and their effects on lipoproteins. *Curr Atheroscler Rep.* 2006;8:466-471.
4. Csallany AS, Seppanen CM, Fritz KL. Effect of high stearic acid containing fat on markers for in vivo lipid peroxidation. *Int J Food Sci Nutr.* 2005;56:567-579.

Appendix

O

Sodium in Your Diet

In my view, it is better to get fed than to avoid salt. My cooking strategies are based on keeping sodium intake around 3,000 to 4,000 milligrams (mg) per day, which is a modest amount. Usual sodium intakes for females are around 3,000 mg per day and for males around 4,000 mg. Differences in energy intake account for the differences in sodium intake.[1] An intake of 3,000 to 4,000 mg of sodium per day is associated with a positive level of dietary variety, and as dietary variety goes up, sodium intake goes up.[2] As with the fat issue, the debate about sodium is at least as much about nutritional politics as it is about science. If you are interested, read "The (Political) Science of Salt."[3]

The nutrition enthusiasts—the ones who currently write nutrition policy in the form of the Dietary Guidelines—acknowledge that not everyone is vulnerable to high blood pressure, but they recommend restricting everyone's sodium intake in order to protect the susceptible. The Dietary Guidelines tell us to consume less than 2,300 mg per day, which is about a teaspoon of salt. That's pretty low. To force your sodium intake down to the 2,300 mg level, you would have to limit salt in cooking; not add salt *after* cooking; virtually eliminate commercially prepared foods such as pizza and spaghetti; avoid canned foods like soups, vegetables, meats, and mixed dinners; and completely avoid luncheon meats and cured foods like ham, bacon, and smoked turkey breasts. Such limitations restrict dietary choices to the point of making it hard to get a meal on the table, and *that* has a serious impact on nutrition and feeding a family.

The Research Is Contradictory

The research on dietary sodium shows, at most, modest decreases in blood pressure and slight changes in cardiovascular disease related to decreases in sodium intake. In fact, a 1996 analysis of 1971 to 1975 National Health and Nutrition Examination Survey (NHANES) participants found the level of cardiovascular disease mortality and all-cause mortality to go *down* as sodium intake went *up*. Based on their data, the researchers concluded that routine, population-wide sodium reductions are not justified.[4] A meta-analysis of 11 trials with more than 3,500 subjects revealed that despite the fact that the interventions used were highly intensive (and therefore unsuited to primary care or population-wide prevention programs), blood pressure changes were minimal (not more than 1 mm of Hg, or mercury) and there was no effect on any cardiovascular events or death. The researchers concluded that reducing salt intake may help hypertensive people stop their medication but that there are no other benefits.[5] On the other hand, *computer modeling*, not to be confused with actual studies, claimed that a 1,300 mg per day lower lifetime sodium intake would translate into an approximately 5 mm Hg smaller rise in systolic blood pressure as individuals advanced from 25 to 55 years of age, a reduction that would presumably save 150,000 lives annually.[6] Keep in mind that the figures are all speculative.

While a 2001 analysis of NHANES data found that dietary intakes of sodium, alcohol, and protein were positively associated with systolic blood pressure, those increases were neutralized by higher intakes of calcium and potassium.[7] Data from more than 5,000 overweight and 5,000 normal weight subjects in the Framingham study show that both normal weight and overweight subjects who consumed more sodium (2,700 mg sodium per day versus 1,200 mg per day) had a *lower* incidence of congestive heart failure.[8] An analysis of 56 research studies showed some blood pressure reduction with a 2,000 milligram per day reduction in urinary sodium intake excretion with older, hypertensive people. (Urinary sodium excretion is roughly equal to dietary intake.) People with normal blood pressure, whose urinary excretion went down by almost *3,000* mg per day, showed no change in blood pressure.[9]

Be Sensible About Salt

Based on the research and my clinical experience working with people who try to restrict their dietary sodium, the target level of 3,000 to 4,000 mg of sodium per day is far more practical and achievable than the 2,300 mg recommended by nutrition policy. Small as it is, that increase in sodium makes a *big* difference with respect to food selection and cooking. This level of sodium allows you to use salt in cooking, use canned soups in moderation, eat canned vegetables and meats, and eat salty snacks occasionally. This level of sodium is appropriate for young children, as well.

If you have high blood pressure, your daily salt intake is a medical matter. About 10 to 25 percent of people suffering from high blood pressure improve when they strictly limit their salt intake—to about 1,000 mg per day. Keep in mind, however, that although drastically cutting down on salt makes blood pressure go down, that doesn't mean that eating salt made it go up in the first place. Excess sodium may not even be the blood-pressure culprit, but rather, insufficient potassium and calcium. It has long

been recognized that we can help prevent high blood pressure by consuming enough potassium (from a variety of fruits and vegetables) and calcium (from dairy products). I prefer the calcium and potassium theory because it encourages *seeking* food, not *avoiding* it.

References

1. Briefel RR, Johnson CL. Secular trends in dietary intake in the United States. *Annu Rev Nutr.* 2004;24:401-431.
2. Murphy SP, Foote JA, Wilkens LR, et al. Simple measures of dietary variety are associated with improved dietary quality. *J Am Diet Assoc.* 2006;106:425-429.
3. Taubes G. The (political) science of salt. *Science.* 1998;281:899-907.
4. Alderman MH, Cohen H, Madhavan S. Dietary sodium intake and mortality: the National Health and Nutrition Examination Survey (NHANES I). *Lancet.* 1998;351:781-785.
5. Hooper L, Bartlett C, Davey Smith G, Ebrahim S. Systematic review of long term effects of advice to reduce dietary salt in adults. *BMJ.* 2002;325:628-637.
6. Dickinson BD, Havas S, for the Council on Science and Public Health AMA. Reducing the population burden of cardiovascular disease by reducing sodium intake: a report of the Council on Science and Public Health. *Arch Intern Med.* 2007;167:1460-1468.
7. Haijjar IM, Grim CE, George V, Dotchen TA. Impact of diet on blood pressure and age-related changes in blood pressure in the US population: analysis of NHANES III. *Arch Intern Med.* 2001;161:589-593.
8. He J, Ogden LG, Bazzano LA, Vupputuri S, Loria C, Whelton PK. Dietary sodium intake and incidence of congestive heart failure in overweight US men and women: first National Health and Nutrition Examination Survey epidemiologic follow-up study. *Arch Intern Med.* 2002;162:1619-1624.
9. Midgley JP, Matthew AG, Greenwood CM, Logan AG. Effect of reduced dietary sodium on blood pressure. *JAMA.* 1996;275:1590-1597.

Appendix
P
Interpreting the News

Here are some questions you can ask yourself when you read or hear about study results.

- What are the *actual* numbers as opposed to the *relative* numbers? Three of the early studies about diet and heart disease claimed a 50 percent reduction in heart attacks with dietary modification. (See appendix L, "Diet and Degenerative Disease: It's Not as Bad as You Think.") However, a look at the actual numbers shows a reduction of from 1.4 to 0.7 deaths per 1,000 men per year, such a modest reduction that it calls into question dietary modification. If the release doesn't give you actual numbers, ignore it.

- What type of study was it? Many media releases are based on epidemiological evidence: observations of large groups of people. Epidemiological studies give *preliminary* results—an educated guess about cause and effect. Such guesses can only be accepted as accurate after they are tested, generally first in animal studies and then in clinical trials with humans. Until then, the evidence is speculative and doesn't give you grounds for making changes in your diet.

- Does the study stand alone, or are its results corroborated by other research? Before a conclusion can be accepted, it has to be supported with evidence from a variety of studies conducted by a number of scientists. A study that stands alone must be regarded as giving preliminary results and therefore doesn't provide grounds for making dietary changes. Responsible nutritional and medical change takes place slowly. If the information is startling and revolutionary and calls into question accepted scientific theory, it is probably preliminary and therefore stands alone. Take it with a grain of salt.

- Was the study published in a peer-reviewed journal? You can find out by asking a medical librarian at your local university or hospital. Peer review sets out to poke holes in a study's design or conclusions. While this isn't foolproof, it helps to ensure that authors haven't distorted data or conclusions. In non-reviewed journals, authors can make poorly substantiated claims without having those claims be challenged

- Are the conclusions of the authors supported by the data presented? Scientific inquiry is more political than we would like to believe, and authors of even peer-reviewed articles draw conclusions that deny the truth of their own data but support or avoid contradicting prevailing thought. For instance, the authors of the study showing those modest reductions in heart disease deaths, from 1.4 to 0.7 per 1,000, describe their results as "striking."

Appendix
Q
Eating Competence and Feeding Dynamics Resources

Your Child's Weight: Helping Without Harming. This groundbreaking book gives clear evidence that children gain too much weight because of *how*, not because of *what* they are fed. Calming, practical and carefully documented, this book empowers readers to feed well, parent well, and let children grow up to get bodies that are right for them. Packed with ever-popular feeding stories, *Your Child's Weight* offers clear guidance for professionals as well as parents.

Child of Mine: Feeding with Love and Good Sense. The gold-standard book on feeding children. Warm, supportive and entertaining for parents. Also used as a solid nutrition, child development and feed dynamics reference for professionals. *Child of Mine* teaches about feeding, growth, and parenting birth through preschool.

How to Get Your Kid to Eat...But Not Too Much. Based on a solid understanding of child development and parent-child relationships, *How to Get Your Kid to Eat* is a problem-solving book that firmly builds the bridge between nutrition and feeding.

ELLYN SATTER'S FEEDING WITH LOVE AND GOOD SENSE: Video and Teacher's Guide. These live action videos (packaged as both VHS and DVD) of real situations touch, move, startle, upset, and inform parents and child care workers and help them take a look at their own feeding behavior. Sometimes feeding goes well, sometimes it doesn't. The hour-long videotape shows what makes the difference. Lesson plans teach nutrition and feeding by observation and experience. Each 15-minute segment comes with a lesson plan, audio script and six reproducible masters.

The Infant. Babies know how much they need to eat, and parents read their messages.

The Older Baby. Babies learn to eat solid foods and communicate with parents.

The Toddler. Toddlers need to explore, but they also need support and limits.

The Preschooler. Preschoolers want to get better at everything—eating included.

ELLYN SATTER'S FEEDING WITH LOVE AND GOOD SENSE: Vignettes and Power-Points. The highly popular *Feeding with Love and Good Sense* video series converted into individual, digitalized vignettes along with informative, turn-key PowerPoint train-the-trainer sessions for professionals and staff that teach the basics of feeding dynamics and demonstrate the use of embedded vignettes. Topics covered include the five developmental stages newborn through preschool as well as basic principles of growth from a feeding-dynamics perspective.

ELLYN SATTER'S FEEDING IN PRIMARY CARE PREGNANCY THROUGH PRE-SCHOOL: Easy-to-Read Reproducible Masters. Written at a 4th-grade reading level for audiences who primarily gather information from being told and by watching others, these illustrated handouts guide and reinforce face-to-face discussion on child feeding. Handouts are formatted on 8 1/2 by 11 paper to make them easy to copy. 55 titles in all including *Eating for Pregnancy, Feed Based on What Your Baby Can Do, Is Your Baby Too Big? Does She Eat Too Much?, Solid Foods, Step by Step, How to Handle the Picky Eater.* Registered purchasers may make up to 300 copies of each master.

ELLYN SATTER'S NUTRITION AND FEEDING FOR INFANTS AND CHILDREN: Handout Masters. Distilled from the pages of both *Child of Mine* and *How to Get Your Kid to Eat,* these ready-to-copy handouts are for parents who gain information by reading as well as by discussion. These readable and engaging handouts tell inquisitive parents not only *what* to do, by *why* to do it. Handouts are used in nutrition, health and education settings. Equally valuable for training nutrition workers. Titles include

Being a Role Model for Your Child's Eating, Breastfeeding Your Baby, If Your Baby Doesn't Eat Enough, What is Normal Growth? If Your Preschooler Seems Fat, If Your Child Won't Eat Vegetables, Should Your Child Drink Milk? Registered purchasers may make up to 300 copies of each master.

Ellyn Satter's Montana FEEDING RELATIONSHIP Training Package. Now available in DVD as well as VHS format, Ellyn Satter gives in-depth staff training on feeding children and preventing feeding problems. Includes five hours of professional quality videos of lecture, demonstration and audience participation. Handouts include a multi-page training outline and materials, references, and informational handouts for parents.

Ellyn Satter and the Ellyn Satter Institute offer a variety of one-, two-, three-, and four-day programs. For a complete listing and overview of these workshops, go to www.EllynSatter.com and click on *Speaking and Training*.

For a current catalog and price list, call Ellyn Satter Associates, 800-808-7976 or see www.EllynSatter.com.

Index

References to the major treatment of a topic are printed in **bold**. Recipe titles are printed in *italic*, as are book titles.